Color Atlas of Oral Diseases
in Children and Adolescents

Color Atlas of Oral Diseases in Children and Adolescents

George Laskaris, D.D.S., M.D.

Consultant in Oral Medicine
Department of Dermatology
"A. Sygros" Hospital, Athens
Associate Professor of Oral Medicine
Medical School
University of Athens, Greece

495 Illustrations

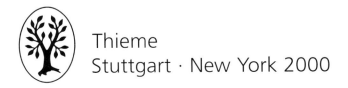
Thieme
Stuttgart · New York 2000

Library of Congress Cataloging-in-Publication Data

Laskaris, George.
   Color atlas of oral diseases in children and adolescents / Georg Laskaris.
   p. cm.
   Includes bibliographical references and index.
   ISBN 0-86577-789-6 (TNY). – ISBN 3-13-111511-4 (GTV)
   1. Pediatric oral medicine Atlases. 2. Pedodontics Atlases.
I. Title.
   [DNLM: 1. Mouth Diseases–Adolescence Atlases. 2. Mouth Diseases–Child Atlases. WU 17 L345c 1999]
RJ460.L37 1999
618.92'097522–dc21
DNLM/DLC
for Library of Congress   99-36035 CIP

© 2000 Georg Thieme Verlag,
Rüdigerstrasse 14,
D-70469 Stuttgart, Germany
Thieme, 333 Seventh Avenue,
New York, NY 10001, USA

Typesetting by
primustype R. Hurler GmbH,
D-73274 Notzingen, Germany
typeset on Textline/HerculesPro

Printed in Germany by
Staudigl-Druck GmbH,
D-86609 Donauwörth

ISBN 3-13-111511-4 (GTV)
ISBN 0-86577-789-6 (TNY)
         1 2 3 4 5 6

This book is dedicated to my three children
Christina, Marina, and *Christos*
for the constant happiness they bring

Foreword

Professor George Laskaris has an international reputation as a clinician with a special interest in diseases of the oral mucosa. An active clinician, he is also a prolific publisher of scholarly works in the field of oral medicine, and this book is a welcome addition to his portfolio. Through his publications, Professor Laskaris offers not only a service to his own patients but, via the wider academic and clinical readers, provides benefit to patients in many other parts of the world.

Professor Crispian Scully
Secretary-General, European Association of Oral Medicine
Dean, Director of Studies and Research
Eastman Dental Institute for Oral Health Care Sciences
and International Centers for Excellence in Dentistry
University of London
London, 1999

Preface

The spectrum of diseases affecting the oral cavity during childhood and adolescence is very broad. Some of the disorders are entirely benign and transient, while others may be painful, severe, and even life-threatening. Like other diseases affecting young patients, oral diseases become a source of anxiety for the parents, and sometimes may adversely affect the normal development of both the body and the mind of the young patients. They also pose diagnostic difficulties for pediatricians, since many of them fall on the borderlines of many specialties, such as dentistry, dermatology, pediatric oncology, plastic and maxillofacial surgery, and oral medicine, each with its own perspective and point of view.

The main purpose of writing this atlas of pediatric oral diseases was to overcome these difficulties by organizing the available information on a uniform basis, combining pictorial material and important clinical, diagnostic, and therapeutic information in a compact format. Some histopathological, immunological, and radiographic pictures have been included where it was thought that they would be helpful. The emphasis is on the brevity and clarity of the written summaries and of course on the quality of the pictorial material, which was collected over a 30-year period.

Gathering and classifying the pictorial material and the disease entities involved considerable difficulties, due to the extremely wide spectrum of conditions concerned and the particular character they take on in pediatric patients. The material of the book has been subdivided into three major parts: local diseases, systemic disorders affecting the oral cavity, and tumors.

The bulk of the pictorial material was collected by the author and photographed using a Nikon medical camera. It is the author's hope that the book will prove useful and will facilitate communication among pediatricians, specialists in oral medicine, orofacial surgeons, dermatologists, otorhinolaryngologists, and pediatric and general dentists—with beneficial results for our young patients.

George Laskaris, D.D.S., M.D.
Athens, 1999

Acknowledgments

My warmest thanks and gratitude are extended to all those who helped in many different ways to make this book possible.

First, I would like to thank C. Kittas, professor of histology, P. Anastasiadis, associate professor of orofacial surgery, A. Katsambas, associate professor of dermatology, and C. Bartsokas, professor of pediatrics, for their useful comments on the text in the subjects of their respective specialties.

Dr. Nikos Lygidakis and Dr. Marina Laskari, pediatric dentist and orthodontist, respectively, wrote the chapter on dental defects, and I thank them for their diligent work.

I am particularly grateful to Stathis S. Papavasiliou, associate professor of endocrinology at the University of Crete, Greece, and Crispian Scully, professor of oral medicine at the University of London, England, for their critical review of the text. I would also like to express my gratitude to the dentists and physicians who entrusted me with their young patients, thus giving me the opportunity to collect the material for the present edition.

Finally, I am grateful to my wife for her constant support, sympathy, and understanding during the efforts involved in writing the book.

The colleagues listed below provided me with transparencies from their personal records, helping to extend the spectrum of disease entities presented in the book. I am most grateful to them for their generosity. Should anyone's name inadvertently have been omitted, please accept my apologies.

- Prof. A. Gianoulopoulos (Greece) for Fig. 462
- Dr. N. Zahariadis (Greece) for Fig. 244
- Dr. E. Kariabas (Greece) for Figs. 460, 461, 484
- Prof. T. Karpathios (Greece) for Fig. 218
- Dr. A. Manderkas (Greece) for Figs. 53, 54, 55
- Prof. H. Moutsopoulos (Greece) for Figs. 314, 315
- Dr. N. Papadogeorgakis (Greece) for Figs. 490, 491
- Dr. A. Parashis (Greece) for Fig. 150
- Dr. G. Siskos (Greece) for Figs. 9, 10, 11, 12, 13
- Dr. A. Tsami (Greece) for Figs. 95, 96, 97, 98, 102, 104, 105, 106
- Dr. C. Castro and Dr. A. Furuse (Brazil) for Figs. 373, 374, 375
- Prof. O. P. Almeida (Brazil) for Fig. 409
- Dr. Mosadomi (Nigeria) for Fig. 483
- Prof. I. van der Wall (Netherlands) for Fig. 492
- Prof. Romero de Leon and Prof. A. Aguirre (USA) for Figs. 141, 142
- Prof. C. Scully (England) for Fig. 327
- Prof. C. Witkop (USA) for Figs. 46, 47

Contents

Part I Local Diseases

Part II   Systemic Diseases

Part III   Tumors

Part I
Local Diseases

1 Dental Defects

Nick A. Lygidakis
Consultant Paediatric Dentist
DDS, MScD, MScM, DrOdont

Marina G. Laskari
Orthodontist, DDS, MSc
Boston University, USA

Defects in Size

These defects result from various etiological factors acting during the stage of dental morphodifferentiation.

Microdontia

Definition
- Refers to teeth that appear smaller in size compared to normal. Pseudomicrodontia refers to all teeth of an individual appearing smaller than normal, as a result of enlarged jaw dimensions. True microdontia refers to teeth of smaller size in a jaw of normal size (Figs. 1.**1,** 1.**2**).

Etiology
- Multifactorial. Generalized microdontia is rare, and may be associated with congenital hypopituitarism or exposure to radiation or chemotherapy during dental development. In contrast, localized microdontia is more common, and is frequently followed by hypodontia; it has therefore been suggested that these two defects are controlled by different mutations in the same genes.
- Syndromes in which microdontia may be seen include the trisomy 21 syndrome, the ectodermal dysplasia syndromes, and the Marshall I, Rieger, focal dermal hypoplasia, Silver–Russell, Williams, Gorlin–Chaudhry–Moss, Coffin–Siris, Salamon, trichorhinophalangeal, odontotrichomelic, neuroectodermal, and dermo-odontodysplasia syndromes.
- Also a frequent finding in cases of cleft lip and palate.

Occurrence in children
- Rare (less than 1%) in primary teeth.
- More common (2.5%) in permanent teeth.
- Females more frequently affected than males.

Localization
- Upper laterals.
- Upper third molars.

Clinical features
- Usual crown shape or sometimes with tapering (peg or conical) crown, but smaller in size than the range of normal variation.

Treatment
- Aesthetic restoration with composites, crowns in severe cases, orthodontic treatment for closure of spaces, if needed.

Macrodontia

Definition
- Refers to teeth that appear larger than the normal size. Some or all teeth may be affected (Fig. 1.**3**).

Etiology
- Multifactorial. Generalized macrodontia is observed in cases of pituitary gigantism, and in individuals with small jaws. Localized macrodontia is observed in cases of unilateral facial hyperplasia, resulting from over-development of tooth buds.
- Macrodontia may also be associated with congenital hemifacial hypertrophy and some genetic syndromes such as craniofacial dysostosis, otodental syndrome, and Sturge–Weber syndrome.

Occurrence in children
- Rare (1.1%) in permanent dentition.

Localization
- Lower third molars and second premolars.
- Upper central incisors.
- Frequent bilateral symmetry.

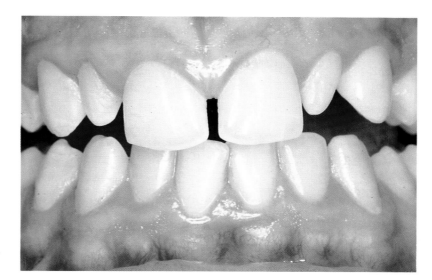

Fig. 1.**1**   Microdontia of the upper lateral incisors

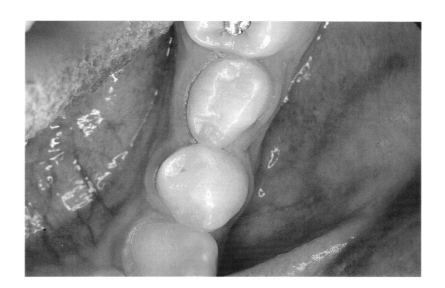

Fig. 1.**2**   Microdontia of a lower premolar

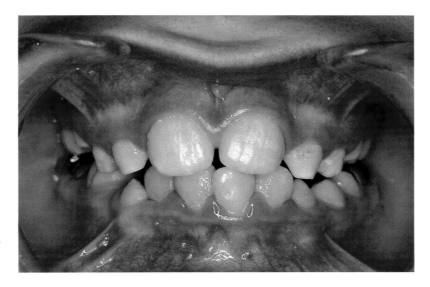

Fig. 1.**3**   Macrodontia of the upper and lower incisors in a patient with otodental syndrome

Clinical features	● Usual tooth morphology with rounded edges, exceeding in size the range of normal variation.
Complications	● Clinically, macrodontia may lead to crowding and potential abnormal teeth eruption as a result of reduced available space in the dental arch.
Treatment	● Aesthetic restoration and orthodontic treatment of the potential crowding.

Conical Teeth

Definition	● Refers to teeth that have a conical shape with a pointed edge.
Etiology	● Frequently followed by hypodontia, and for this reason it has been suggested that these two anomalies are controlled by different mutations in the same genes (Fig. 1.**4**). ● In the majority of the cases, conical teeth are found in patients with genetic disorders such as ectodermal dysplasia, Rieger, dento-onychodermal and incontinentia pigmenti syndromes.
Occurrence in children	● Rare in both permanent and primary teeth (0.2%).
Localization	● Upper incisors.
Clinical features	● Characteristic conical shape with sharp, pointed edge.
Treatment	● Aesthetic restoration with composites, crowns.

Defects in Shape

These defects manifest as a result of various etiological factors acting during the initiation/proliferation and the morphodifferentiation stages of dental development.

Gemination

Definition	● Refers to incomplete division of the tooth bud, resulting in the formation of two partially or completely independent crowns with a shared root (Fig. 1.**5**). If the division is complete, the anomaly is termed twinning, and results in the formation of a supernumerary tooth, which appears as a minor image of its normal partner.
Etiology	● This defect can be found in both the primary and permanent dentitions, and results from various degrees of invagination of the developing dental organ caused by local, systemic, and genetic factors. ● The genetic factors involved are probably similar to those affecting the dental lamina in cases of hyperdontia.
Occurrence in children	● Including fusion, rare in both primary (0.5–1.6%) and in permanent (0.1–0.2%) teeth. ● Males and females equally affected. ● 30–50% of the primary cases are followed by defects in the permanent successors.
Localization	● Upper and lower incisors.
Clinical features	● Variable, from a minor notch in the incisal edge of a wide crown to almost two separate crowns. Similarly, the pulp chamber and the root canal may be common to both elements, or separate for each one.
Complications	● Potential crowding of the dental arch. Difficulty in the differential diagnosis between gemination and fusion of a normal and supernumerary tooth.
Treatment	● Aesthetic restoration with composites, or surgical removal of the supernumerary in cases of twinning. Orthodontic treatment of the potential crowding.

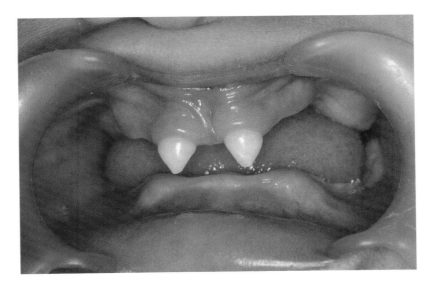

Fig. 1.**4** Conical teeth in a patient with hypohidrotic ectodermal dysplasia

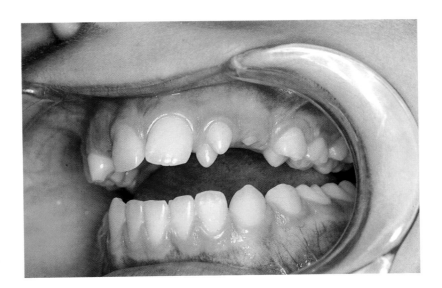

Fig. 1.**5** Gemination of an upper lateral incisor

Fusion

Definition
- Refers to the union of two discrete tooth buds, resulting in the formation of a tooth with an anomalous shape.

Etiology
- The defect is a result of interdental lamina persistence during dental organ development, caused by local factors.
- Genetic factors have also been implicated, such as autosomal dominant inheritance with reduced penetrance.

Occurrence in children
- Including gemination, it is rare in both primary (0.5–1.6%) and permanent (0.1–0.2%) teeth.
- Ethnic variations result in a higher incidence in some populations.
- 30–50% of the primary cases are followed by defects in the permanent successors.

Localization
- Anterior teeth.

Clinical features
- If fusion occurs early during the tooth development, the defect affects the total length of the tooth, resulting in a single tooth of almost normal size.
- If fusion occurs later, the defect only affects the root (Fig. 1.**6**), resulting in shared dentine and cementum, and one large tooth or a tooth with bifid crown.

Complications
- Fusion most often leads to a reduced number of teeth in the dental arch, although occasionally a normal and a supernumerary tooth may be fused. In the latter case, there is difficulty in the differential diagnosis between this defect and gemination. Fusion in the primary dentition may be followed by aplasia of the permanent successor.

Treatment
- Aesthetic restoration with composites, or surgical separation and removal of the fused supernumerary tooth. Orthodontic treatment of the potential crowding.

Concrescence

Definition
- Refers to a type of fusion in which the formed teeth are joined only along the line of cementum.

Etiology
- This defect can happen before or after the teeth erupt, and is most probably a result of local trauma, dental crowding, and dislocation of tooth germs during root formation.

Occurrence in children
- Rare.

Localization
- Upper second and third molars.

Clinical features
- Diagnosis of the alteration can be definite only with radiographs.

Complications
- The defect does not have any clinical significance except in cases in which extractions are needed and appropriate surgical manipulations should be followed.

Treatment
- No treatment is required, since the affected teeth are asymptomatic.

Dilaceration

Definition
- Refers to an extensive bend in the root on the cervical area of the affected teeth.

Etiology
- The defect results from disruption of the Hertwig epithelial root sheath due to eccentric dislocation of the already formed crown in relation to the developing adjacent soft tissues (Figs. 1.**7**, 1.**8**).
- Dilaceration has been associated with trauma of the predecessor primary teeth during the developmental period of the permanent tooth, or with therapeutic irradiation of the area.

Occurrence in children
- Rare.
- 3% of the successors in cases of traumatized primary teeth.

Localization
- Anterior teeth.

Clinical features
- Malformed crown, frequently hypoplastic, and severe deviation of the long axis of the crown or root segment of the tooth.

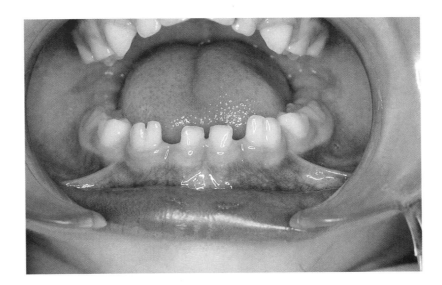

Fig. 1.**6**   Fusion of lower primary lateral incisors and canines

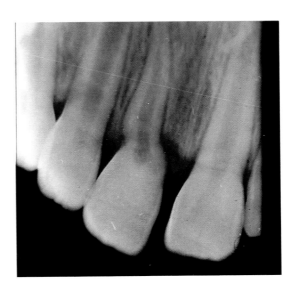

Fig. 1.**7**   Dilaceration, mesial–distal, of an upper central incisor due to trauma in the predecessor primary tooth

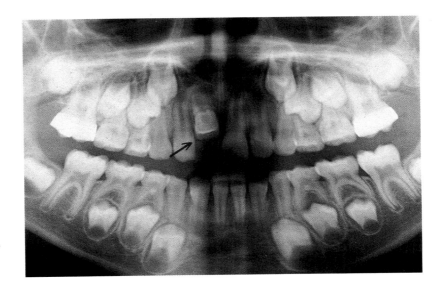

Fig. 1.**8**   Dilaceration, buccal–palatal, of an upper central incisor due to trauma in the predecessor primary tooth

Complications	• Clinical problems caused by the defect include difficulties in case of extraction, and the frequent impaction of these teeth.
Treatment	• In case of normal eruption, aesthetic or prosthetic restoration. In case of impaction, combined surgical and orthodontic treatment in order to align the tooth in the dental arch, followed by aesthetic restoration.

Dens Invaginatus (Dens in Dente)

Definition	• Refers to a defect characterized by a prominent lingual cusp and a centrally located pit (Fig. 1.**9**).
Etiology	• The defect results from early invagination of the enamel epithelium into the dental papilla of the underlying tooth germ. Local and genetic factors have been implicated.
Occurrence in children	• Rare in primary teeth. • More common in permanent teeth (1–5%).
Localization	• Upper permanent lateral incisors, usually bilateral.
Clinical features	• The defect may not be clinically apparent, and does not frequently cause problems. If present, the labial surface of the tooth is normal, whereas the defect in the lingual surface may vary from a deep cingulum pit to a tooth with grossly distorted crown and root. • Three types of the defect are recognized, depending on the extension of the cavity into the root.
Complications	• Increased frequency of caries in the lingual pits of the affected teeth due to the thin and incomplete layer of enamel, followed occasionally by pulp inflammation and necrosis, as a result of improper brushing and cleaning of the involved area.
Treatment	• Preventive filling of the pit. In case of odontogenic infection, endodontic treatment of the tooth.

Dens Evaginatus

Definition	• Refers to a defect characterized by an elevated, tuberculated appearance of the occlusal surface of the affected teeth. Evaginations contain enamel, dentine, and pulp (Fig. 1.**10**).
Etiology	• The defect results from focal hyperplasia of the ectomesenchyme of the primitive dental papilla. Genetic factors acting during the developmental period of the teeth have been implicated.
Occurrence in children	• Rare (less than 1%). • Frequent finding in individuals of Mongolian origin (1–4%).
Localization	• Premolars and molars, usually bilaterally.
Clinical features	• The affected teeth have a conical, tuberculated projection from the central fissure of the occlusal surface.
Complications	• Pulp may extend into the tubercula, resulting in an increased risk of pulp exposure after mild mechanical trauma to the occlusal surface.
Treatment	• Reduction of the occlusal tubercula (cusp) in order to induce formation of secondary dentine, or reduction of the opposing tooth in order to eliminate possible traumatic occlusion.

Taurodontism

Definition	• Refers to a dental defect usually found in multirooted teeth. It is characterized by a prolonged crown and more apically located root furcation, resulting in the creation of enlarged pulpal chambers with increased occlusal–apical length (Fig. 1.**11**). Three types of the defect have been recognized, termed *hypotaurodontism*, *mesotaurodontism*, and *hypertaurodontism* according to the extension of the pulp chamber into the root. • The defect has also been classified among pulp dysplasias.

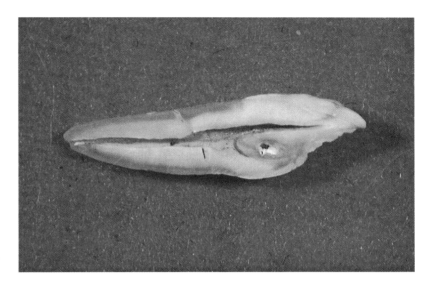

Fig. 1.9 Dens in dente (dens invaginatus) of an upper central incisor, resulting in pulpal necrosis

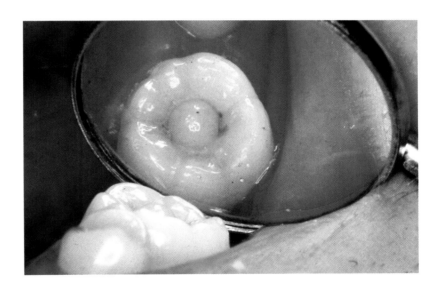

Fig. 1.10 Dens evaginatus in an upper molar

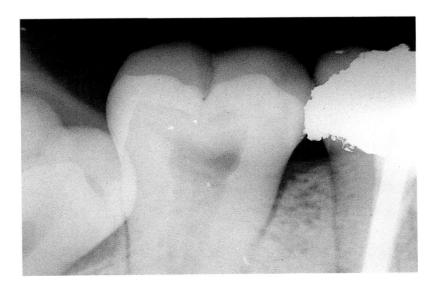

Fig. 1.11 Radiological features of taurodontism in a lower second molar

Etiology	• Polygenic, with additional implication of local factors. The defect has been attributed to the failure of the Hertwig's epithelial root sheath to invaginate below the crown at the proper time during dental development. • Taurodontism is frequently found in patients with trisomy 21 and Klinefelter syndromes, as well as other chromosomal anomalies involving an abnormal number of X chromosomes. • It is also found in cases of type IV amelogenesis imperfecta, trichodentoosseous syndrome types I, II, III, Down's syndrome, ectodermal dysplasia, and some other syndromes.
Occurrence in children	• Rare in primary teeth. • More common in permanent molars (6–10%).
Localization	• First and second molars. • Frequently a bilateral finding.
Clinical features	• Definite diagnosis only with radiographs revealing vertical enlargement of the coronal pulp chamber extending below the cervical area of the tooth. The bifurcation or the trifurcation of the root is displaced apically.
Complications	• Needs special care in case of endodontic treatment.
Treatment	• No treatment is required, since the affected teeth are asymptomatic.

Enamel Pearls

Definition	• Refers to ectopic nodular deposits of enamel observed at the roots of the involved teeth (Figs. 1.**12,** 1.**13**). Two types have been recognized: extradental and intradental.
Etiology	• Unknown. These defects arise from local activity of the Hertwig's epithelial root sheath remnants.
Occurrence in children	• Rare. • Higher incidence in Mongoloid and Eskimo populations.
Localization	• Upper molars.
Clinical features	• Diagnosis of the defect is only possible with radiographs. • They are usually found near the root furcations of single or multirooted teeth, and their size varies from a pinhead to a cusp. Occasionally, they contain dentine as well as enamel, and the pulp usually extends into them.
Treatment	• No treatment is required, since the affected teeth are asymptomatic.

Odontomas

Definition	• Refers to odontogenic hamartomatous "tumors" containing dental calcified tissues.
Etiology	• Unknown. These structures are malformations rather than tumors, originating from the dental tissues or their formative elements.
Occurrence in children	• Rare (0.15 per thousand). • These are the most frequent odontogenic "tumors" (67%).
Localization	• Compound and mixed odontomas more frequently in the anterior maxilla. • Complex odontomas more frequently in the premolar/molar region of both jaws. • Primary dentition is rarely involved (2% of the cases).
Clinical features	• Odontomas are asymptomatic and frequently diagnosed radiographically (Fig. 1.**14**). • They are classified in two major types. Compound odontomas are masses composed of multiple, discrete, small, tooth-like formations with well-recognized dental hard tissues, whereas complex odontomas are a more homogeneous mass of disorganized different anomalous dental tissues. Sometimes both types exist simultaneously, and the defect is termed mixed odontoma.

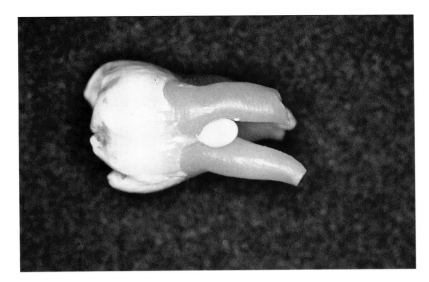

Fig. 1.**12**   Enamel pearl in the cervical furcation of an upper first molar

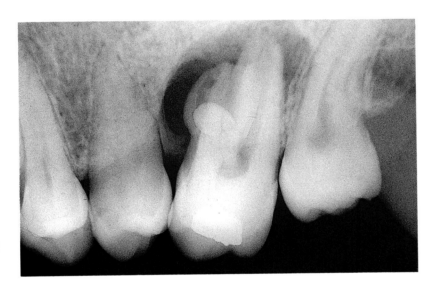

Fig. 1.**13**   Radiological features of enamel pearl in the root of an upper first molar

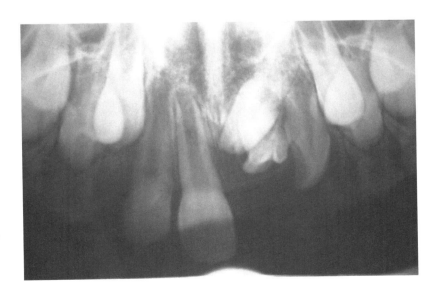

Fig. 1.**14**   Radiological features of odontomas in the upper anterior region resulting in eruption failure of the adjacent tooth

Complications
- Frequently (30–50%), they cause disturbance or total failure of eruption of the adjacent permanent teeth.

Treatment
- Surgical removal of the odontoma and, in case of eruption disturbances of the adjacent permanent teeth, orthodontic treatment.

Defects in Location

These defects result from etiological factors acting during the initiation and proliferation stages of dental development.

Ectopic Localization, Eruption

Definition
- Refers to a defect characterized by the eruption of a normal tooth into another location in the dental arch.

Etiology
- The defect results from ectopic placement of the tooth bud, or an irregular eruption path (Fig. 1.**15**). This is either caused by congenital migration of the tooth bud at the start of embryogenesis, related to genetic and environmental factors, or by displacement of the tooth during eruption, related to local factors.
- Local factors implicated are tooth–dental arch size discrepancy, prolonged primary tooth retention, presence of clefts, ankylosis, cystic or neoplastic formations, trauma. Generalized factors implicated are endocrine deficiency, febrile disease and irradiation.

Occurrence in children
- Ectopic location, rare.
- Ectopic eruption, 0.9–2.0%.
- Females more frequently affected than males (2 : 1).

Localization
- Canines and incisors.
- First permanent molars.
- Maxillary teeth more frequently affected than mandibular (3 : 1).

Clinical features
- A radiographically normal tooth located or erupting at an abnormal site.

Complications
- Frequently, ectopic localization/eruption is followed by impaction of the tooth concerned. Resorption of the adjacent teeth can also be found in some cases, particularly in the case of permanent molars.

Treatment
- Orthodontic treatment. Combined surgical–orthodontic approach in case of impaction.

Defects in Number

These defects result from the action of various etiological factors during the initiation and proliferation stages of the dental development.

Anodontia, Hypodontia

Definition
- Refers to a defect characterized by congenital absence from the dental arch of some teeth (hypodontia) or all of them (anodontia) (Figs. 1.**16**, 1.**17**). Severe hypodontia is also termed oligodontia.
- Anodontia and hypodontia may affect both the primary and permanent dentition. Pseudohypodontia is characterized by the absence of teeth from the dental arch due to impaction, delay of eruption, or early exfoliation.

Etiology
- The defect results from dental lamina obstruction or disruption during the early stages of embryogenesis, caused by abnormal activity of local, systemic, and genetic factors. Genetic factors, usually multigenic, have been strongly implicated.
- Hypodontia and anodontia are frequently associated with more than 70 genetic disorders and syndromes, primarily with those characterized by ectodermal involvement, such as the ectodermal dysplasias and the following syndromes: Rieger's, incontinentia pigmenti, Robinson's, Seckel's, orofaciodigital, focal dermal hypoplasia, Hallermann–Streiff, oculodentodigital, Russell–Silver, chondroectodermal dysplasia, frontometaphyseal dysplasia, craniofacial dysplasia, and others. It is also a frequent finding in patients with cleft lip and cleft palate.

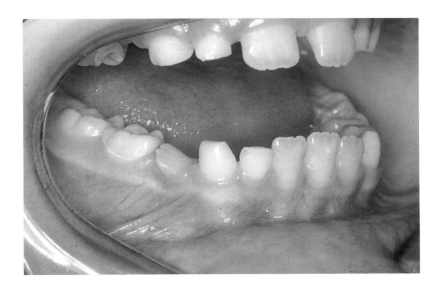

Fig. 1.**15**   Ectopic location and eruption of a lower lateral incisor

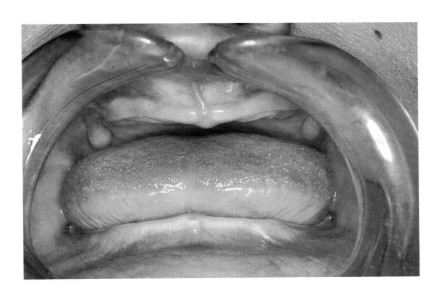

Fig. 1.**16**   Anodontia in a patient with hypohidrotic ectodermal dysplasia

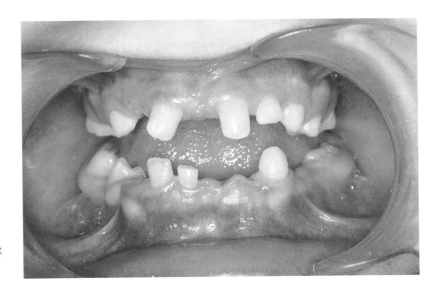

Fig. 1.**17**   Hypodontia in a patient with hypohidrotic ectodermal dysplasia

Occurrence in children
- Anodontia: rare.
- Hypodontia of primary teeth: 0.1–0.7%.
- Hypodontia of permanent teeth, excluding third molars: 3.0–7.5%.
- In hypodontia, two or more teeth are involved in 50% of the cases.
- Considerable ethnic variation.

Localization
- Third molars, upper lateral incisors, second premolars.

Clinical features
- Missing teeth, spacing, and occasionally abnormal location in the remaining teeth.

Complications
- Aesthetic and mastication problems.

Treatment
- Orthodontic and prosthetic treatment, implants.

Supernumerary Teeth

Definition
- Refers to a condition characterized by the presence of supernumerary teeth in the dental arch. These teeth may be either of normal morphology (supplemental) or, more frequently, are anomalous, with irregular size and shape (accessory).

Etiology
- The defect results from continuing abnormal activity of the dental lamina, which leads to the formation of supernumerary tooth buds. The etiology of the defect is multifactorial, although there is a strong genetic background under the control of several different loci.
- Frequent finding in patients with Gardner's syndrome, cleidocranial dysplasia, Hallermann–Streiff syndrome, and orofaciodigital syndrome type I.

Occurrence in children
- Primary dentition 0.3–0.6%, permanent dentition 1.0–3.5%.
- More frequently observed in the maxilla, by a ratio of 9 : 1.
- Supernumeraries in the primary dentition may be followed by supernumeraries in the permanent dentition in 30–50% of cases.
- Males more frequently affected than females (2 : 1).
- Ethnic variation.

Localization
- Near the middle line in the incisal region of the maxilla (mesiodens).
- Beyond the third molar (distomolars) or in the molar area (paramolars).

Clinical features
- Supplemental or conical, tuberculate, and odontoma-like shape (Figs. 1.**18**, 1.**19**).
- 75% of these teeth remain impacted in the bone, and are diagnosed only radiographically.

Complications
- In the case of impacted supernumerary teeth, there is an increased possibility of inhibited or delayed eruption of adjacent teeth. If the supernumeraries erupt in the dental arch, they usually cause functional and aesthetic problems.

Treatment
- Removal of the supernumerary teeth and orthodontic treatment of the affected area.

Defects of Eruption and Exfoliation

These defects result from the action of various etiological factors during the eruption stage of the dental development.

Eruption Defects

Early eruption

Definition
- This refers to accelerated eruption of either the primary or permanent teeth. In addition, the term "natal teeth" refers to primary teeth that have already erupted at birth (Fig. 1.**20**), whereas neonatal teeth are teeth erupting within one month after birth. These two defects usually represent regular primary teeth with imperfect roots, although sometimes they are supernumerary.

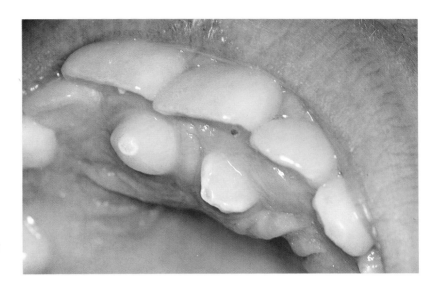

Fig. 1.**18**   Erupted supernumerary teeth (mesiodens) in the upper anterior area

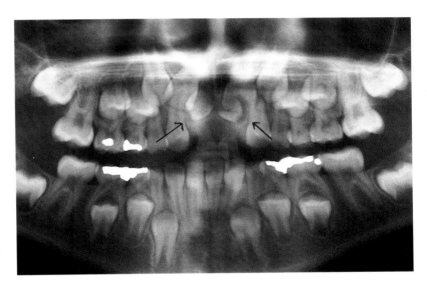

Fig. 1.**19**   Radiological features of upper anterior supernumerary teeth, resulting in eruption delay of the adjacent central incisors

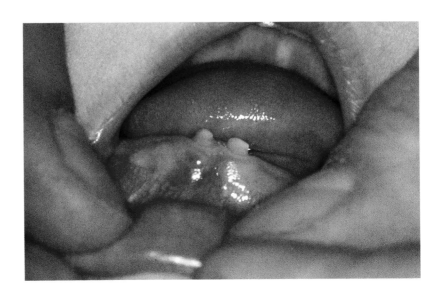

Fig. 1.**20**   Natal teeth in a new-born baby

Etiology	• Multifactorial, implicating local, systemic, and strong genetic factors. Early eruption of primary and permanent teeth can be found in the following syndromes: pycnodysostosis, hemihypertrophy, holoprosencephaly, Sotos, Klippel–Trenaunay–Weber, Sturge–Weber.
	• Excluding cases of isolated random occurrence of natal teeth, this defect may be associated with certain genetic disorders, such as the following syndromes: Ellis–van Creveld, Hallermann–Streiff, Saldino–Noonan, odonto-onychodysplasia, pachonychia congenita, X-linked ectodermal dysplasia.
Complications	• Frequently, natal teeth cause great difficulties in breast feeding, since they are usually lower central incisors.
Treatment	• In case of early eruption, no treatment is required. In case of natal teeth, extraction because of feeding problems is indicated.

Delayed eruption

Definition	• This refers to delay of eruption by more than six months for primary teeth, or more than 6–10 months for permanent teeth (Figs. 1.**21**, 1.**22**).
Etiology	• Delayed eruption can be caused by either local or systemic factors and genetic disorders.
Local factors	• Space loss and dental crowding
	• Trauma, radiation
	• Supernumerary teeth, odontomas
	• Delay of primary teeth exfoliation
	• Early primary teeth exfoliation
	• Dentigerous cyst, eruption cyst
	• Dilaceration
	• Pathological local defects of bone or soft tissues
Genetic/systemic disorders	• Vitamin D–resistant rickets
	• Hypothyroidism
	• Fibrous dysplasia
	• Pycnodysostosis
	• Cleidocranial dysplasia
	• Down's syndrome
	• Incontinentia pigmenti
	• Gardner's syndrome
	• Focal dermal hypoplasia (Goltz syndrome)
	• Osteopetrosis
	• Pseudohypoparathyroidism (Albright hereditary osteodystrophy)
	• Apert syndrome
	• Growth retardation, alopecia, pseudo-anodontia, and optic atrophy (GAPO) syndrome
	• Mucopolysaccharidosis I, II, VI
	• Mucolipidosis II
	• Faciogenital dysplasia (Aarskog's syndrome)
	• Cornelia de Lange syndrome
	• Schinzel–Giedion syndrome
	• Prader–Willi syndrome
	• Otodental syndrome
	• Robinson's syndrome
	• Amelo-onychohypohidrotic dysplasia
Complications	• Usually, severe dental crowding in the affected area.
Treatment	• In case of delayed tooth eruption caused by local etiological factors, removal of the factor and orthodontic evaluation followed by surgical or orthodontic treatment, or both, when needed.

Ankylosis

Definition	• Ankylosis appears clinically as an eruption defect, frequently followed by irregular occlusion. It is characterized by occlusal surface retention of the affected teeth, at a level at least 1 mm or more cervical to the adjacent teeth (Fig. 1.**23**).

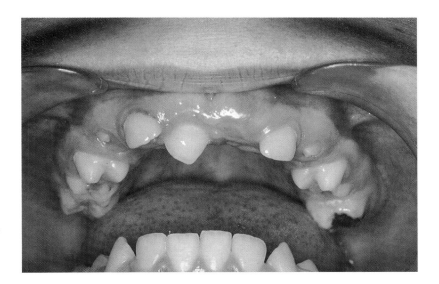

Fig. 1.**21**   Eruption delay of upper central incisors due to impacted odontomas and supernumerary teeth

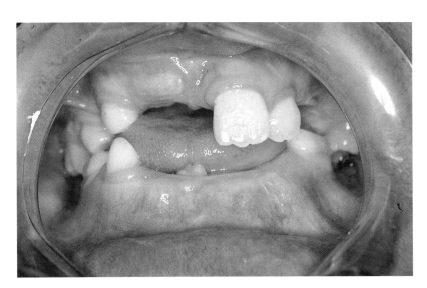

Fig. 1.**22**   Eruption delay of upper and lower anterior teeth due to impacted supernumerary teeth in a patient with cleidocranial dysplasia

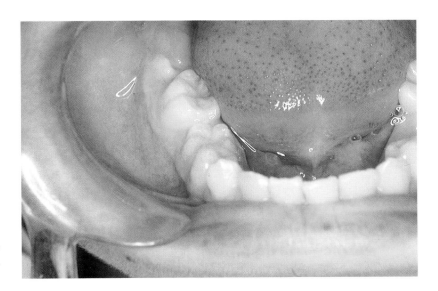

Fig. 1.**23**   Radiological features of moderate ankylosis of a lower second primary molar

Etiology
- The defect is caused by local traumatic and metabolic factors, whereas genetic factors have also been implicated. It is the result of continuing eruption of the adjacent teeth in contrast to the immobilization of the affected teeth.

Occurrence in children
- Primary teeth 1.3–9.9%.
- Coexistence of missing successors 11–20%.
- Permanent teeth, rare compared to primary (1 : 10).

Localization
- Primary and permanent molars.
- More frequently in the mandible.
- Frequently a bilateral finding.

Clinical features
- Occlusal surface at least 1 mm cervically compared to adjacent teeth.
- Sharp, clear sound on percussion.
- Absence of regular mobility.
- Three clinical forms: mild, moderate, severe.

Radiological features
- Break of periodontal membrane continuity.
- Absence of findings in ankylosed buccal and lingual surfaces.
- Findings in 30% of the cases with ankylosed proximal surfaces (Figs. 1.**24,** 1.**25**).

Complications
- In moderate and severe cases, the defect usually causes orthodontic disturbances in the involved area, resulting from malalignment of the adjacent and opponent teeth.

Treatment
- Depending on the severity of the ankylosis, a) follow-up of the resorption rate of the ankylosed tooth and possible build-up; b) mechanical luxation; c) extraction and orthodontic treatment.

Early Exfoliation

Definition
- Refers to early loss of either primary or permanent teeth.

Etiology
- The condition results frequently from trauma, periodontal disease, and extraction due to caries. However, some genetic and systemic disorders may cause early loss of teeth as a result of damage to either soft periodontal tissue or bone (Fig. 1.**26**).

Genetic/systemic disorders
- Prepubertal periodontitis
- HIV periodontitis
- Hypophosphatasia
- Acatalasia
- Papillon–Lefèvre syndrome
- Gingival fibromatosis and hypertrichosis
- Oculodentodigital syndrome, type I
- Ehlers–Danlos syndrome, type VIII
- Progeria
- Vitamin D–resistant rickets
- Diabetes mellitus
- Glycogen storage disease, type Ib
- Langerhans cell histiocytosis
- Cyclic neutropenia
- Leukemia
- Inherited immunodeficiencies
- Acrodynia
- Neoplasms
- Hajdu–Cheney syndrome
- Chediak–Higashi syndrome
- Ellis–van Creveld syndrome

Enamel Defects

These defects result from the action of various etiological factors during the apposition and mineralization stages of dental development.

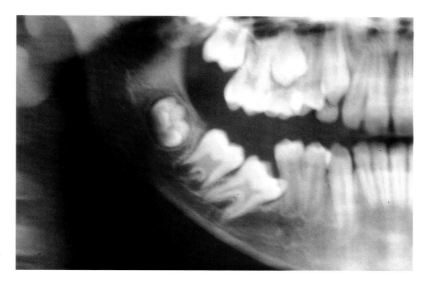

Fig. 1.**24** Radiological features of severe ankylosis of a lower first permanent molar

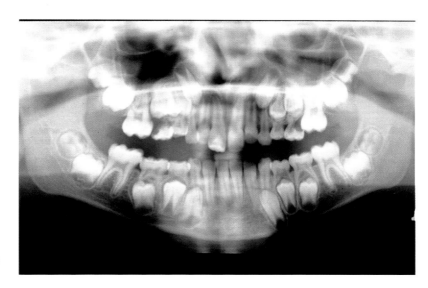

Fig. 1.**25** Radiological features of mild and moderate ankylosis of the upper and lower primary molars

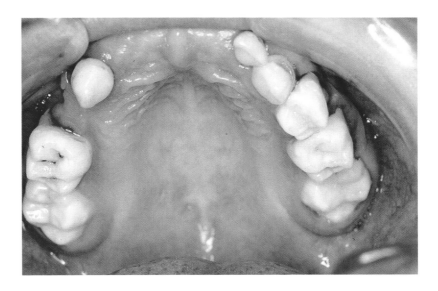

Fig. 1.**26** Early exfoliation of an upper primary molar due to periodontitis in a patient with cyclic neutropenia

Definition	• The range of enamel defects covers a group of defects clinically recognized as enamel hypoplasia, hypocalcification, hypomaturation (demarcated and diffuse enamel opacities), or a combination of the former, depending on the phase of amelogenesis that the etiological factor acts on.
Etiology	• Defective formation of the enamel matrix results in hypoplasia; defective calcification of an otherwise normal quantity of organic matrix results in hypocalcification; and defective formation of the crystallites in various areas of the enamel rods and sheaths results in hypomaturation (opacities). • The whole range of enamel defects may be attributed to local, systemic, and genetic etiological factors. The clinical features are similar, although in defects of local etiology, single teeth are involved, whereas in those of systemic etiology all the teeth developing during the time of action of the etiological factor are affected (chronological defect). The genetic defects represent a separate nosological entity, usually affecting all the teeth, primary and permanent, and they are further divided into *isolated* enamel defects, termed amelogenesis imperfecta, and enamel defects associated with genetic disorders or syndromes.
Local factors	• Trauma, chronic infection, local surgery, cleft lip and palate, radiation, burns, osteomyelitis, jaw fracture.
Systemic etiological factors	*Prenatal (defects in primary teeth)* • Various maternal diseases such as Vitamin A and D deficiency, diabetes mellitus, infections such as syphilis, rubella, cytomegaloviral infection, maternal alcoholism, toxemia, hypertension, malnutrition, hypoparathyroidism, cardiac, renal and pulmonary diseases, anemia, prolonged taking of medicines. *Perinatal and neonatal (defects in primary and permanent teeth)* • Neonatal hypocalcemia, severe perinatal and neonatal hypoxic injury, prolonged delivery, prematurity, low birth weight, twins, cerebral injury, neurological disorders, hyperbilirubinemia, prolonged neonatal diarrhea and vomiting, severe neonatal infections, high fever. *Postnatal (defects in permanent teeth)* • Nutritional and gastrointestinal disturbances resulting in hypocalcemia and vitamin D deficiency, bacterial and viral infections (particularly those with high fever), exanthematous diseases, juvenile hypothyroidism, hypoparathyroidism, hypogonadism, phenylketonuria, alcaptonuria, renal disorders, congenital heart disease, congenital allergy, oxalosis, mercury poisoning (acrodynia), fluorosis, prolonged use of medicines, prolonged diarrhea and vomiting, radiation and cytotoxic therapy.
Occurrence in children	• Frequent in primary dentition (33%). • Frequent in cases of local etiology; 12–23% in permanent teeth following trauma or chronic inflammation in the predecessor primary teeth. • Frequent in cases of systemic etiology; 71% in children with a history of prenatal insult. • Approximately 70 genetic disorders are associated with enamel defects.
Localization	• In cases of local etiology, mainly in permanent incisors and premolars. • In cases of systemic etiology, mainly in the primary molars and permanent incisors and molars, but also in all the teeth developing during the period of action of the etiological factor. • In cases of genetic etiology, all teeth in both primary and permanent dentitions may be involved.
Clinical features	• Hypoplasia, pits, grooves, and lines in the whole enamel surface or in certain areas. Possible reduction of the enamel thickness (Figs. 1.**27**–1.**29**).

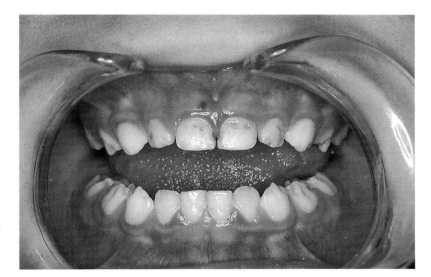

Fig. 1.**27**   Enamel hypoplasia and hypomineralization of all the primary teeth (chronological) resulting from prolonged use of muscle-relaxing medicines during pregnancy

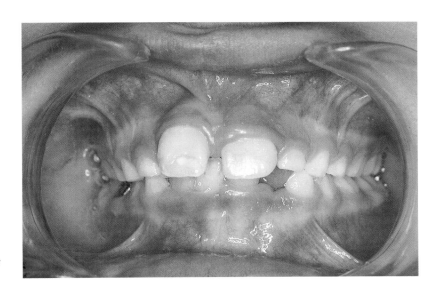

Fig. 1.**28**   Enamel hypoplasia and hypomineralization of an upper central incisor due to mechanical trauma of the predecessor primary tooth

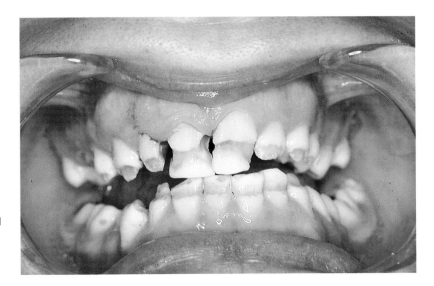

Fig. 1.**29**   Enamel hypoplasia of all the permanent teeth (chronological), resulting from prolonged use of medicines for chronic nephrotic syndrome

- Hypocalcification, soft enamel of yellow-brownish color, easily removed by probing in isolated areas of the enamel, enamel attrition, sensitivity in thermal stimuli (Figs. 1.**30,** 1.**31**).
- Hypomaturation (opacities), dull enamel with mottled, white, opaque appearance and regular thickness, reduced hardness and possible microfractures (Fig. 1.**32**).

Complications

- Occasional occlusal distortion, aesthetic problems, sensitivity.

Treatment

- Conservative aesthetic restorations, prosthetic rehabilitation.

Amelogenesis Imperfecta

Definition

- The term "amelogenesis imperfecta" characterizes isolated defects of the enamel resulting exclusively from genetic factors and not associated with generalized genetic disorders and syndromes. This proposed terminology has been questioned recently, since other local abnormalities associated with amelogenesis imperfecta have been found, such as skeletal anterior open bite. In addition, the assumption of an isolated enamel defect in amelogenesis imperfecta may not be correct, since it depends on the clinician's ability to diagnose other abnormalities elsewhere in the body.

Etiology

- The defect results from genetic factors acting during embryogenesis, particularly in the phases of enamel formation.
- Recently, it has been suggested that the anomaly results from a defect in the enamel matrix proteins amelogenin and enamelin. The amelogenin gene has been located in the p22.1–22.3 region of the X chromosome and in the pericentromeric region of the Y chromosome. The X-linked types of amelogenesis imperfecta are therefore strongly associated with a molecular defect in this locus.
- They are classified into many types, according to their clinical features and mode of inheritance.

Classification

Type I, hypoplastic
- Ia: pitted hypoplastic, autosomal dominant (Fig. 1.**33**)

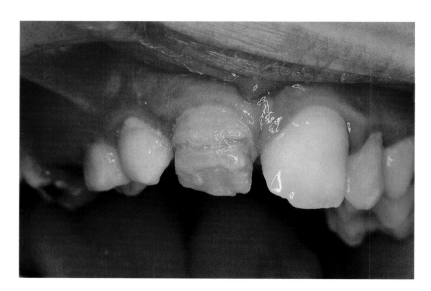

Fig. 1.**30** Enamel hypoplasia and hypomineralization of an upper central incisor, resulting from surgical intervention in the area when the patient was aged two

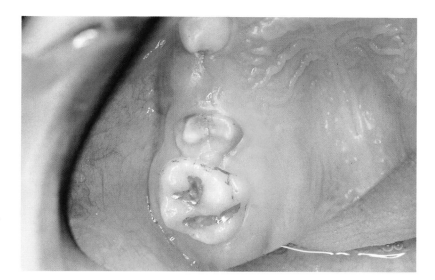

Fig. 1.**31**   Enamel hypomineralization and hypomaturation of an upper premolar, resulting from chronic pulpal infection of the predecessor primary molar

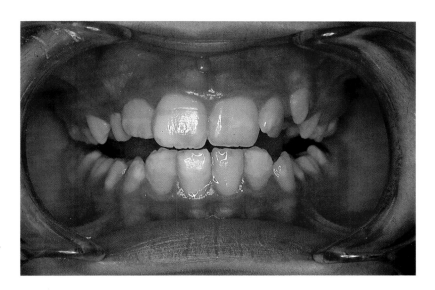

Fig. 1.**32**   Hypomineralization and hypomaturation (opacities) of the permanent incisors and molars, resulting from prolonged use of antibiotics for chronic infection in the neonate

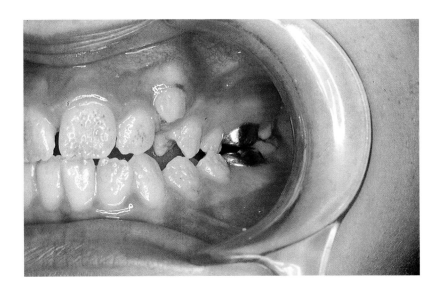

Fig. 1.**33**   Hypoplastic pitted amelogenesis imperfecta (type Ia)

- Ib: local hypoplastic, autosomal dominant (Fig. 1.**34**)
- Ic: local hypoplastic, autosomal recessive
- Id: smooth hypoplastic, autosomal dominant (Fig. 1.**35**)
- Ie: smooth hypoplastic, X-linked dominant
- If: rough hypoplastic, autosomal dominant (Fig. 1.**36**)
- Ig: rough hypoplastic (enamel agenesis), autosomal recessive

Type II, hypomature
- IIa: hypomature pigmented enamel, autosomal recessive
- IIb: hypomature enamel, X-linked recessive (Fig. 1.**37**)
- IIc: snow-capped enamel, autosomal dominant

Type III, hypocalcified
- IIIa: hypocalcified enamel, autosomal dominant (Fig. 1.**38**)
- IIIb: hypocalcified enamel, autosomal recessive (Fig. 1.**39**)

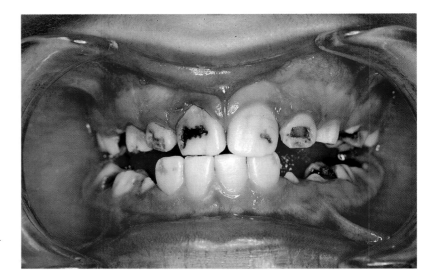

Fig. 1.**34** Hypoplastic amelogenesis imperfecta with local hypoplasias (type Ib)

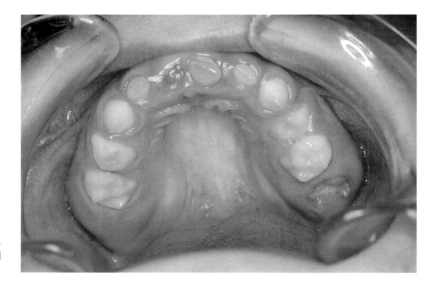

Fig. 1.**35** Hypoplastic amelogenesis imperfecta with smooth enamel (type Id)

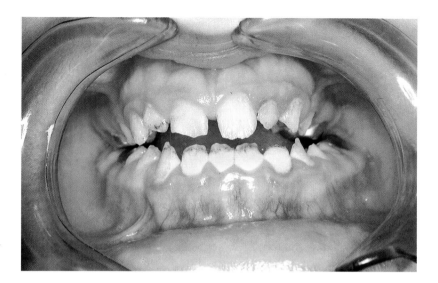

Fig. 1.**36** Hypoplastic amelogenesis imperfecta with rough enamel (type If).

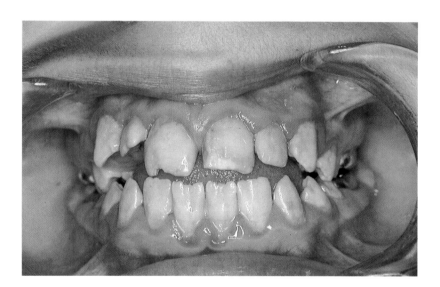

Fig. 1.**37** Hypomature amelogenesis imperfecta (type IIb)

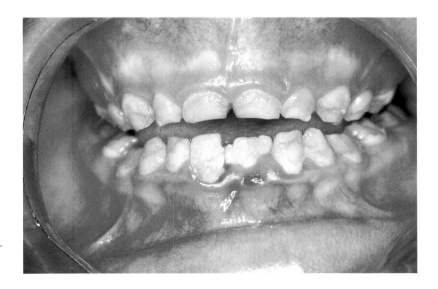

Fig. 1.**38** Hypomineralized amelogenesis imperfecta. Autosomal dominant (type IIa)

Type IV, hypomature–hypoplastic with taurodontism
- IVa: hypomaturation–hypoplasia with taurodontism, autosomal dominant
- IVb: hypoplasia–hypomaturation with taurodontism, autosomal dominant

Occurrence in children
- One per 4000–8000, all types
- 60–73% of the total hypoplastic types, 20–40% hypomaturation types, 7% hypocalcified types

Localization
- All teeth, primary and permanent

Clinical features

Hypoplasia
- Normal or reduced enamel thickness throughout the whole surface, or in isolated areas.
- Enamel pits, grooves, fissures and linear depressions randomly distributed over the entire enamel surface.
- Hard enamel with a normal or slightly yellow-brown color.
- Frequent microfractures of the enamel, and possible attrition.
- Types Id, Ie, and If appear clinically as teeth to have been prepared for jacket crowns.

Hypocalcification
- Regular enamel thickness at the time of tooth eruption.
- Soft enamel easily removed.
- Gradual reduction of the thickness resulting from easy attrition.
- Only dentine remains in severe forms of the defect.
- Increased sensitivity in thermal stimuli.
- Yellow-brownish color of the enamel, with pigment deposition.
- Associated occasionally with anterior skeletal open-bite.

Hypomaturation
- Opaque mottled enamel of normal thickness.
- Enamel approaches the radiodensity of dentine.
- Relatively soft enamel with frequent microfractures.
- Mottled brownish-yellow to white appearance.

Complications
- Occasional occlusal distortion, aesthetic problems, sensitivity.

Treatment
- Conservative aesthetic restorations; in severe cases, prosthetic rehabilitation.

Enamel Defects Associated with Genetic Disorders

Definition
- Many genetic disorders or syndromes may be associated, with variable incidences, with a wide variety of enamel defects. In these cases, the defect is not termed "amelogenesis imperfecta" but "enamel hypoplasia," "enamel hypocalcification," or "enamel hypomaturation," depending on the clinical features of the defects (Figs. 1.**40, 1.41**).

Genetic disorders
- Tricho-odonto-onychial dysplasia
- Oculodentodigital syndrome, types I and II
- Orofaciodigital syndrome (type I)
- Amelo-onychohypohidrotic dysplasia
- Ectodermal dysplasia with syndactyly
- Amelocerebrohypohidrotic syndrome
- Acrorenal ectodermal dysplasia, lipoatrophic diabetes
- Enamel renal syndrome
- Epidermolysis bullosa, dystrophic
- Focal dermal hypoplasia (Goltz syndrome)
- Hypomelanosis of Ito
- Corneodermato-osseous syndrome
- Naegeli–Franceschetti–Jadassohn syndrome
- Trichodento-osseous syndrome (types I, II, III)
- Seckel's syndrome
- Arthrogryposis and ectodermal dysplasia
- Prader–Willi syndrome
- Singleton–Merton syndrome
- Congenital insensitivity to pain with anhydrosis

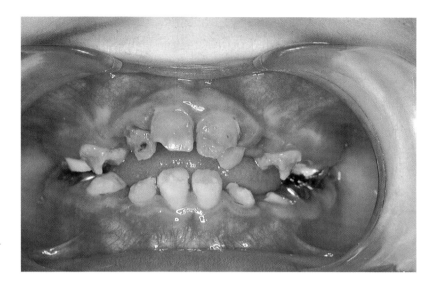

Fig. 1.**39** Hypomineralized amelogenesis imperfecta. Autosomal recessive (type IIb)

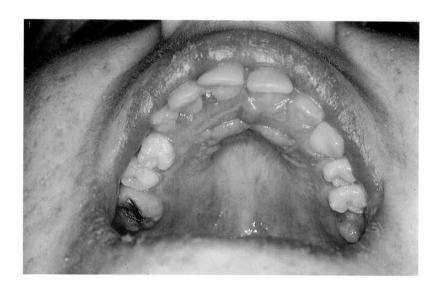

Fig. 1.**40** Enamel hypoplasia in a patient with Goltz syndrome

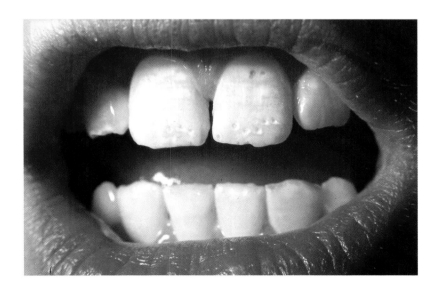

Fig. 1.**41** Enamel hypoplasia in a patient with tuberous sclerosis

- Faciogenital dysplasia (Aarskog's syndrome)
- Mucopolysaccharidosis IV A, B (Morquio–Ullrich syndrome)
- Lipoid proteinosis
- Mucolipidosis II (Leroy I syndrome)
- Vitamin D–dependent rickets
- Pseudohypoparathyroidism (Albright hereditary osteodystrophy)
- Tuberous sclerosis
- Pycnodysostosis

Dentine Defects

Dentinogenesis Imperfecta

Definition
- Dentinogenesis imperfecta is a genetic disorder affecting dentine collagen during embryogenesis, and particularly in the phases of tissue differentiation and organic matrix formation.

Etiology
- Dentinogenesis imperfecta can be found either isolated, characterized as type II, or as type I simultaneously with other features of osteogenesis imperfecta, a group of genetic collagen disorders characterized by anomalies in bones, joints, eyes and teeth.
- The gene responsible for type II has been found on the 4q chromosome, whereas in type I (osteogenesis imperfecta), mutant genes have been found in chromosomes 7q and 17q.

Occurrence in children
- Type I, one per 2500–5000 (osteogenesis imperfecta).
- Type II, one per 8000.

Localization
- All teeth, primary and permanent.

Clinical features
- Striking amber translucent and discolored teeth (Fig. 1.**42**).
- Enamel suffering from non-accidental fractures, resulting not only from dentine defect, but also from the presence of defect in the enamel–dentine junction.
- Fragile roots and loose teeth.
- Gradual attrition or non-accidental fractures of the entire crown (Figs. 1.**43**, 1.**44**), resulting in decreased occlusal height.
- Type I may present a wide range of clinical features in the same patient, varying from easily detectable defects in all teeth, primary and permanent, to only mild pigmentation of few teeth.
- Type II shows greater uniformity, with more severe clinical features.

Radiological features
- Characteristic short roots.
- Obliteration of pulp chambers and root canals (Fig. 1.**45**).

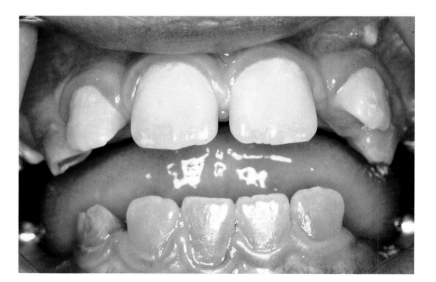

Fig. 1.**42** Isolated dentinogenesis imperfecta of the primary and permanent teeth (type II)

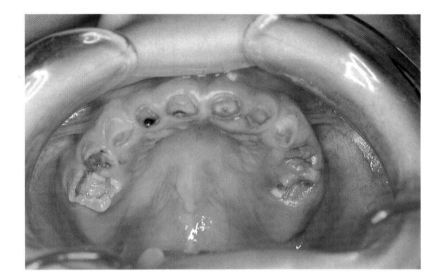

Fig. 1.**43**   Dentinogenesis imperfecta (type I) of the primary teeth, revealing severe attrition in a patient with osteogenesis imperfecta type I

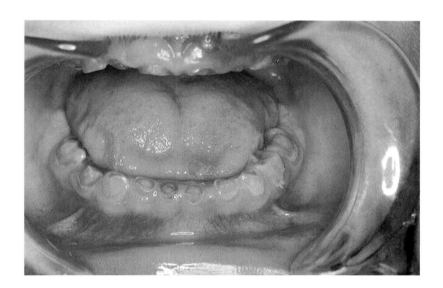

Fig. 1.**44**   Dentinogenesis imperfecta (type I) of the primary teeth, revealing less severe attrition in a patient with osteogenesis imperfecta type I (the brother of the patient in Fig. 1.**43**)

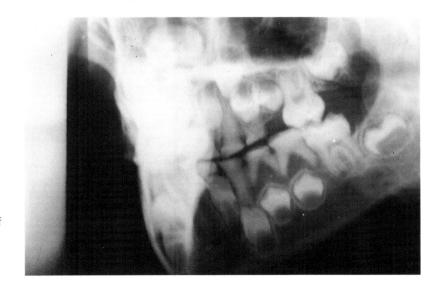

Fig. 1.**45**   Radiological features of primary and permanent molars in dentinogenesis imperfecta (type I) in a patient with osteogenesis imperfecta type I

- Reduced cervical diameter and radiographic contrast of dentine.
- Frequent periapical radiolucencies.

Complications
- Occlusal distortion, fragile teeth, abscesses.

Treatment
- Prosthetic rehabilitation, overdentures.

Dentine Dysplasia

Definition
- Dentine dysplasia is usually divided into two distinct types: type I, or radicular dysplasia, and type II, or coronal dysplasia.

Etiology
- The defect results from epithelial invagination of the dental organ cells into the dental papilla, producing ectopic formation of dentine.
- The condition is transmitted an as autosomal dominant trait.

Occurrence in children
- One per 100 000.

Localization
- In both types, all teeth, primary and permanent.

Clinical features
- Type I, teeth with normal crowns of regular or slightly amber translucency. Tendency toward complete obliteration of pulp cavities. Abnormal spaces between the teeth, malalignment, malposition, and severe mobility as a result of poor root formation (Fig. 1.**46**).
- Type II, semi-transparent opalescent primary teeth, similar to those in dentinogenesis imperfecta, and normal clinical appearance in the permanent teeth. Incomplete obliteration of pulp cavities, particularly in the primary teeth, and frequently pulp stones (Fig. 1.**47**).

Radiological features

Type I
- Extremely short roots.
- Obliterated pulp chambers and root canals before eruption.
- Frequently periapical radiolucencies around the defective roots.

Type II
- Complete obliteration of pulp chambers and root canals after eruption.
- Frequently, pulp stones.
- Absence of periapical radiolucencies.

Complications
- Occlusal distortion, abscesses.

Treatment
- Prosthetic rehabilitation, overdentures.

Dentine Defects Associated with Genetic Disorders or Syndromes

Definition
- Some genetic disorders or syndromes may be associated, with variable incidences, with dentine defects. In these cases, the defect is not termed "dentinogenesis imperfecta."

Genetic disorders, syndromes
- Hypophosphatasia
- Osteogenesis imperfecta types I, III, IV (dentinogenesis imperfecta type I)
- Unger–Trott syndrome
- Vitamin D–resistant rickets
- De Toni–Debré–Fanconi syndrome
- Albright hereditary osteodystrophy (pseudohypoparathyroidism)
- Mucopolysaccharidosis III (Sanfilippo syndrome)
- Tumoral calcinosis
- Ehlers–Danlos syndrome
- Epidermal nevus syndrome
- Brachioskeletogenital (BSG)syndrome
- Dentine–osseous dysplasia

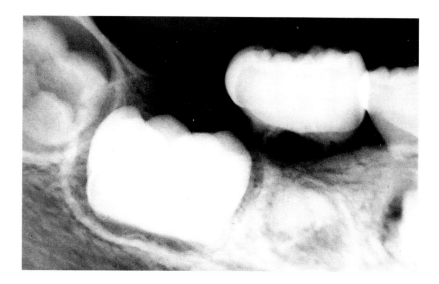

Fig. 1.**46**   Radiological features of radicular dentine dysplasia (type I)

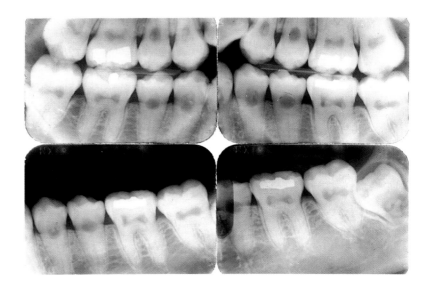

Fig. 1.**47**   Radiological features of coronal dentine dysplasia (type II)

Defects Involving the Whole Tooth Structure

Odontodysplasia

Definition
- The term refers to a severe dental defect involving all dental tissues of both ectodermal and mesodermal origin.

Etiology
- The etiology is still unknown, although local, systemic, and genetic factors have been implicated. Recently, reports have suggested that the defect is caused by local vascular deficiency, resulting from a local developmental anatomic defect, such as a vascular nevus.
- The alteration has occasionally been associated with the epidermal nevus syndrome.

Occurrence in children
- Rare, but underreported.
- More common in females.

Localization
- Both primary and permanent dentitions are affected.
- Maxilla more frequently affected than mandible (2 : 1).
- The whole or part of a quadrant is involved. The defect crosses the midline in only 16% of the cases, affecting also anterior teeth.

Clinical features
- Tooth eruption is delayed and painful. Occasionally, teeth fail to erupt (Fig. 1.**48**).
- Frequent abscesses.
- Gingival enlargement and inflammation.
- Discolored yellow teeth with rough and small crowns and gross hypoplastic and hypocalcified enamel and dentine.

Radiological features
- Ghost-like appearance of the teeth with periapical radiolucencies (Fig. 1.**49**).
- Short roots with very wide pulp canals and open apices.

Complications
- Occlusal distortion, painful teeth, abscesses.

Treatment
- In cases of less affected teeth, prosthetic restoration. In severe cases, removal of the affected teeth and prosthetic rehabilitation of the involved area.

Tooth Discoloration

Definition
- Refers to color changes in the teeth.

Etiology
- The defects result from the deposition of various pigmented elements either on the enamel surface (extrinsic pigmentation) or in the inner layers of the dentine and pulp (intrinsic pigmentation).
- These defects are associated either with systemic factors and involve all the teeth, or with local factors, mainly trauma, involving certain teeth (Fig. 1.**50**).

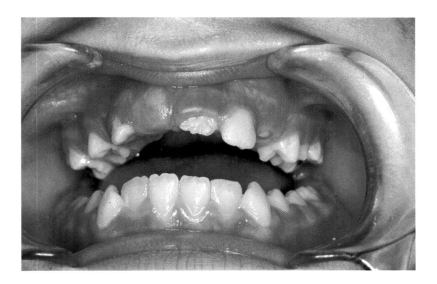

Fig. 1.**48**   Clinical features of regional odontodysplasia

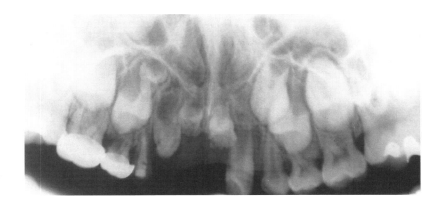

Fig. 1.**49**   Radiological features of regional odontodysplasia

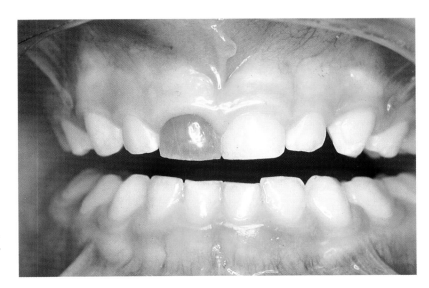

Fig. 1.**50**   Intrinsic brown pigmentation, resulting from pulpal necrosis of the primary incisor due to trauma

Occurrence in children

- Rare.

Clinical features

Extrinsic pigments may involve all or some of the teeth, and result from an excess of various chemical elements in the saliva, which may or may not be metals, including the following (Fig. 1.**51**):

- Iron, magnesium, silver: black pigmentation.
- Mercury: gray or green-black pigmentation.
- Lead: gray pigmentation.
- Copper: brown or green pigmentation.
- Bromides: brown pigmentation.
- Nickel, antimony: green pigmentation.
- Cadmium: yellow pigmentation.
- Potassium: violet pigmentation.
- Enamel hypoplasia/hypocalcification: yellow-brown pigmentation.

Intrinsic pigments. This group includes the following, apart from local discoloration due to trauma:

- Erythroblastosis fetalis (incorporation of bilirubin into the developing dentition): yellow-green and blue-green color of teeth, gradually reducing with age; particularly noticeable in the anterior teeth.
- Tetracyclines (incorporation of tetracycline into the hydroxyapatite of the calcified areas of the dentine and in smaller amounts in the enamel): initially light yellow, and later a darker gray-brown color in the teeth, with horizontal bands.
- Erythropoietic porphyria, congenital (incorporation of porphyrin in developing dentition): reddish-brown or pinkish discoloration of the teeth.
- Alcaptonuria (deposition of homogentisic acid in the developing dentition): brown color of the teeth.
- Oxalosis (incorporation of oxalate crystals into the developing dentition): slate-gray discoloration of the teeth.
- Fluorosis (defective mineralization of the enamel organic matrix, resulting from defective ameloblasts during enamel maturation, due to high levels of fluoride): chalky and opaque white or gray stains and patches (Fig. 1.**52**).
- Cystic fibrosis (discoloration of the teeth results from the disease alone or medication, particularly tetracyclines): dark teeth, ranging from yellowish-grey to dark brown.
- Dentinogenesis imperfecta (genetic abnormality of the dentine collagen during the phase of histodifferentiation and organic matrix formation): brownish, semi-transparent opalescent teeth.

Treatment

- Vital and non-vital bleaching techniques.
- Conservative aesthetic restorations, prosthetic rehabilitation.

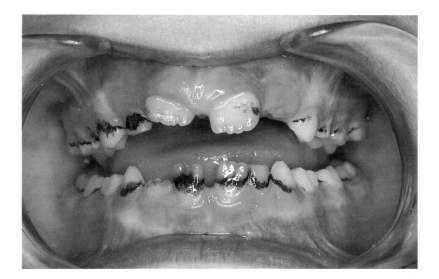

Fig. 1.**51** Extrinsic black pigmentation, resulting from increased levels of iron in the saliva

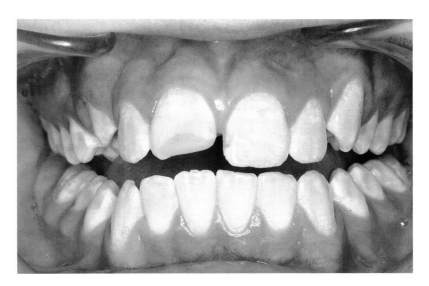

Fig. 1.**52** Intrinsic pigmentation of the permanent teeth, resulting from fluorosis

2 Developmental Anomalies

Orofacial Clefts

Definition
- Orofacial clefts are developmental malformations of multiple tissue maturation processes of the oral cavity and face.

Etiology
- The etiology remains obscure. Genetic and environmental factors may be related to isolated defects.
- Several developmental syndromes may be associated with orofacial clefts.
- In 15–30% of patients, there is a family history of similar congenital defects.

Occurrence
- The prevalence of cleft palate varies from 0.29 to 0.56 per 1000 births in children, while the prevalence of cleft lips is about one per 9000 births.
- A considerable ethnic association with the prevalence of orofacial clefts has been reported.
- Cleft lip and cleft palate occur in 0.52–1.34 per 1000 births.

Localization
- Lips, hard and soft palate, uvula, maxilla, mandible.

Clinical features
- Cleft lip is characterized by a defect that usually involves the upper lip (Figs. 2.**1**, 2.**2**). About 75–80% of cleft lips are unilateral, and the left side is more often affected than the right. Isolated cleft lip occurs less often than a combination with cleft palate and cleft jaw defects. Missing and, rarely, supernumerary teeth may be observed.
- Cleft palate is characterized by a defect in the midline of the palate that varies in severity and may involve the hard palate, soft palate, or both (Fig. 2.**3**).
- Maxillary anterior alveolar clefts are characterized by a bony defect in the maxilla, usually between the central and lateral incisors (Fig. 2.**4**).

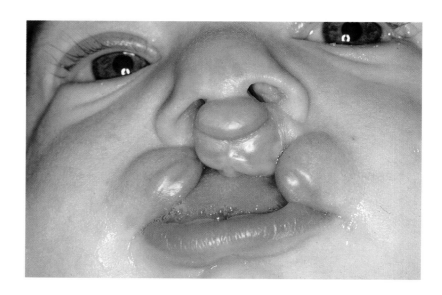

Fig. 2.**1**   Cleft lip, bilateral

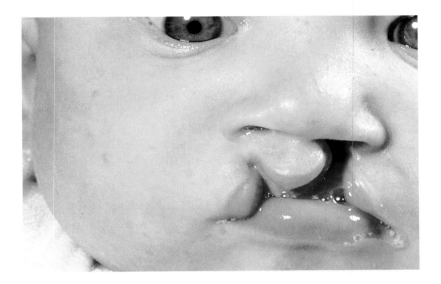

Fig. 2.**2**   Cleft lip, bilateral

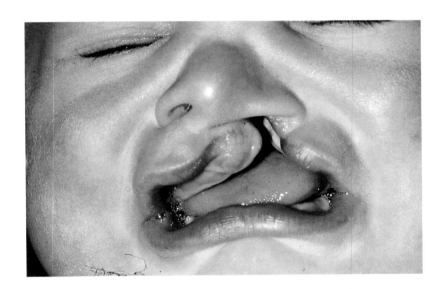

Fig. 2.**3**   Cleft lip and palate

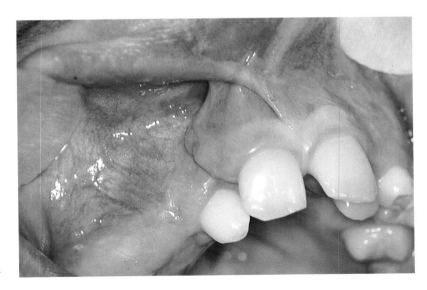

Fig. 2.**4**   Maxillary anterior alveolar cleft

- Bifid uvula is a minor expression of cleft palate, and may occur alone or in combination with more severe defects (Fig. 2.**5**).

Treatment

- Plastic surgical repair. Prosthetic and orthodontic appliances are also necessary.

Bifid Tongue

Definition

- Bifid tongue is a developmental malformation of the tongue caused by lack of fusion of the lateral halves and resulting in cleavage of the tongue.

Occurrence

- Rare.

Localization

- Tip of the tongue, midline of the dorsum of the tongue.

Clinical features

- The complete form is very rare, and may result in the formation of two complete tongues.
- The incomplete form appears either as an asymptomatic deep groove in the midline of the dorsum of the tongue, or as a double ending of the tip of the tongue (Fig. 2.**6**). Neither form has any clinical significance.
- Bifid tongue may coexist with the orofaciodigital syndrome.

Treatment

- The incomplete form requires no treatment.
- The complete form needs surgical reconstruction.

Ankyloglossia

Definition

- Ankyloglossia or tongue-tie is a developmental malformation in which the tongue is abnormally fixed to floor of the mouth or lingual aspect of the gingiva, due to a short and malpositioned lingual frenulum.

Occurrence

- Rare. Approximately one per 1000 births.

Clinical features

- The lingual frenulum is short, thick or thin, and fibrous (Figs. 2.**7**, 2.**8**).
- The malformation may cause partial or complete immobility of the tongue.

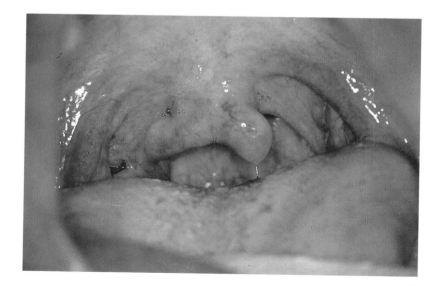

Fig. 2.**5** Bifid uvula

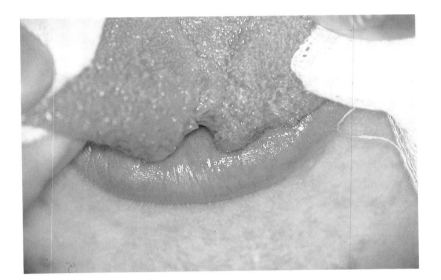

Fig. 2.**6**   Bifid tongue

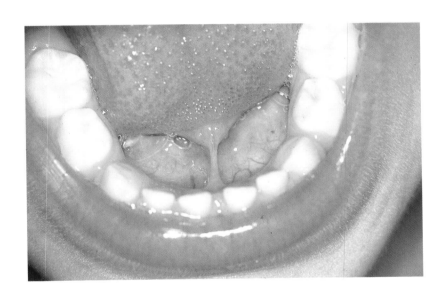

Fig. 2.**7**   Ankyloglossia

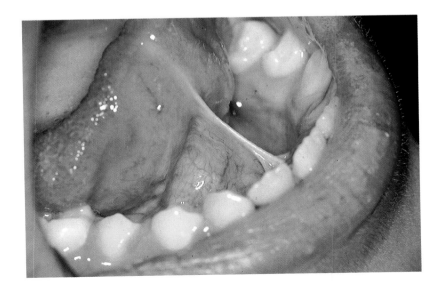

Fig. 2.**8**   Ankyloglossia

- Mild cases are asymptomatic, and may go unnoticed for a long time. Severe cases may cause problems with speaking, eating and breast-feeding.

Treatment
- Surgical clipping of the frenulum in severe cases.

Lip Frenulum Anomalies

Definition
- Lip frenulum is a normal connective tissue structure extending from the lips to the alveolar process of the teeth.

Clinical features
- Rarely, the central frenulum of the upper and lower lips may be thick, broad and long, with an adhesion to the marginal gingiva.
- In severe cases, a large gap between the central incisors, or gingival regression or tooth movement may occur (Figs. 2.**9**, 2.**10**).

Treatment
- Surgical correction.

Congenital Lip Pits

Definition
- Congenital lip pits or paramedian lip pits are developmental invaginations, which may occur alone or in combination with commissural pits, cleft lip, or cleft palate.

Etiology
- They may be inherited as an autosomal dominant trait.
- They develop through incomplete regression of the lateral sulci of the lower lip during embryonic development.

Occurrence
- Rare.

Localization
- A few millimeters from the midline of the vermilion border of the lower lip, usually bilateral.
- Labial commissures.

Clinical features
- Clinically, they present as bilateral or unilateral depressions (Fig. 2.**11**).
- The size varies from 1 mm to 10 mm, and the depth of blind sinuses may extend to 1 cm or more.
- A small amount of mucous secretion may accumulate at the depth of the pits, and the lip may be enlarged and swollen.
- Occasionally, a fistula may coexist.
- The diagnosis is based on clinical criteria.

Treatment
- Surgical correction for cosmetic purposes.

Double Lip

Definition
- Double lip is a malformation that may be present at birth or later in life.

Etiology
- It may be congenital due to the failure of the pars glabrosa and the pars villosa to fuse along the horizontal sulcus during lip formation.
- Acquired double lip is one of the main components of Ascher's syndrome (double lip, blepharochalasis and goiter).

Occurrence
- Rare.

Localization
- Often the upper lip, and less frequently the lower lip.

Clinical features
- Clinically, it is characterized by an asymptomatic, protruding horizontal fold on the mucosal surface of the lip.

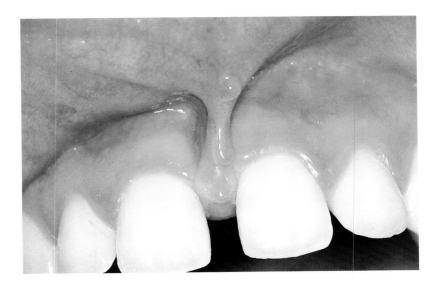

Fig. 2.**9**   Thick and long central frenulum of the upper lip

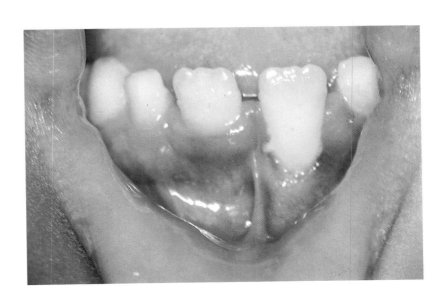

Fig. 2.**10**   Thin and long central frenulum of the lower lip

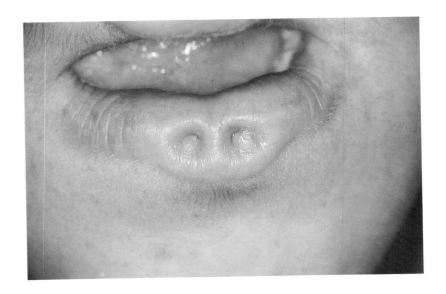

Fig. 2.**11**   Bilateral congenital lip pits

- Typically, the double lip is visible during speech or smiling, or when the lips are tensed (Figs. 2.**12**, 2.**13**).
- The diagnosis is based on clinical criteria.

Treatment

- Mild cases require no treatment.
- Severe cases require surgical correction for cosmetic purposes.

Fordyce's Granules

Definition

- Fordyce's granules are a normal anatomical variation, characterized by the presence of ectopic sebaceous glands in the oral mucosa.

Etiology

- Developmental.

Occurrence

- They present in about 20–30% of children and adolescents.
- About 80% of adults have Fordyce's granules.

Localization

- Upper lip, buccal mucosa, retromolar area, anterior tonsillar pillar.

Clinical features

- Clinically, Fordyce's granules present as multiple yellow or whitish-yellow, slightly raised, tiny pinhead-sized spots that are well circumscribed (Fig. 2.**14**).
- Solitary enlarged Fordyce's granules may also be seen (Fig. 2.**15**).
- The granules are asymptomatic, and come to the patient's attention by chance.
- The diagnosis is usually based on clinical criteria.

Laboratory tests

- Histopathological examination reveals normal collections of sebaceous glands without hair follicles.

Differential diagnosis

- Candidiasis
- Lichen planus
- Leukoplakia

Treatment

- No treatment is required.

Exostoses

Definition

- Exostoses are developmental harmless bony overgrowths that may affect the jaws.

Etiology

- Unknown. Genetic and environmental factors may be involved in their development.

Occurrence in children

- Rare. The lesions are usually first noticed after 20 years of age.

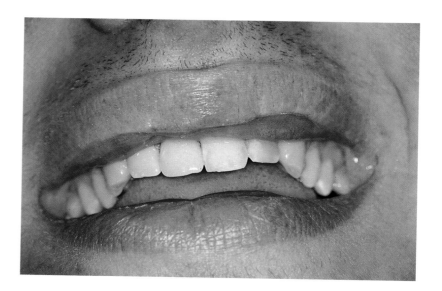

Fig. 2.**12** Double upper lip

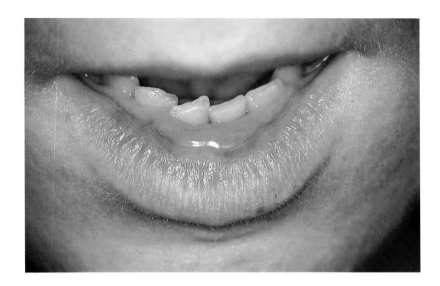

Fig. 2.**13** Double lower lip

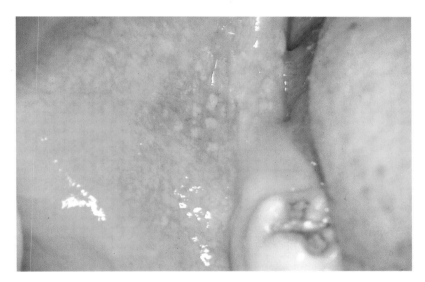

Fig. 2.**14** Multiple Fordyce's granules on the buccal mucosa and retromolar area

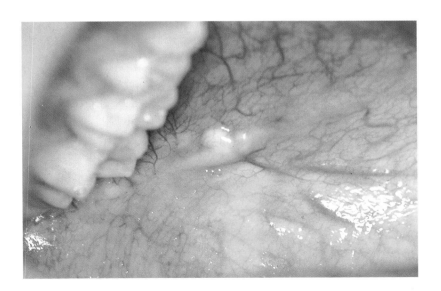

Fig. 2.**15** Solitary hypertrophic Fordyce's granules on the buccal mucosa

Localization
- Midline of the hard palate (torus palatinus).
- Lingual surfaces of the mandible, usually in the premolar region (torus mandibularis).
- Buccal surface of the maxillary and/or mandibular alveolar ridge (buccal exostoses).

Clinical features
- Clinically, exostoses present as bony, hard nodules covered by normal mucosa (Fig. 2.**16**).
- The number and size of the lesions vary considerably.
- Rarely, the overlying mucosa may be ulcerated due to mechanical trauma.
- The lesions grow slowly, and are asymptomatic.
- The diagnosis is based on clinical criteria.

Treatment
- No treatment is required. Surgical excision is indicated only when it is necessary to fit a prosthesis.

Facial Hemiatrophy

Definition
- Facial hemiatrophy, or Parry–Romberg syndrome, is a degenerative disorder characterized by atrophic changes of the deeper structures (e.g. fat, muscle, cartilage, and bone) involving one side of the face.

Etiology
- Unknown.

Occurrence
- Rare. The disease usually starts in childhood, and girls are affected more frequently than boys (ratio 3 : 2).

Localization
- One side of the face, lips, tongue, maxilla, mandible, teeth.

Clinical features
- The affected side appears atrophic, and the skin is wrinkled, shriveled and often shows hyperpigmentation or hypopigmentation (Fig. 2.**17**). Rarely, bilateral facial atrophy may occur.
- Unilateral atrophy of the lips and tongue is the most common oral manifestation. Hypoplasia of the maxilla and mandible, delayed eruption of the teeth, and malocclusion may also occur.
- Enophthalmos, alopecia, sweat gland disorders, trigeminal neuralgia, facial paresthesia, and epilepsy may develop.
- The atrophic process progresses slowly for several years and then becomes stable.
- Diagnosis is based on clinical criteria.

Differential diagnosis
- Scleroderma
- Facial hemihypertrophy
- Lipodystrophy

Treatment
- Plastic reconstruction
- Orthodontic treatment, if there is malocclusion.

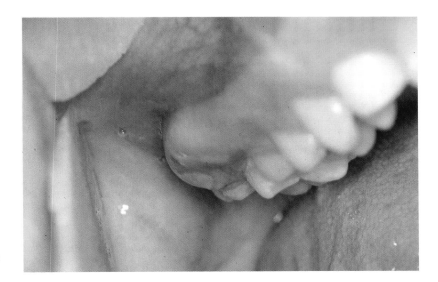

Fig. 2.**16**   Buccal exostoses of the maxilla

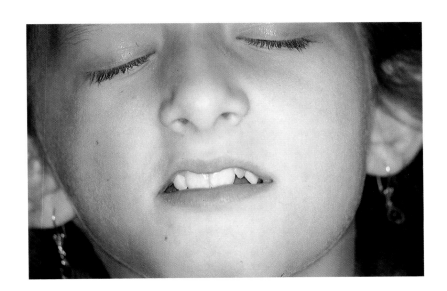

Fig. 2.**17**   Facial hemiatrophy. Atrophy of the right side of the face

3 Mechanical and Electrical Injuries

Traumatic Ulcer

Definition
- Traumatic ulcer is a form of acute or chronic mechanical injury to the oral mucosa leading to loss of all epithelial layers.

Etiology
- It can result from a sharp or broken tooth, an ill-fitting amalgam restoration, orthodontic materials, accidental biting during mastication, sharp foreign bodies and clumsy use of dental instruments.

Occurrence in children
- Common.

Localization
- Tongue, buccal mucosa, lips, gingiva, mucobuccal fold.

Clinical features
- Traumatic ulcer usually presents as a single, ill-defined painful ulceration, with a smooth surface and erythematous or whitish borders (Figs. 3.**1**–3.**4**).
- The size may range from a few millimeters to several centimeters.
- There is a close relationship between the ulcer and the irritating cause.
- The ulcer may persist for a long time, but usually heals within 7–10 days after elimination of the cause.
- The diagnosis is based on the history and clinical features.

Laboratory tests
- Biopsy and histopathological examination only to rule out malignancies or other specific ulcerations.

Differential diagnosis
- Aphthous ulcers
- Necrotizing ulcerative gingivitis and stomatitis
- Eosinophilic ulcer
- Squamous-cell carcinoma
- Necrotizing sialadenometaplasia

Treatment
- Removal of the etiological factors.
- Symptomatic.

Bite Injuries

Definition
- Bite injuries are common lesions caused by chronic manipulation of the oral mucosa.

Etiology
- Continuous mild chewing, sharp teeth.
- In children under stress, or in those with psychological problems.

Occurrence in children
- Common.

Localization
- Lateral borders and tip of the tongue.
- Buccal mucosa, lower lip.

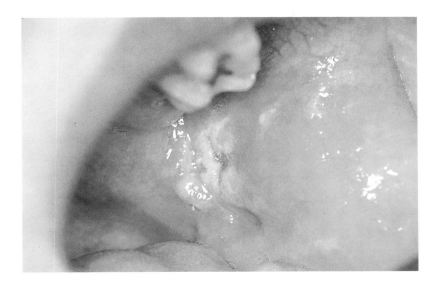

Fig. 3.**1** Traumatic ulcer of the buccal mucosa

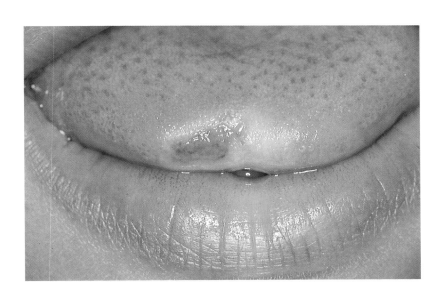

Fig. 3.**2** Traumatic ulcer of the tongue

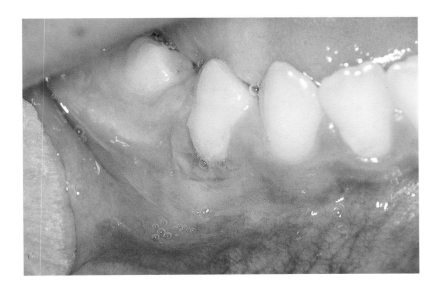

Fig. 3.**3** Traumatic ulcer of the gingiva (first premolar area)

Clinical features

- The lesions usually present as macerated, irregular thickened, shredded, painless, white areas with characteristic desquamation of the affected epithelium (Figs. 3.**5**–3.**8**).
- Superficial erosions may also be seen.
- The lesions may be unilateral or bilateral, localized or diffuse.
- Diagnosis is based on the history and the clinical features.

Differential diagnosis

- Candidiasis
- White sponge nevus
- Leukoedema
- Hairy leukoplakia
- Lichen planus
- Leukoplakia

Treatment

- No treatment is required.
- Elimination of the habit.

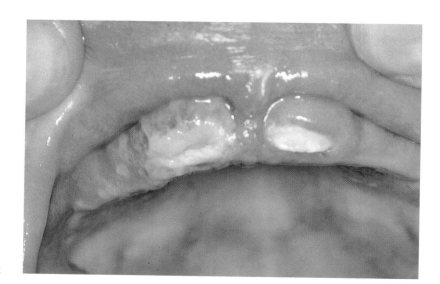

Fig. 3.**4**   Traumatic ulcer of the upper alveolar mucosa in an infant

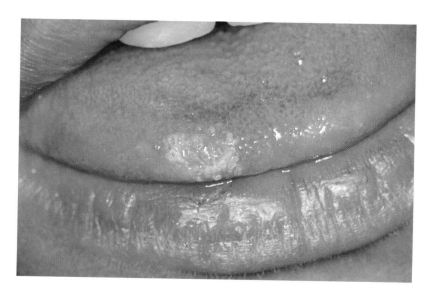

Fig. 3.**5**   Chronic biting of the tip of the tongue

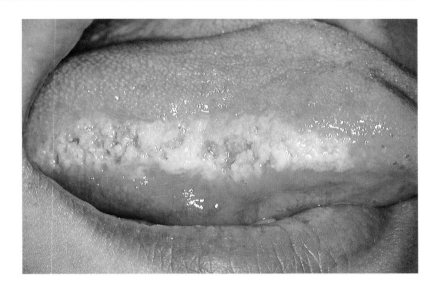

Fig. 3.**6**   Chronic biting of the right lateral border of the tongue

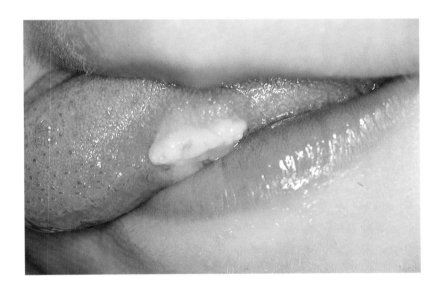

Fig. 3.**7**   Chronic biting, resulting in a tumor-like lesion on the left lateral border of the tongue

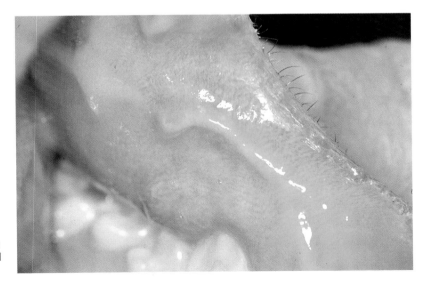

Fig. 3.**8**   Chronic mild biting, resulting in a linear mucosal elevation along the occlusal line of the buccal mucosa

Self-Induced Injury

Definition
- Self-induced injury, or factitious trauma, is deliberate injury to the oral mucosa by the patients themselves.

Etiology
- In children with serious psychological problems who want to attract attention, or are mentally retarded.
- The trauma is usually inflicted through repeated biting of the fingernails, or with toothpicks, pencils, knives, and other hard, sharp objects.

Occurrence in children
- Relatively common.

Localization
- Tongue, gingiva, lips, buccal mucosa.

Clinical features
- The lesions vary from erythema, to a deep, ill-defined, painful oral ulceration with sharp borders (Figs. 3.**9**–3.**11**).
- Similar lesions may be seen on the skin (Fig. 3.**12**).
- The lesions are slow to heal, due to perpetuation of the injury by the patient.
- The diagnosis is based on the history and on clinical suspicion.
- The patients usually deny that they produce the lesions themselves.

Laboratory tests
- Biopsy and histopathological examination only to rule out other specific lesions.

Differential diagnosis
- Traumatic ulcer from other causes
- Aphthous ulcers
- Tuberculosis
- Syphilis
- Neoplasms

Treatment
- Discontinuation of the habit.
- Collaboration with a pediatrician and a psychologist.

Electrical Burns

Definition
- Electrical burns are collectively the most common burns seen in the oral cavity in children.

Etiology
- Biting into an electric cable, or inappropriate use of a faulty electrical appliance.

Occurrence in children
- Fairly common.
- Most electrical burns occur in children below six years of age.

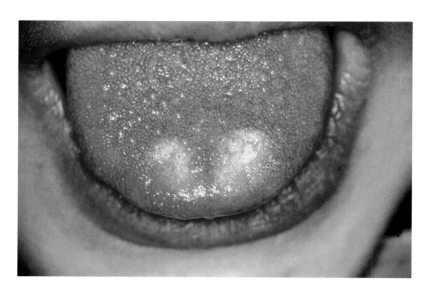

Fig. 3.**9** Two minor factitious injuries on the dorsum of the tongue

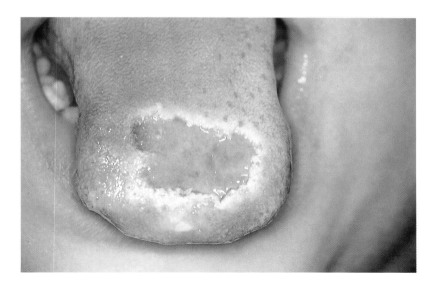

Fig. 3.**10** Large factitious ulcer on the dorsum of the tongue

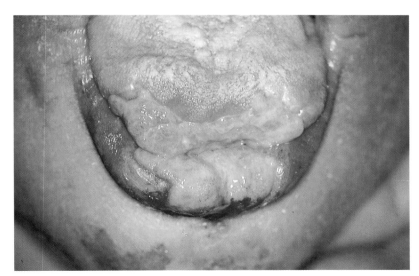

Fig. 3.**11** Huge factitious ulcers on the tongue and the lower lip in a young boy with serious psychological problems

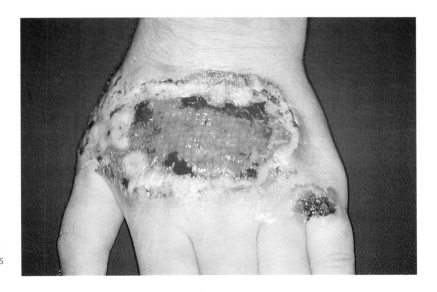

Fig. 3.**12** Huge factitious ulcer on the skin in a young girl with serious psychological problems

Localization

- Lips, commissures, and perioral areas are most frequently affected.
- Tongue, gingiva, alveolar ridge, floor of the mouth and mucobuccal folds may also be less frequently affected.

Clinical features

- Clinically, electrical burns in the oral mucosa present as a painless, white-gray, coagulated lesion with no bleeding and surrounded by a narrow rim of erythema. Progressively, the white-gray surface evolves into brown-black charred tissues and finally sloughs, leaving a deep ulcer that may hemorrhage (Fig. 3.**13**).
- The adjacent teeth may become non-vital.
- Scarring and microstomia are common complications.
- The diagnosis is based on the history and the clinical features.

Differential diagnosis

- Traumatic ulcers
- Severe thermal burn
- Noma

Treatment

- It is supportive.
- Surgical reconstruction may be necessary in severe cases.

Other Lesions

Various lesions caused by mechanical injury are frequently observed in children's oral mucosa. Hyperplasia after continuous mild injury caused by orthodontic or prosthetic materials, traumatic hematoma, traumatic hemorrhagic bullae, erythema, and small erosions produced by the toothbrush are some of the most frequent oral lesions that may cause diagnostic problems (Fig. 3.**14**).

In such cases, the diagnosis is based on a detailed history, which helps to exclude oral lesions due to other causes, and biopsy and histological examination may rarely be necessary.

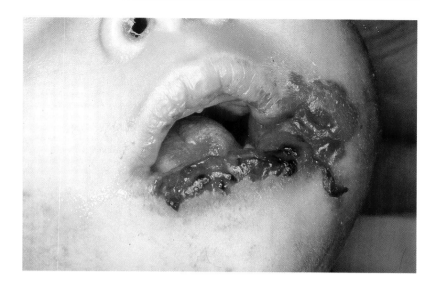

Fig. 3.**13**   Electrical burn on the lower lip and left commissure

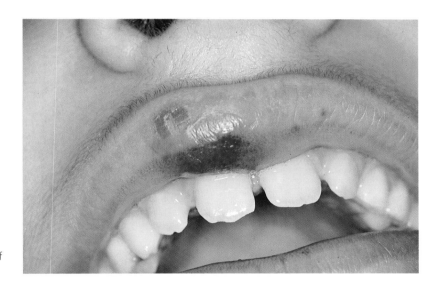

Fig. 3.**14**   Traumatic hematoma of the upper lip

4 Chemical Burns and Allergies

Chemical Burns

Definition
- Chemical burns are oral lesions caused by direct contact between various chemicals and drugs and the oral mucosa.

Etiology
- The chemicals come into direct contact with the oral mucosa because of improper use.
- Common chemicals and drugs that may be placed in the mouth include aspirin, trichloroacetic acid, sodium perborate, hydrogen peroxide, silver nitrate, phenol, paraformaldehyde, alcohol, battery acid, chlorine, and other detergents and agricultural drugs.

Occurrence in children
- Common.

Localization
- Lips, tongue, buccal mucosa, floor of the mouth, gingiva, vestibular sulcus.

Clinical features
- The extent and severity of the lesions depend on the kind of the caustic agent, its concentration, and the duration of the exposure.
- The lesions may be mild or severe, and they usually have similar clinical features.
- Clinically, the lesions present as white or erythematous wrinkled plaques, erosions or ulcerations, which are often covered by whitish pseudomembranes (Figs. 4.**1**–4.**4**).
- The use of the rubber dam has significantly reduced iatrogenic burns.
- The diagnosis is based on the history, the clinical features, and exclusion of other lesions or diseases.

Differential diagnosis
- Traumatic lesions
- Thermal burns
- Electric burn
- Erosions seen in lichen planus and bullous diseases

Treatment
- Symptomatic. The lesions usually disappear within a week on removal of the chemical or the drug.
- Topical and, rarely, systemic steroids in severe cases.

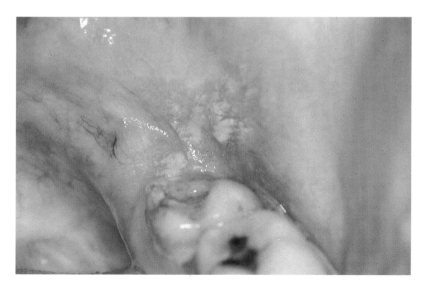

Fig. 4.**1** Aspirin burn on the buccal mucosa and retromolar area

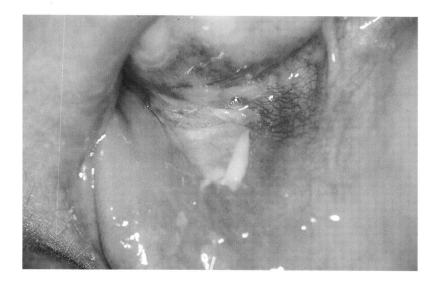

Fig. 4.**2**   Trichloroacetic acid burn on the lower labial mucosa

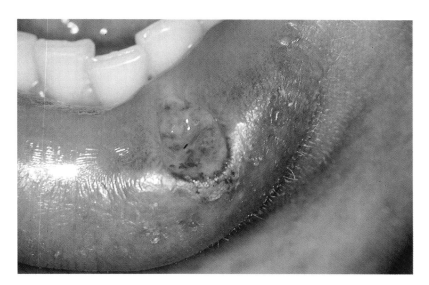

Fig. 4.**3**   Chlorine compound burn on the lower lip

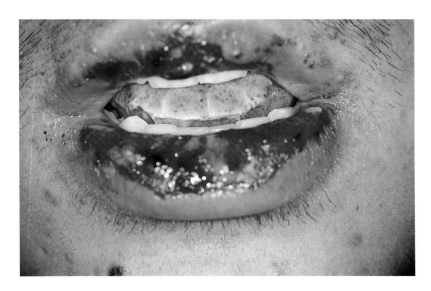

Fig. 4.**4**   Severe and extensive erosions of the lips and tongue due to accidental contact with an agricultural compound

Angioneurotic Edema

Definition
- Angioneurotic edema is a relatively common diffuse allergic reaction of the soft tissues. The disorder may be hereditary (rare) or acquired (common).

Etiology
- The acquired form may be caused by local anesthetics, drugs, foods, infections, emotional stress, etc.
- The hereditary form is inherited as an autosomal dominant trait.
- The great majority of angioneurotic edemas are idiopathic.

Occurrence in children
- Relatively rare.

Localization
- Oral mucosa (lips, tongue, soft palate, buccal mucosa).
- Skin (face, hands, arms, legs, genitals).
- Respiratory and gastrointestinal tract occur mainly in the hereditary form.

Clinical features
- Acute, painless soft-tissue swelling, with a smooth, shiny surface (Fig. 4.5).
- The enlargement resolves within 24–72 hours.
- The swelling may be solitary or multiple, and the size be up to several centimeters in diameter.
- Edema of the epiglottis represents a severe complication that may result in death.

Differential diagnosis
- Glandular cheilitis
- Cheilitis granulomatosa
- Melkersson–Rosenthal syndrome
- Lymphedema
- Surgical emphysema
- Acute abscess of the soft tissues
- Traumatic swelling

Treatment
- Antihistamines, systemic corticosteroids.
- In severe cases, intramuscular epinephrine.

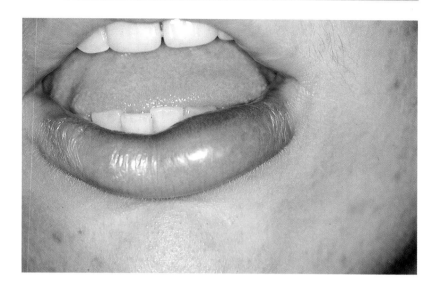

Fig. 4.**5**   Acquired form of angioneurotic edema on the lower lip

5 Foreign-Body Deposits

Amalgam Tattoo

Definition
- Amalgam tattoo is a submucosal implantation of dental amalgam.

Etiology
- The most common ways that amalgam can be incorporated into the oral mucosa are: continuous contact between an amalgam filling and the oral soft tissues, and embedding of amalgam fragments into the oral tissues during dental filling or surgery.

Occurrence in children
- Relatively rare.

Localization
- The most common sites are the gingiva, alveolar mucosa, buccal mucosa, palate, and floor of the mouth.

Clinical features
- Clinically, amalgam tattoo presents as a black or dark-blue asymptomatic macule or plaque (Fig. 5.**1**). The borders of the lesion may be well defined or irregular, and the size varies from a few millimeters to several centimeters.
- Adjacent teeth usually have amalgam restorations.
- The diagnosis is usually based on the clinical features.

Laboratory findings
- Amalgam fragments may be visible on the radiograph as a densely radiopaque lesion.
- Microscopically scattered dark-brown granules are seen in the connective tissue.

Differential diagnosis
- Pigmentation from other metals
- Melanocytic nevus
- Freckle and ephelis
- Malignant melanoma
- Pigmentation due to drugs

Treatment
- Treatment is not required.
- Excisional biopsy is required only for diagnostic purposes.

Other Foreign-Body Implantations

Definition
- Incorporation of foreign body materials into the oral mucosa, such as silver, pencil graphite, metal dust, fish bone, wood pieces and other solid material.

Occurrence in children
- Common.

Localization
- Gingiva, alveolar mucosa, tongue, buccal mucosa, palate, lips.

Clinical features
- Clinically, the lesions present as an asymptomatic, grayish or melanotic macule or plaque, or even as an inflammatory swelling (Figs. 5.**2**, 5.**3**).
- The diagnosis is based on the history, clinical features, and occasionally on histopathological features.

Laboratory tests
- Radiographic examination.
- Biopsy and histopathological examination.

Differential diagnosis
- Amalgam tattoo
- Melanocytic nevus
- Pyogenic granuloma
- Soft-tissue abscess

Treatment
- Surgical excision of the foreign body.

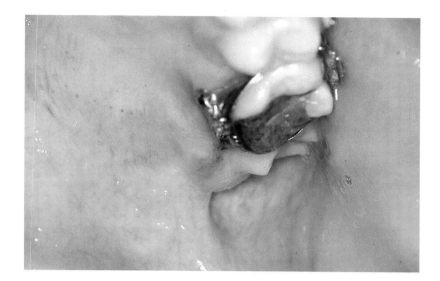

Fig. 5.**1**   Amalgam tattoo on the palatal alveolar mucosa

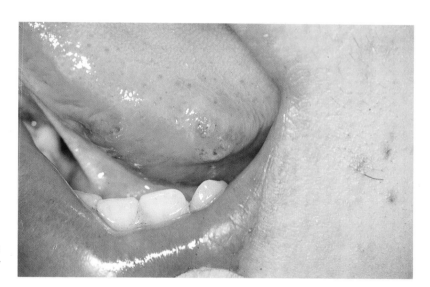

Fig. 5.**2**   Fish bone implantation on the lateral border of the tongue, resulting in an inflammatory swelling

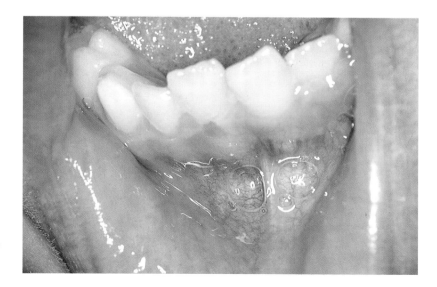

Fig. 5.**3**   Pencil graphite implantation into the dentogingival sulcus of the lateral incisor

Materia Alba of the Gingiva

Definition
- Materia alba is the result of necrotic epithelial cells, bacteria, and accumulation of food debris on the oral mucosa.

Etiology
- It is usually seen in patients with poor oral hygiene who neglect toothbrushing, or in cases in which painful oral lesions make oral hygiene difficult.

Occurrence in children
- Common.

Localization
- Dentogingival margins, attached gingiva, alveolar vestibular mucosa.

Clinical features
- Clinically, a white or yellow-whitish plaque is seen, which can be easily removed with slight rubbing, leaving an erythematous surface (Fig. 5.**4**).
- The plaque is painless, and is usually accompanied by halitosis.
- The diagnosis is based on the clinical features.

Differential diagnosis
- Candidiasis
- Leukoplakia
- Lichen planus
- Chemical burn

Treatment
- Good oral hygiene.

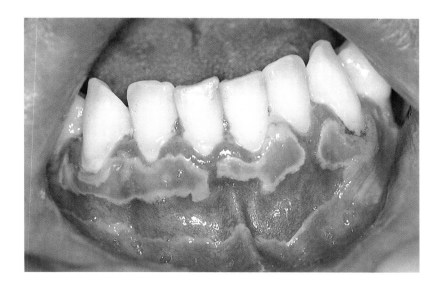

Fig. 5.**4**   Materia alba on the attached lower gingiva

6 Periodontal Diseases

Gingivitis

Definition
- Gingivitis is an inflammatory disease of the marginal gingiva, either localized or generalized.

Etiology
- It is primarily caused by bacterial plaque accumulation due to inadequate oral hygiene.
- Calculus, mechanical irritation, and irregularities in the position of the teeth may be contributory factors.

Occurrence in children
- Common.

Localization
- Free and interdental gingiva. Mainly observed during the mixed dentition, and more rarely in the primary dentition.
- Sometimes in areas of tooth eruption (eruption gingivitis).

Clinical features
- Redness and edema, usually without pain (Fig. 6.**1**).
- Gingival hyperplasia may sometimes be observed (Fig. 6.**2**).
- Bleeding may occur spontaneously, or after light probing.
- There is often halitosis.
- The diagnosis is made clinically.

Differential diagnosis
- Desquamative gingivitis
- Drug-induced gingival hyperplasia
- Gingivitis due to mouth breathing
- Acute leukemia

Treatment
- Plaque control and good oral hygiene.
- Gingivectomy, in cases of severe gingival hyperplasia.

Periodontitis

Definition
- Periodontitis is the result of progression of the inflammatory process from the gingiva to the deeper periodontal structures.

Etiology
- Bacterial plaque is important for the initiation of the disease.
- The same factors as in chronic gingivitis, which usually evolve into periodontitis.
- Systemic predisposing factors include: diabetes mellitus, human immunodeficiency virus (HIV) infection, immune diseases, metabolic diseases, etc.
- Host factors are also important, and appear to be influenced by genetic and environmental factors such as smoking.

Occurrence in children
- Rare, mainly in adolescents.

Localization
- Localized or generalized.

Clinical features
- The consequences of periodontitis are alveolar bone resorption and loss of attachment, followed by periodontal pocket formation.
- Inflammation and edema of the gingiva, pockets deeper than 3 mm (Fig. 6.**3**).
- Bleeding and malodorous breath, teeth migration, tooth movement.
- The diagnosis is usually made clinically.

Radiographic features
- Alveolar bone resorption.

Differential diagnosis
- Papillon–Lefèvre syndrome
- Langerhans' cell histiocytosis
- Acatalasia
- Hypophosphatasia
- Leukemia
- Glycogen storage disease type Ib
- Scurvy

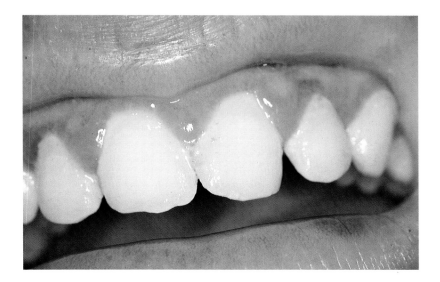

Fig. 6.**1**   Chronic gingivitis

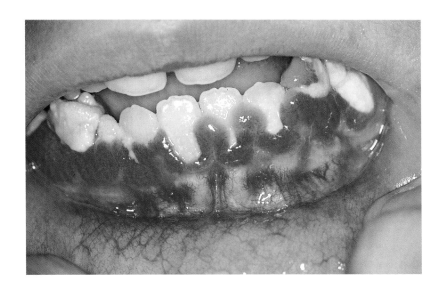

Fig. 6.**2**   Chronic hyperplastic gingivitis

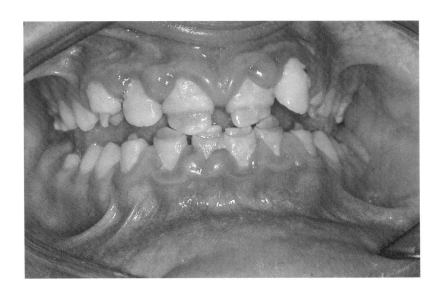

Fig. 6.**3**   Periodontitis

Treatment	• Plaque control and good oral hygiene.
	• Scaling and root planing and/or surgery.
	• Maintenance therapy is very important.

Juvenile Periodontitis

Definition
• Juvenile periodontitis is a specific type of early-onset periodontitis, which usually affects adolescents, and is characterized by severe alveolar bone loss.

Etiology
• *Actinobacillus actinomycetemcomitans* and probably other pathogens may be involved.
• Reduced immune response to endotoxins of bacterial plaque or genetic immune insufficiency have been proposed.

Occurrence in children
• Only in adolescents.
• Familial occurrence.

Localization
• Affects only permanent teeth.
• Localized or generalized.
• Selectively affects incisors and first molars.

Clinical features
• Mild gingival inflammation (Fig. 6.**4**).
• Rapid and severe destruction of alveolar bone.
• Deep periodontal pockets, bleeding, malodorous breath.
• Absence of local factors (bacterial plaque, calculus).
• Tooth mobility and migration (Fig. 6.**5**).

Radiographic features
• Severe and rapid bone loss (Fig. 6.**6**).

Differential diagnosis
• Prepubertal periodontitis
• Adult periodontitis
• Papillon–Lefèvre syndrome
• Ehlers–Danlos syndrome, type VIII
• Crohn's disease
• Chediak–Higashi syndrome
• Ulcerative necrotizing periodontitis in HIV infection
• Langerhans' cells histiocytosis
• Glycogen storage disease type Ib
• Cyclic neutropenia and agranulocytosis
• Juvenile diabetes mellitus (type I)
• Down's syndrome

Treatment
• Conservative mechanical treatment or surgery.
• Systemic antibiotics, local antiseptics.

Desquamative Gingivitis

Definition
• Desquamative gingivitis is a relatively common clinical manifestation of various mucocutaneous diseases on the gingiva (a non-specific disease entity), with a well-defined clinical pattern.

Etiology
• The most common disorders that cause desquamative gingivitis are cicatricial pemphigoid, lichen planus, bullous pemphigoid, pemphigus, linear IgA disease and, rarely, other mucocutaneous diseases.

Occurrence in children
• Very rare.

Localization
• Buccal anterior gingiva of the maxilla and mandible.
• Usually localized and rarely generalized.

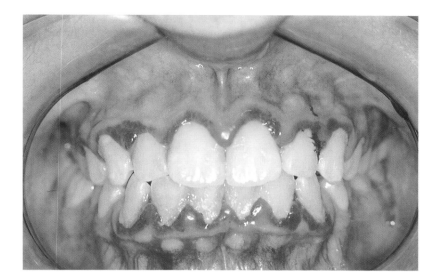

Fig. 6.**4**   Juvenile periodontitis, early stage

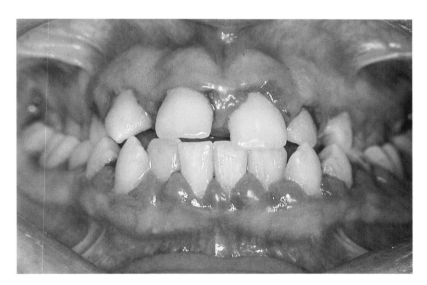

Fig. 6.**5**   Juvenile periodontitis, late stage and tooth migration

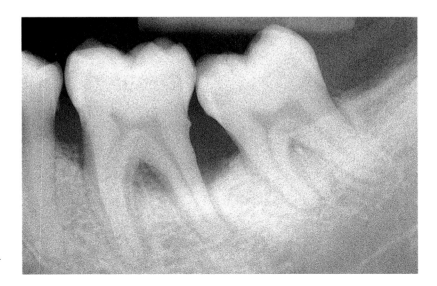

Fig. 6.**6**   Juvenile periodontitis, extensive bone loss

Clinical features	• Red gingiva, edematous with erosions (Figs. 6.**7**, 6.**8**). • Characteristic desquamation of the epithelium or bleeding bullous formation after rubbing with the spatula. • Painful gingiva during mastication and brushing. • Rarely, bleeding. The disease has periods of remission and exacerbation. • Searching for other signs and symptoms of the underlying disease is important for the diagnosis.
Laboratory examinations	• Histopathological examination. • Direct immunofluorescence. • Indirect immunofluorescence.
Differential diagnosis	• Recognition of the diseases that cause desquamative gingivitis • Erythema multiforme • Plasma-cell gingivitis • Psoriasis with gingival involvement • Mechanical trauma • Allergic gingivitis
Treatment	• The same as the treatment of the underlying disease. • Local or systemic corticosteroids. • Avoidance of excessive mechanical pressure with the toothbrush.

Plasma-Cell Gingivitis

Definition	• Plasma-cell gingivitis is a unique type of gingival disorder with characteristic clinical and histopathological features.
Etiology	• Unknown. An allergic reaction to exogenous allergens, bacteria, *Candida albicans* has been proposed.
Occurrence in children	• Rare; mainly in adolescents.
Localization	• Free and attached gingiva. • Localized or generalized. • Similar lesions have been observed on the tongue and lips.
Clinical features	• Intense redness, with burning sensation of the gingiva (Fig. 6.**9**). • Sudden occurrence, without systemic symptoms. • Duration of months or years, with frequent recurrences.
Histopathology	• Dense infiltration of the connective tissue, mainly by plasma cells. • Spongiosis of the epithelium and infiltration by inflammatory cells.
Differential diagnosis	• Desquamative gingivitis • Erythematous candidiasis • Erythroplakia • Systemic lupus erythematosus • Porphyria and psoriasis of the gingiva • Drug-induced gingivitis or stomatitis
Treatment	• Symptomatic, usually with poor results. • Local or systemic use of antifungal drugs. • Systemic administration of antihistamines. • Local corticosteroid ointments.

Hereditary Gingival Fibromatosis

Definition	• Hereditary gingival fibromatosis is a gingival enlargement that occurs in children, either alone or as a manifestation of several hereditary syndromes.
Etiology	• Genetic. Hereditary transmission, usually autosomal dominant and rarely autosomal recessive.
Occurrence in children	• Exclusively in children, usually with the initiation of permanent dentition.
Localization	• Maxilla and mandible. Buccal, lingual, and palatal. • Usually generalized, with more severe enlargement in the maxilla.

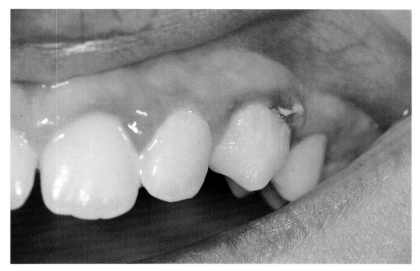

Fig. 6.**7** Desquamative gingivitis in a young girl with cicatricial pemphigoid

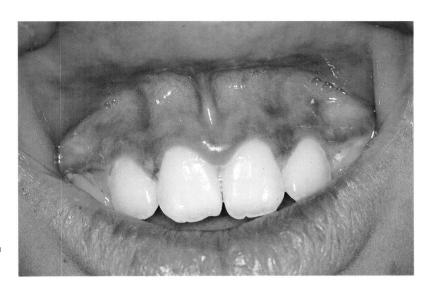

Fig. 6.**8** Desquamative gingivitis in a young boy with cicatricial pemphigoid

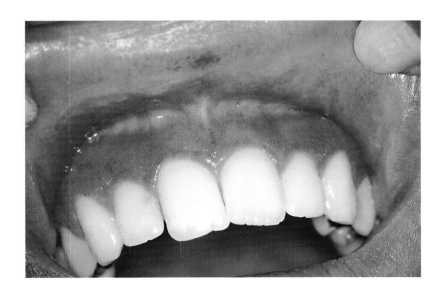

Fig. 6.**9** Plasma-cell gingivitis

Clinical features
- Severe enlargement of the gingiva, which cover the teeth partially or completely (Figs. 6.**10**–6.**12**).
- The gingiva are smooth, with a firm consistency.
- Fibrous proliferation in later stages.
- Normal or slightly red gingival color.

Differential diagnosis
- Drug-induced gingival hyperplasia (cyclosporine, nifedipine and other calcium-channel blockers, diphenylhydantoin)
- Laband, Ramon, Cross, and Rutherford syndromes
- Leukemia, amyloidosis, Crohn's disease

Treatment
- Gingivectomy.
- Good oral hygiene.

Drug-Induced Gingival Hyperplasia

Definition
- Gingival hyperplasia leading to various degrees of enlargement.

Etiology
- The drugs that cause gingival hyperplasia are usually: diphenylhydantoin, cyclosporine, nifedipine, and other calcium-channel blockers.
- Bacterial plaque, poor oral hygiene, calculus, and gingival inflammation are predisposing factors.

Occurrence in children
- Frequent, especially in epileptic children taking diphenylhydantoin. Rare in children receiving treatment with immunosuppressive agents or receiving calcium-channel blockers.

Localization
- Free and interdental maxillary and mandibular gingiva, usually anteriorly.

Clinical features
- Asymptomatic enlargement of the interdental papillae.
- Progression of the enlargement in the free gingiva, with partial or complete coverage of the teeth (Figs. 6.**13**–6.**15**).
- Normal color.
- Firm and painless gingiva on palpation.
- Usually absence of bleeding and pseudopockets formation.

Differential diagnosis
- Hereditary gingival fibromatosis
- Genetic syndromes causing gingival enlargement
- Gingival enlargement due to mouth breathing
- Leukemia, amyloidosis, Crohn's disease

Treatment
- Good oral hygiene.
- Removal of bacterial plaque and calculus.
- Gingivectomy.
- Replacement or removal of the responsible drug, if possible.

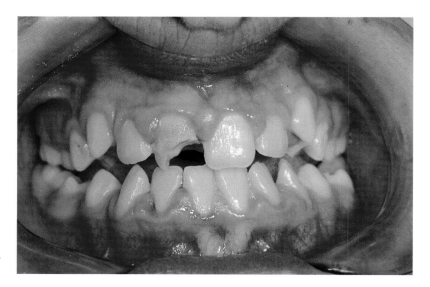

Fig. 6.**10**   Hereditary gingival fibromatosis

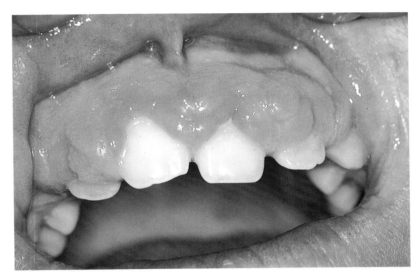

Fig. 6.**11**   Hereditary gingival fibro-matosis

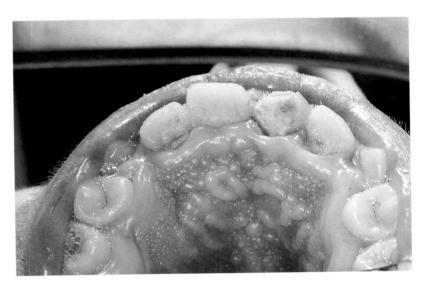

Fig. 6.**12**   Hereditary gingival fibro-matosis

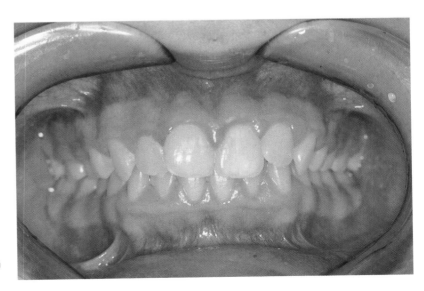

Fig. 6.**13**   Mild gingival hyperplasia caused by phenytoin

Gingivitis Due to Mouth Breathing

Definition
- This is a chronic form of gingivitis that leads to gingival hyperplasia and enlargement.

Etiology
- Caused by mouth breathing, usually because irregularities of the nasal septum or incomplete lip closure result in dryness of the oral mucosa and lead to bacterial plaque accumulation.

Occurrence in children
- Common.

Localization
- Anterior maxillary, usually buccal gingiva.

Clinical features
- Painless enlargement of the interdental gingiva.
- Usually, partial coverage of the crown (Fig. 6.**16**).
- Normal or slightly red gingival color, and usually large and incomplete lip closure (Fig. 6.**17**).
- Dry, shiny gingival surface, with stippling.
- The diagnosis is made clinically.

Differential diagnosis
- Drug-induced gingival hyperplasia
- Hereditary gingival fibromatosis, leukemia

Treatment
- Gingivectomy
- Restoration of nasal breathing.

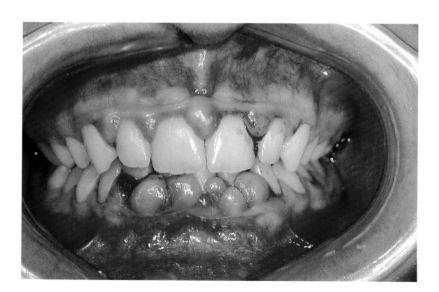

Fig. 6.**14** Severe gingival hyperplasia caused by phenytoin

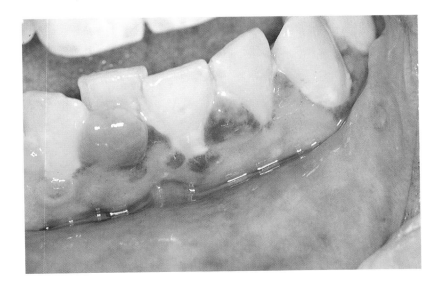

Fig. 6.**15**   Gingival hyperplasia caused by cyclosporine

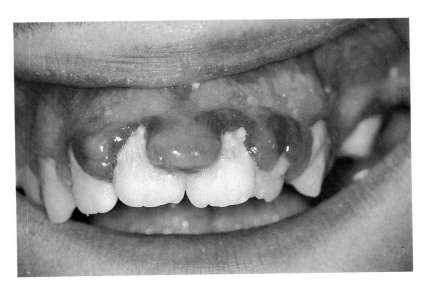

Fig. 6.**16**   Gingival hyperplasia due to mouth breathing

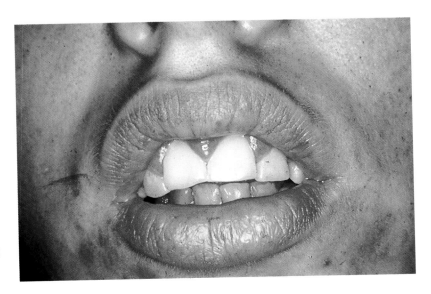

Fig. 6.**17**   Gingival hyperplasia and large, incompletely closed lips, due to mouth breathing

7 Diseases of the Lips

Exfoliative Cheilitis

Definition

- Exfoliative cheilitis is a chronic, mild, inflammatory disorder of the vermilion border of the lips.

Etiology

- The exact etiology remains unknown.
- It is more common in individuals with psychological problems, stress, and a history of atopic dermatitis.
- It is a common complication of systemic retinoid agents.
- Secondary *Candida albicans* infection may occur.

Occurrence in children

- Relatively common, particularly in adolescents.
- Girls are more often affected.

Localization

- The vermilion border of the lips.
- Involvement is usually more severe on the lower than the upper lip.

Clinical features

- Dryness, mild edema, and inflammation.
- Scaling and occasionally cracking in a vertical dimension is the prominent clinical feature (Fig. 7.**1**).
- Progressively, the vermilion border may become covered with a thickened whitish-brown crust (Fig. 7.**2**).
- Superficial erosions and a burning sensation are common.
- The lesions can last for weeks, months, or even years, with periods of remission and exacerbation.
- The aesthetic problem is major for the patient.
- The diagnosis is usually made clinically.

Differential diagnosis

- Contact cheilitis
- Lip-licking cheilitis
- Infectious cheilitis
- Actinic cheilitis

Treatment

- Symptomatic. Topical steroid ointment, topical antifungal agents.
- Topical moisturizing ointments.
- Removal of underlying causes, if known.
- Psychological support, and in severe cases mild tranquilizers.

Contact Cheilitis

Definition

- Contact cheilitis is an acute inflammatory disorder of the lips resulting from an allergic chemical contact.

Etiology

- Topical allergens e.g., lipstick, toothpaste, mouthwashes, topical medications, food products, musical instruments, cigarette filter tips, etc.

Occurrence in children

- Rare; more common in adolescents.
- Girls are more commonly affected.

Localization

- The vermilion border of the lips, with perioral skin spread occasionally.
- Less often, cheilitis may be part of an allergic contact stomatitis.

Clinical features

- Mild edema, erythema, dryness, and scales are the early signs of the disease.
- Fissures and persistent, thickened, whitish-yellow crusts may occur in severe cases (Fig. 7.**3**).
- Angular and perioral spread may be seen.
- Pustules and bullous formation may rarely occur periorally.
- A burning sensation is a common symptom.
- The diagnosis is usually based on the history and the clinical features.

Laboratory tests

- A patch test may be helpful diagnostically.

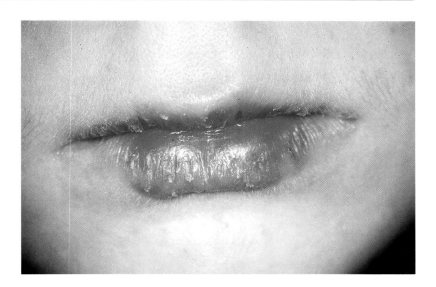

Fig. 7.**1**   Mild exfoliative cheilitis and edema of the lower lip

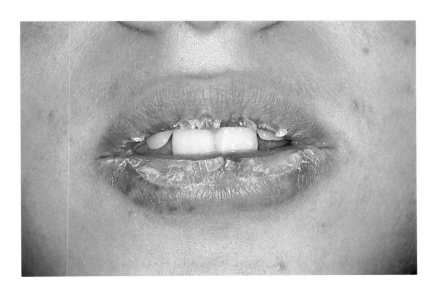

Fig. 7.**2**   Severe exfoliative cheilitis

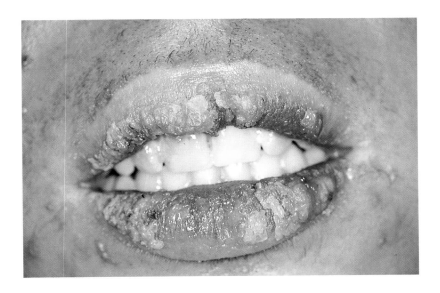

Fig. 7.**3**   Severe contact cheilitis

Differential diagnosis	• Exfoliative cheilitis • Lip-licking cheilitis • Perioral dermatitis
Treatment	• The cornerstone of treatment is elimination of the allergen, if known. • Systemic steroids in low doses for a short time are usually helpful in severe cases. • Topical steroids for one to two weeks are also indicated in less severe cases.

Lip-Licking Cheilitis

Definition	• This is a unique irritant inflammatory disorder of the lips and perioral skin.
Etiology	• Continual habitual licking of the lips and of the perioral area. • Atopy is a common predisposing condition.
Occurrence in children	• Common.
Localization	• Lips, commissures, perioral skin.
Clinical features	• Erythema, mild edema, and thin scaling formation (Fig. 7.**4**). • Characteristically, an erythematous wide border encircling the lips, with a normal skin area just around the vermilion border (Fig. 7.**5**). • In chronic cases, fissures in a vertical direction may occur. A burning sensation is a common symptom. • The diagnosis is made clinically.
Differential diagnosis	• Exfoliative cheilitis • Contact cheilitis • Perioral dermatitis
Treatment	• The most important step is to stop the habit. • Topical steroid treatment, with or without antifungals, for a short time is helpful.

Cheilitis Glandularis

Definition	• Cheilitis glandularis is a rare chronic inflammatory disorder of the minor salivary glands of the lips.
Etiology	• Unknown.
Occurrence in children	• Rare.
Localization	• Mainly the lower lip, and rarely the upper lip.
Clinical features	• It is characterized by asymptomatic swelling of the lower lip (Fig. 7.**6**). • Characteristically, squeezing of the lip may produce droplets of mucin secretion from the dilated ductal openings. • Rarely, crusting, superficial erosions, and microabscesses may occur.
Histopathology	• Hypertrophy of minor salivary glands and ductal dilatation. • Chronic inflammation and dilated lymphatic vessels.
Differential diagnosis	• Infectious cheilitis • Cheilitis granulomatosa • Crohn's disease • Angioedema • Cystic fibrosis
Treatment	• Topical steroids and antibiotics in cases of infection are of limited value. • In severe persistent cases, vermilionectomy.

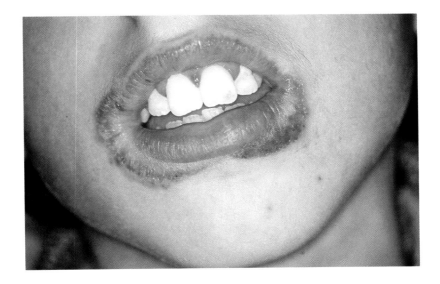

Fig. 7.**4**   Mild lip-licking cheilitis

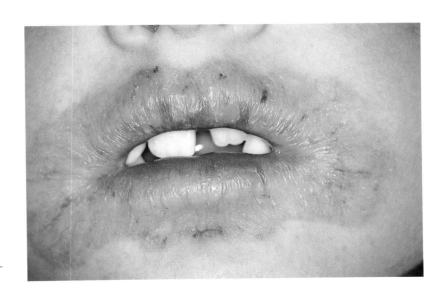

Fig. 7.**5**   Severe and extensive lip-licking cheilitis

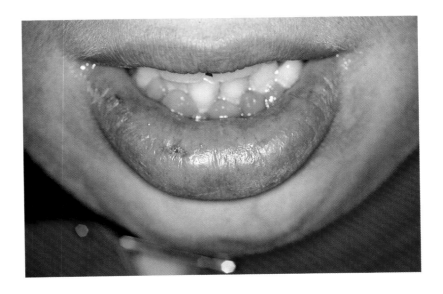

Fig. 7.**6**   Cheilitis glandularis

Cheilitis Granulomatosa

Definition
- Cheilitis granulomatosa, or Miescher's cheilitis, is a rare chronic disorder that may occur alone, or as part of systemic diseases that produce orofacial granulomatous lesions.

Etiology
- Unknown.

Occurrence in children
- Rare. It occurs more often in adolescents.
- Girls are slightly more commonly affected than boys.

Localization
- One or both lips.

Clinical features
- Non-tender swelling that may totally resolve between attacks.
- It has a sudden onset and chronic course. After a period of remission and exacerbation, the swelling becomes permanent and extreme (Fig. 7.**7**).
- Small vesicles, superficial erosions, scaling, and microabscesses may occasionally occur.
- It may appear alone, or as part of orofacial granulomatosis.
- The enlargement of the lips is distressing to the patient.
- The clinical diagnosis should be confirmed by biopsy.

Histopathology
- Edema of the lamina propria with dilation of the lymphatic vessels.
- Granulomatous inflammation consisting of epithelioid histiocytes, and lymphocytes with or without multinucleated giant cells.
- There is no caseation necrosis or severe fibrosis.

Differential diagnosis
- Cheilitis glandularis
- Melkersson–Rosenthal syndrome
- Crohn's disease
- Sarcoidosis
- Tuberculosis
- Cystic fibrosis
- Angioedema

Treatment
- Intralesional injection of corticosteroids. In persistent cases, systemic steroids.
- Antibiotics in cases of infection.
- In severe cases with aesthetic problems, surgical reconstruction of the lips.

Angular Cheilitis

Definition
- Angular cheilitis, or perlèche, is a common disorder that occurs at the corner of the mouth.

Etiology
- Multifactorial.
- In children, the most common causes are mechanical irritation, malocclusion, atopic dermatitis, candidiasis, bacterial infection, habitual licking and maceration of the commissures, deficiency anemia, nutritional deficiencies, acquired immune deficiency syndrome (AIDS).

Occurrence in children
- Relatively common.

Localization
- The angles of the mouth.

Clinical features
- Erythema, fissuring, scaling, erosions, and maceration (Figs. 7.**8,** 7.**9**).
- Occasionally, the lesions may spread from the corner of the mouth to the adjacent skin.
- Dryness, a burning sensation and sometimes mild pain may occur.
- Untreated, the lesions may last for a long time, with remissions and exacerbations.
- The diagnosis is made clinically.

Differential diagnosis
- Rarely, systemic diseases that may involve the corner of the mouth, e.g. herpes simplex, pemphigus vulgaris, acanthosis nigricans.

Treatment
- The most important step is to identify and treat the predisposing factors.
- Topical corticosteroid with an antifungal agent and antibiotics is the best.

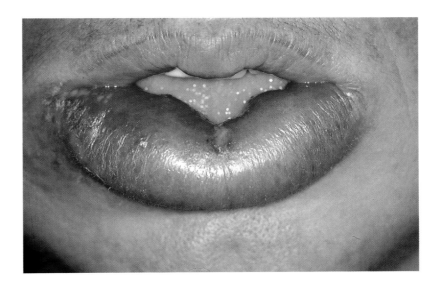

Fig. 7.**7**   Cheilitis granulomatosa

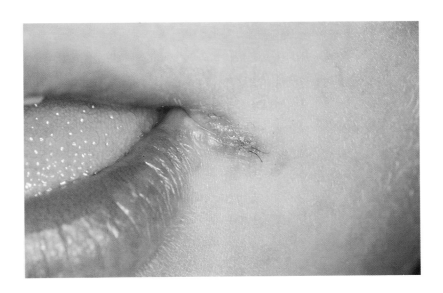

Fig. 7.**8**   Angular cheilitis

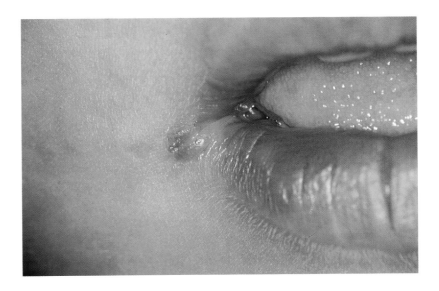

Fig. 7.**9**   Angular cheilitis

Median Lip Fissure

Definition
- Median lip fissure is a relatively rare, chronic disorder that may appear in the lower or upper lip.

Etiology
- The exact etiology remains unclear.
- Predisposing factors are mechanical irritation, maceration, cold, windy and dry weather, continuous licking and biting, atopic dermatitis, human immunodeficiency virus (HIV) infection.
- Recently, a hereditary predisposition has been suggested.

Occurrence in children
- Rare.

Localization
- More often the midline of the lower lip, and less often the upper lip.

Clinical features
- It presents as a deep inflammatory painful vertical fissure (Fig. 7.**10**).
- Spontaneous bleeding, discomfort, and pain are common.
- The lesion is usually infected by bacteria and *Candida albicans*.
- Characteristically, the lesion is chronic, with a cycle of splitting and partial healing. The recurrence rate is high.
- The diagnosis is made clinically.

Differential diagnosis
- Actinic cheilitis
- Herpes labialis
- Mechanical trauma

Treatment
- Topical corticosteroids, with or without antibiotics and antifungals, may be helpful.
- In severe and persistent fissures, the therapy of choice is deep surgical excision.

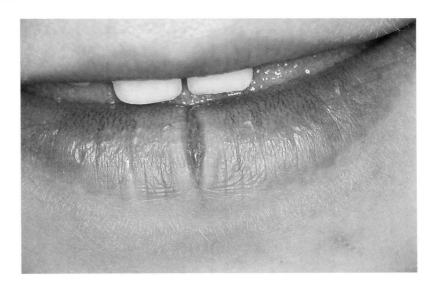

Fig. 7.**10**   Median lip fissure

8 Diseases of the Tongue

Median Rhomboid Glossitis

Definition
- Median rhomboid glossitis a benign disorder with characteristic morphology.

Etiology
- In the past, it was regarded as a developmental anomaly, due to the persistence of the tuberculum impar (the median tongue bud) as a result of a failure of the two lateral parts of the tongue to fuse.
- It has recently been suggested that it is an inflammatory lesion caused primarily or secondarily by *Candida albicans*.

Occurrence in children
- Very rare.

Localization
- On the dorsal surface of the tongue along the midline, just anterior to the foramen cecum.

Clinical features
- Typical rhomboid or oval, well-demarcated shape.
- Characteristically, the lesion is reddish, flat, or slightly multilobulated, with a smooth, depapillated surface (Fig. 8.**1**).
- The size varies from 1 cm to 3 cm. The condition is usually asymptomatic. Rarely, however, patients may complain of discomfort.
- The diagnosis is made clinically.

Differential diagnosis
- Erythematous candidiasis
- Thyroglossal duct cyst
- Lymphangioma
- Hemangioma
- Leiomyoma

Treatment
- There is no treatment.
- In cases of *Candida albicans* infection, topical or systemic antifungal drugs are helpful.
- Reassuring the patient that the lesion is harmless.

Geographic Tongue

Definition
- Geographic tongue, or erythema migrans, is a harmless common disorder that primarily affects the tongue and is characterized by atrophy or temporary loss of the filiform papillae.

Etiology
- Unknown. It is often seen in more than one member of the same family, although an inheritance pattern is not clear.
- It occurs with increased frequency in children with atopy and seborrheic dermatitis, and in patients with psoriasis, often pustular.

Occurrence in children
- Common. The disorder is four to five times more frequent in children and adolescents than in adults.
- It occurs in about 2% of the population, and females are more frequently affected than males.

Localization
- Usually, the dorsal surface and lateral borders of the tongue.
- Rarely, other oral mucosa sites may be involved (labial, buccal, soft palate, gingiva).

Clinical features
- It is characterized by an erythematous, well-demarcated smooth, round, or circinate patch, due to atrophy or loss of the filiform papillae.
- The erythematous areas are characteristically surrounded partially or totally by a slightly raised, whitish margin (Figs. 8.**2**, 8.**3**).
- Sometimes, the lesions start as a small whitish plaque, quickly followed by a central red zone that increases centrifugally.
- The size varies from a few millimeters to several centimeters.

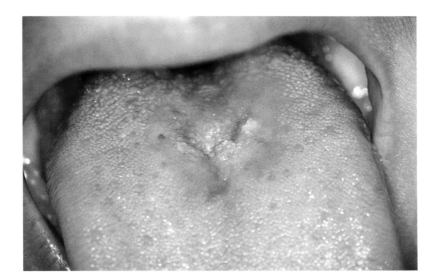

Fig. 8.**1**   Median rhomboid glossitis

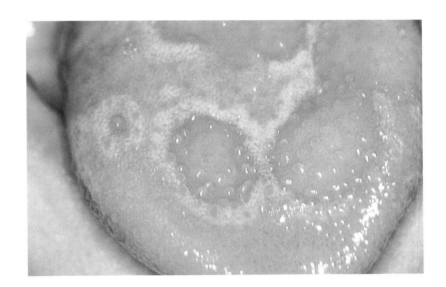

Fig. 8.**2**   Geographic tongue

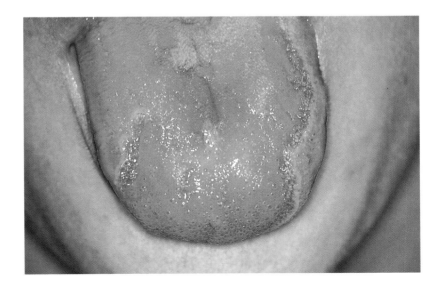

Fig. 8.**3**   Geographic tongue

- The lesions are usually multiple and asymptomatic, although a slight burning sensation may be involved.
- The typical course is the rapid appearance of lesions in one area, which disappear within a short time and develop again in another area, or rarely in the same area.
- The lesions last for about two weeks or more. A few patients develop lesions lasting several years.
- Geographic tongue more often appears in patients with fissured tongue.
- When similar lesions occur in other oral mucosal areas, the disorder is termed "geographic stomatitis" (Fig. 8.**4**).
- The diagnosis is made clinically.

Differential diagnosis

- Lichen planus
- Oral psoriasis
- Reiter's syndrome
- Candidiasis
- Transient loss of filiform papillae
- Pachyonychia congenita

Treatment

- No treatment is needed. Reassuring the patient that the disorder is harmless is enough.

Fissured Tongue

Definition

- Fissured tongue, or scrotal tongue, is a relatively common developmental disorder.

Etiology

- The exact cause remains unclear. However, an autosomal dominant trait with incomplete penetrance may be involved.
- Xerostomia and aging may also be responsible for the disorder.

Occurrence in children

- Relatively uncommon; more common in adolescents.
- Usually seen in children with Down's syndrome.
- The prevalence ranges from 0.5% to 5% of the population.

Localization

- The dorsal surface and the borders of the tongue.

Clinical features

- Several variations may be seen.
- Multiple fissures, covered with normal mucosa and coursing in various directions, are one of the most common variations (Fig. 8.**5**).
- A central median fissure with transverse smaller multiple folds is also another common variant (Fig. 8.**6**).
- The number, direction, and depth of the fissures varies considerably.
- The disorder is usually asymptomatic, although food debris may rarely lodge between the fissures, leading to mild inflammation and burning.
- Geographic tongue may also be seen in about 10–20% of patients with fissured tongue.
- The diagnosis is made clinically.

Differential diagnosis

- Melkersson–Rosenthal syndrome
- Down's syndrome
- Acromegaly
- Sjögren's syndrome

Treatment

- No treatment is needed. Reassuring the patients that the disorder is benign is sufficient.
- Brushing the tongue is sometimes suggested in order to remove food debris from the grooves.

Furred Tongue

Definition

- Furred tongue, or coated tongue, is a transient benign condition, unusual in healthy individuals.

Etiology

- It is due to reduced desquamation of the epithelium, food debris, and bacterial accumulation. However, the exact etiology remains unclear.
- Predisposing factors are acute febrile oral and systemic infections, painful oral ulcerations, dehydration, soft diet, and poor oral hygiene.

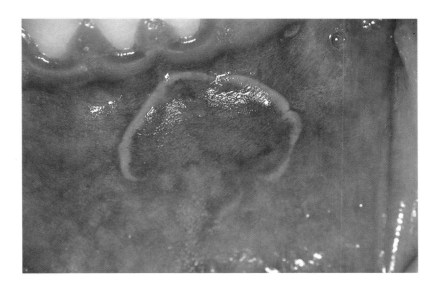

Fig. 8.**4** Geographic stomatitis, solitary lesion on the lower lip mucosa

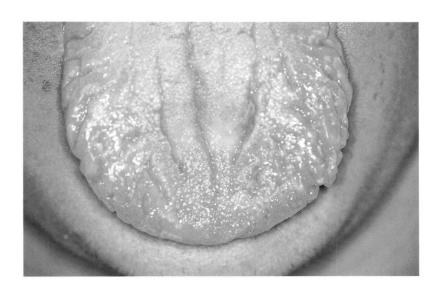

Fig. 8.**5** Fissured tongue

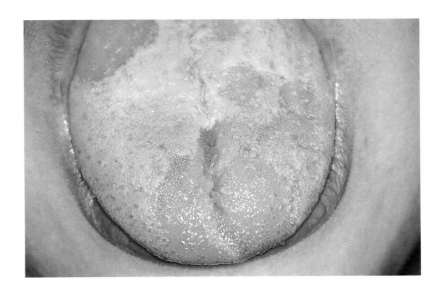

Fig. 8.**6** Fissured tongue with a deep medial fissure, associated with geographic tongue lesions

Occurrence in children	• Relatively common.
Localization	• Exclusively on the dorsal surface of the tongue.
Clinical features	• White or yellow thick coating as a result of lengthening of the filiform papillae, usually less than 3–4 mm (Figs. 8.**7**, 8.**8**).
	• Accumulation of food debris, bacteria, and epithelial-cell desquamation also contributes to the development of the disorder.
	• Typically, the coating is asymptomatic and appears and disappears within a short period of time.
	• The diagnosis is made clinically.
Differential diagnosis	• Hairy tongue
	• Pseudomembranous candidiasis
	• Hairy leukoplakia
	• White sponge nevus
Treatment	• Good oral hygiene.
	• Brushing the dorsum of the tongue (or mechanical debridement).
	• Treatment of the underlying disease.

Hairy Tongue

Definition	• Hairy tongue is a relatively common condition due to marked accumulation of keratin and elongation and hypertrophy of the filiform papillae.
Etiology	• The exact cause is unclear.
	• Several predisposing factors are associated with the disorder, such as heavy smoking, emotional stress, poor oral hygiene, long use of oxidizing and sodium perborate-containing mouthwashes, metronidazole and other antibiotics, radiation of the neck area, *Candida albicans*.
Occurrence in children	• Very rare. More common in adolescents.
Localization	• The middle of the dorsal surface of the tongue, sparing the lateral margin, mainly on the anterior two-thirds.
Clinical features	• The filiform papillae are elongated (1–2 mm) and lengthened (0.5–3 cm).
	• The color is usually brown, brown-yellowish or black (Figs. 8.**9**, 8.**10**).
	• The disorder is usually asymptomatic. However, occasionally an unpleasant feeling and bad taste may be present.
	• The condition lasts for weeks or months.
	• The diagnosis is made clinically.
Differential diagnosis	• Furred tongue
	• Candidiasis
	• Familial acanthosis nigricans
Treatment	• Removal of the predisposing factors.
	• Good oral hygiene.
	• Brushing of the dorsum of the tongue with a toothbrush.
	• In severe cases, topical application by a specialist of keratolytic agents (trichloroacetic acid, salicylic acid, podophyllin, urea 40% in water) is very helpful.

Crenated Tongue

Definition	• Crenated tongue is a harmless condition of the tongue.
Etiology	• It is due to the abnormal pressure or thrusting of the tongue onto the teeth, leading to the formation of tongue impressions.
	• Malpositioned teeth.
	• Edema and enlargement of the tongue are also predisposing factors.
Occurrence in children	• Relatively common.
Localization	• On the lateral borders and the tip of the tongue.
Clinical features	• Multiple, scalloped impressions on the lateral margins of the tongue.

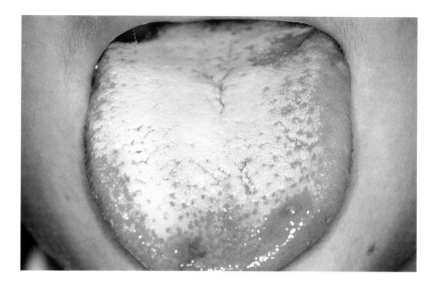

Fig. 8.**7**   Furred tongue

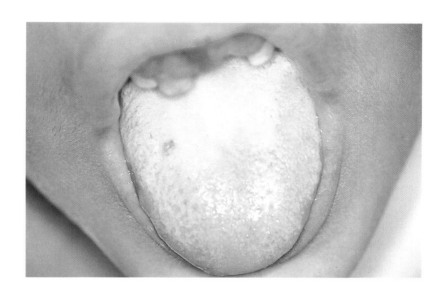

Fig. 8.**8**   Furred tongue

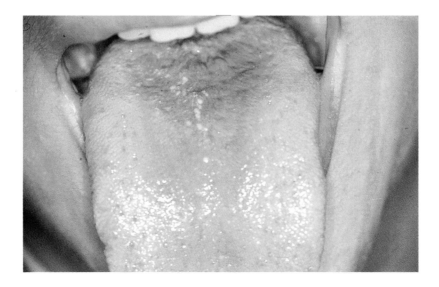

Fig. 8.**9**   Hairy tongue

- The overlying oral mucosa is normal, and the lesions are asymptomatic.
- If there is pathological tongue enlargement, inflammation and pain may be present.
- The diagnosis is made clinically.

Differential diagnosis
- Acromegaly
- Myxedema
- Lipoid proteinosis
- Amyloidosis
- Macroglossia

Treatment
- No treatment is needed.

Hyperplastic Foliate Papillae

Definition
- Hyperplasia of the foliate papillae is a relatively common phenomenon.

Etiology
- Local chronic irritation, infection of the upper respiratory tract.
- Hyperplasia of the lymphoid tissue of the papillae.

Occurrence in children
- Rare.

Localization
- Posterolateral border of the tongue.

Clinical features
- Inflamed, red, swelling nodules, two to five in number.
- The condition may be lateral or bilateral.
- The patient may complain of a burning sensation and mild pain. Occasionally, the condition is asymptomatic.
- The condition lasts for a few weeks or months.
- The diagnosis is usually made clinically.

Differential diagnosis
- Lymphangioma
- Lymphoepithelial cyst

Treatment
- Reassuring the patient.
- Elimination of the irritating factor(s).

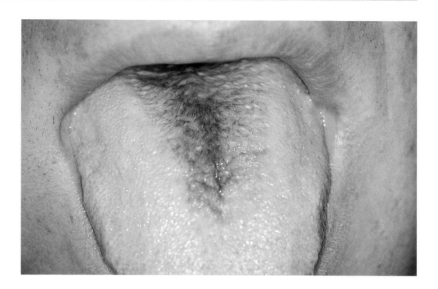

Fig. 8.**10**   Hairy tongue

9 Non-Odontogenic Cysts

Mucocele

Definition
- Mucocele is a common lesion of the oral mucosa, originating from the minor salivary gland ducts.

Etiology
- Commonly (90–95%), the lesion is induced by local minor trauma and duct rupture, followed by mucin spillage into the surrounding soft tissues (mucous extravasation phenomenon).
- Rarely, it is due to obstruction, probably caused by a mucous plug or a sialolith (mucous retention cyst).
- Occasionally, a transient ductal obstruction at the epithelial surface may occur (superficial mucocele).

Occurrence in children
- Common, particularly after 10 years of age.

Localization
- The lower lip, lateral to the midline, is the most common site of involvement (75–80%).
- Less frequently, the mucocele may occur on the buccal mucosa, floor of the mouth, ventral surface of the tongue, soft palate, or upper lip.
- Superficial mucocele develops usually on the soft palate and retromolar area.

Clinical features
- Painless, dome-shaped, slightly bluish or translucent, fluctuating swelling (Figs. 9.**1**–9.**3**).
- Deeper lesions may have a normal color.
- A common sign is a periodical reduction of the swelling due to rupture and partial release of the fluid, soon followed by new accumulation.
- The size varies from a few millimeters to several centimeters.
- The duration of the lesion at the time of diagnosis varies from a few days to several weeks, or even months.
- The diagnosis is usually made clinically.

Histopathology
- Mucin accumulation surrounded by granulation and fibrous tissue (mucous extravasation phenomenon).
- A cyst cavity, filled with mucin and lining by the ductal epithelium (mucous retention cyst).
- Chronic inflammation of the cyst wall is present. Infiltration by numerous neutrophils, histiocytes, and plasma cells is common.

Differential diagnosis
- Lymphangioma
- Pyogenic granuloma
- Lymphoepithelial cyst
- Lipoma
- Mucoepidermoid carcinoma

Treatment
- Surgical excision.

Ranula

Definition
- Ranula is a form of mucocele located on the floor of the mouth.

Etiology
- Leakage of mucin due to trauma or obstruction of the duct of a salivary gland.
- Usually, ranula originates from the sublingual gland, and less commonly from the submandibular gland, or from the minor salivary glands of the floor of the mouth.

Occurrence in children
- Relatively common. It may occur congenitally.

Localization
- Exclusively on the floor of the mouth, usually lateral to the midline.

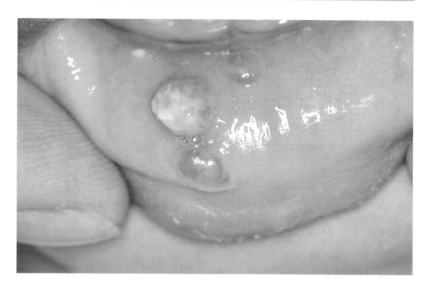

Fig. 9.**1**   Multiple mucoceles of the lower lip

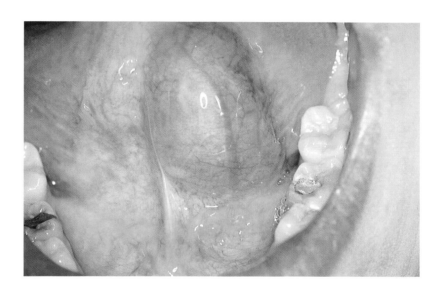

Fig. 9.**2**   Large mucocele of the ventral surface of the tongue

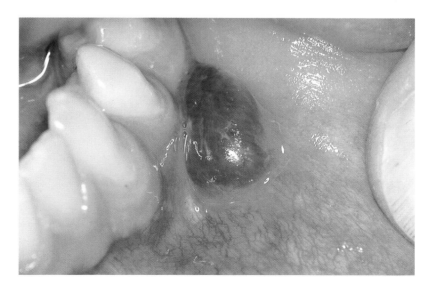

Fig. 9.**3**   Mucocele of the buccal mucosa

Clinical features	• Smooth, dome-shaped, fluctuating and painless swelling (Fig. 9.**4**).
	• The color is usually bluish, but deep lesions may have a normal color.
	• The size varies from a few to several centimeters in diameter. Very large lesions, which may occupy the floor of the mouth, can also occur.
	• It usually appears unilaterally.
	• The diagnosis is usually made clinically.
Histopathology	• Similar to that of a mucocele.
Differential diagnosis	• Dermoid cyst
	• Lymphoepithelial cyst
	• Lymphangioma
	• Cystic hygroma
	• Lipoma
	• Abscess of the floor of the mouth
Treatment	• Surgical removal or marsupialization.
	• Recurrence is common.

Lymphoepithelial Cyst

Definition	• Lymphoepithelial cyst is a unique, uncommon, developmental soft-tissue cyst.
Etiology	• Probably, cystic degeneration of the surface mucosal epithelium or the glandular epithelium entrapped in lymphoid tissue during embryogenesis.
Occurrence in children	• Rare. It usually presents after 40 years of age.
	• By contrast, cervical lymphoepithelial cyst is relatively common.
Localization	• On the floor of the mouth (50–60%). Other sites of occurrence include the posterior lateral border and ventral surface of the tongue and soft palate.
	• Extraorally along the upper lateral neck, along the anterior border of the sternocleidomastoid muscle (cervical lymphoepithelial cyst).
Clinical features	• Asymptomatic, submucosal, mobile, well-defined and elevated nodule (Fig. 9.**5**).
	• It has a yellowish or whitish color, and is usually firm on palpation.
	• The size ranges from 0.5 cm to 2.0 cm in diameter.
	• The clinical diagnosis should always be confirmed by biopsy.
Histopathology	• The cyst lumen is lined by thin stratified squamous epithelium.
	• Characteristically, the cystic wall consists of lymphoid tissue.
	• Germinal centers may also be present.
Differential diagnosis	• Lipoma
	• Granular-cell tumor
	• Small dermoid cyst
	• Mucocele
	• Lymphoid tissue aggregation
Treatment	• Surgical excision.

Thyroglossal Duct Cyst

Definition	• Thyroglossal duct cyst is a rare developmental lesion that may form along the thyroglossal tract.
Etiology	• Cystic degeneration of remnants of the thyroglossal duct epithelium.
Occurrence in children	• Relatively common.
	• Intraoral lesions are rare.
	• About 50% of the cases are diagnosed before adulthood.
Localization	• Along the midline, from the suprasternal notch to the foramen cecum of the tongue.
	• Intraorally, on the midline of the dorsum of the tongue close to the foramen cecum.

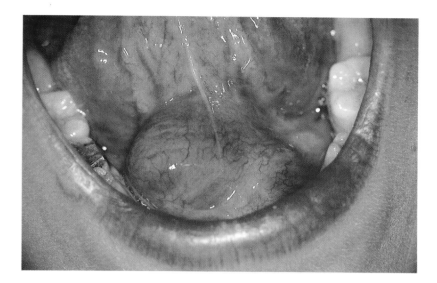

Fig. 9.**4**   Ranula

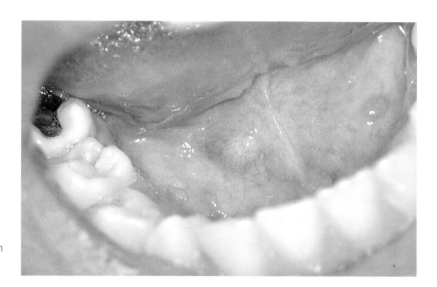

Fig. 9.**5**   Lymphoepithelial cyst,
presenting as a yellowish nodule on
the right side of the floor of the
mouth

Clinical features
- It appears as a painless, fluctuating swelling, either intraorally (Fig. 9.**6**), or along the midline of the neck (Fig. 9.**7**). Occasionally, a fistula may form.
- The size varies from 1 cm to 3 cm or more in diameter.
- Rarely, a carcinoma may arise from the epithelium of the cyst.
- The clinical diagnosis should be confirmed histologically.

Histopathology
- The cyst lumen is lined by stratified squamous ciliary or transitional epithelium.
- The cyst wall consists of lymphoid and thyroid tissue.

Differential diagnosis
- Median rhomboid glossitis
- Benign and malignant tumors
- Lingual thyroid
- Osseous choristoma
- Cervical lymphoepithelial cyst

Treatment
- Surgical removal.

Dermoid Cyst

Definition
- Dermoid cyst is an uncommon developmental cystic lesion.

Etiology
- Cystic degeneration of embryonic epithelial remnants.

Occurrence in children
- Rare, relatively more common in adolescents.
- Congenital cysts in infants may rarely occur.

Localization
- Along the midline of the floor of the mouth (often).
- The lower lip, tongue, and bones of the jaws (less often).

Clinical features
- Slow-growing, painless swelling, with a normal or yellowish-red color and a characteristic soft, dough-like consistency on palpation.
- If the cyst develops above the geniohyoid muscle, it may displace the tongue upward and create problems in mastication, speech, and swallowing (Fig. 9.**8**).
- When the cyst occurs below the geniohyoid muscle, it may protrude submentally (Fig. 9.**9**).
- The size varies from a few millimeters to 10 cm in diameter.
- The clinical diagnosis should be confirmed histologically.

Histopathology
- The internal surface of the cyst is lined by orthokeratinized stratified squamous epithelium. Keratin is often present in the cyst lumen.
- The cystic wall consists of connective tissue without dermal appendages (epidermoid cyst), or may contain skin appendages, e.g., sebaceous glands, hair follicles, sweat glands (dermoid cyst), or rarely bone, teeth, and endodermal elements (teratoid cyst).

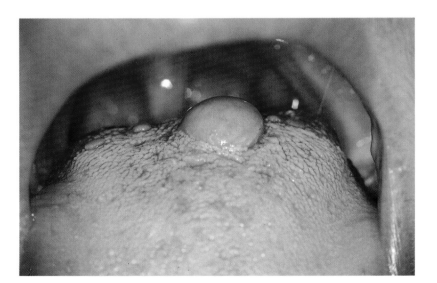

Fig. 9.**6** Thyroglossal duct cyst on the dorsum of the tongue

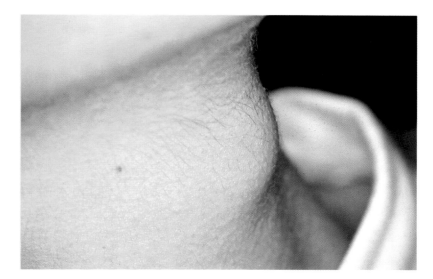

Fig. 9.**7**   Thyroglossal duct cyst on the midline of the neck

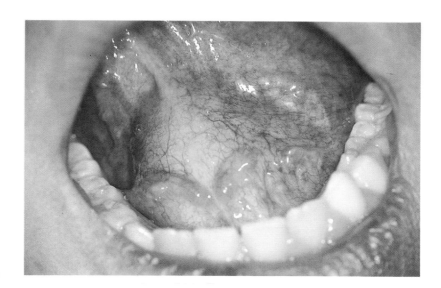

Fig. 9.**8**   Dermoid cyst, midline swelling in the floor of the mouth

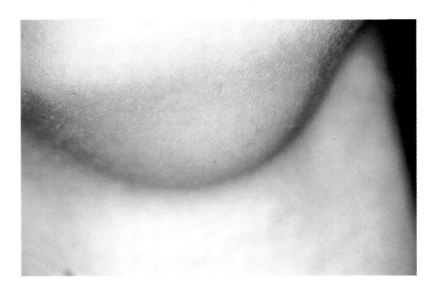

Fig. 9.**9**   Dermoid cyst, submental swelling

Differential diagnosis	• Ranula • Lymphoepithelial cyst • Thyroglossal duct cyst • Lymphangioma • Cystic hygroma • Soft-tissue abscess
Treatment	• Surgical removal.

Incisive Papilla Cyst

Definition	• Incisive papilla cyst is a soft-tissue variant of a nasopalatine duct cyst.
Etiology	• Epithelial rests of the nasopalatine duct.
Occurrence in children	• Rare.
Localization	• Incisive papilla.
Clinical features	• Soft swelling, usually covered by normal mucosa (Fig. 9.**10**, 9.**11**). • Occasionally, it displays bluish-red discoloration due to the fluid contents of the cyst. • Often, the cyst may become inflamed and painful due to infection. • There are no findings on radiographic examination. • The clinical diagnosis should be confirmed histologically.
Histopathology	• The lining of the cyst consists of stratified squamous epithelium (often), pseudostratified columnar epithelium, cuboidal epithelium, or a combination of these. • The cystic wall consists of connective tissue, blood vessels, nerve bundles, cartilage, and nests of salivary glands. Chronic inflammation is common.
Differential diagnosis	• Trauma and inflammation of the incisive papilla • Dental and periodontal abscess • Fibroma • Pyogenic granuloma • Dentigerous cyst
Treatment	• Surgical removal.

Parasitic Cyst (Cysticercosis)

Definition	• Parasitic cysts in the oral cavity are a very unusual phenomenon. • Cysticercosis is a chronic parasitic infection. • The infection is endemic in Mexico, India, Africa, Eastern Europe, and South America.
Etiology	• *Taenia solium* larvae from raw or inadequately cooked pork. • Ingestion of *Taenia* eggs through fecally contaminated vegetables, food, water, or direct contact with another human carrier.
Occurrence in children	• Oral involvement is very rare.
Localization	• Subcutaneous tissues, brain, and skeletal muscles are most commonly affected. • The oral mucosa is rarely affected (buccal mucosa, lips, tongue).
Clinical features	• The clinical manifestations are dependent on the organ involved. • The oral soft-tissue lesions present as a painless, well-circumscribed, mobile nodule. The size varies from 0.5 cm to 2.0 cm, and the lesion is soft on palpation (Fig. 9.**12**). • Diagnosis of the oral lesion should always be confirmed by biopsy and histopathological examination.

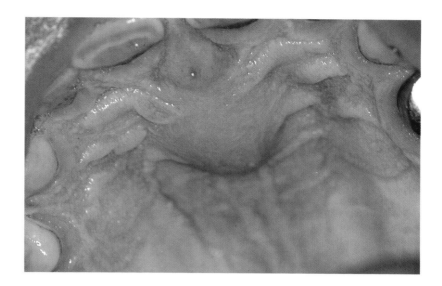

Fig. 9.**10**   Incisive papilla cyst

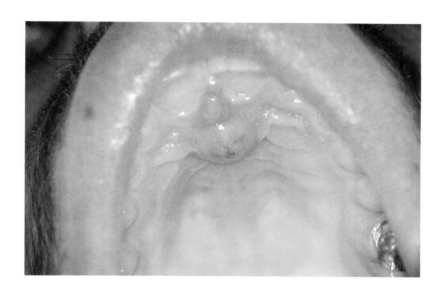

Fig. 9.**11**   Incisive papilla cyst

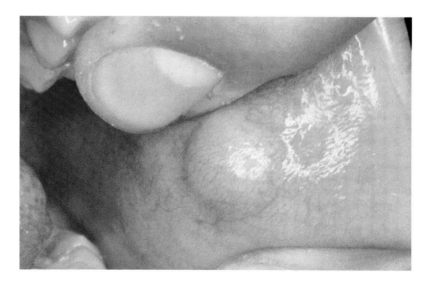

Fig. 9.**12**   Parasitic cyst (cysticercosis) on the buccal mucosa

Laboratory tests

- Histopathological examination of the oral lesion reveals a cystic cavity that is lined by a delicate membrane and contains a larval form of *Taenia solium* (Fig. 9.**13**).
- Direct smear examination of feces, radiography, computed tomography (CT), magnetic resonance imaging (MRI), and serological tests are necessary to diagnose systemic lesions.

Differential diagnosis

- Lipoma
- Fibroma
- Neurofibroma
- Mucocele
- Lymphoepithelial cyst

Treatment

- Surgical excision of the oral lesion.
- Systemic drugs, e.g., praziquantel, albendazole, flubendazole.

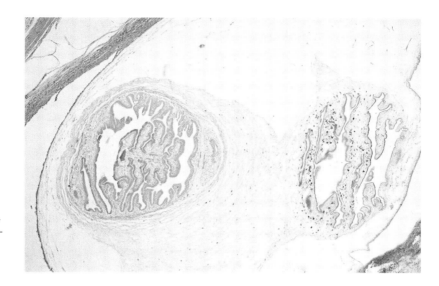

Fig. 9.**13**   Cysticercosis. Histological image of the buccal mucosa lesion, showing two cystic cavities containing larval forms of *Taenia solium*

10 Odontogenic Cysts

Gingival Cysts of the Newborn

Definition
- Gingival cysts of the newborn are small, keratin-filled cysts.

Etiology
- Remnants of the dental lamina.

Occurrence in children
- Very common, exclusively in newborns.

Localization
- Usually on the alveolar mucosa of the maxilla.

Clinical features
- Multiple or solitary asymptomatic, whitish nodules on the alveolar processes of neonates (Figs. 10.**1**, 10.**2**).
- They are approximately 1–3 mm in diameter.
- The cysts regress spontaneously within a few weeks.
- Similar lesions are: Epstein's pearls (which occur on the midline of the hard palate), and Bohn's nodules (which occur scattered over the hard palate, near the border with the soft palate).

Histopathology
- The cystic cavity is lined by a thin stratified squamous epithelium.
- The lumen is filled with keratin.

Differential diagnosis
- Granular-cell tumor of infancy
- Lymphangioma
- Candidiasis

Treatment
- No treatment is indicated.

Eruption Cyst

Definition
- Eruption cyst is a soft-tissue variant of the dentigerous cyst, associated with an erupting deciduous or permanent tooth.

Etiology
- Separation of the dental follicle from around the tooth crown.

Occurrence in children
- Common.

Localization
- Any erupting tooth.
- Molars and canines are more frequently involved.

Clinical features
- It presents as a well-demarcated, translucent, soft swelling directly overlying the crown of an erupting tooth.
- The color is blue or dark red, depending on the amount of blood in the cyst fluid (Figs. 10.**3**, 10.**4**).

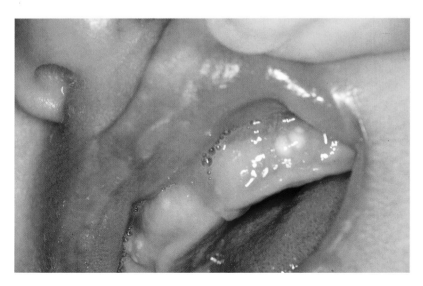

Fig. 10.**1** Gingival cysts of the newborn. Multiple whitish nodules on the maxillary alveolar mucosa

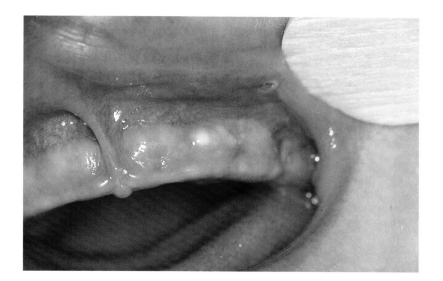

Fig. 10.**2** Gingival cysts of the newborn. Solitary whitish nodule on the maxillary alveolar mucosa

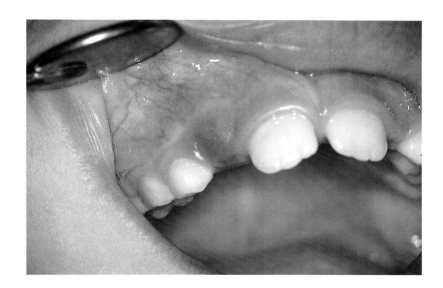

Fig. 10.**3** Eruption cyst

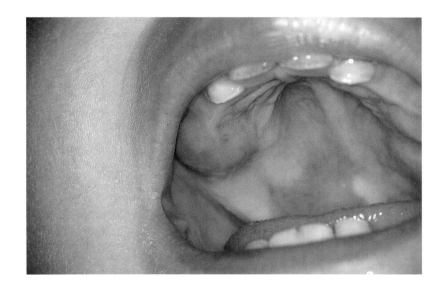

Fig. 10.**4** Eruption cyst

- It is more common with premature eruption of the teeth.
- The diagnosis is usually made clinically.

Histopathology
- The cystic cavity is lined by a thin layer of non-keratinizing squamous epithelium.
- A variable inflammation may be present in the lamina propria.

Differential diagnosis
- Hematoma
- Hemangioma
- Tooth abscess
- Amalgam tattoo
- Pigmented nevi
- Malignant melanoma

Treatment
- Not usually required, as the cyst often ruptures spontaneously.
- Excision of the roof of the cyst may encourage eruption of the tooth.

Periapical Cyst

Definition
- Periapical or radicular cyst is the most common odontogenic cyst, and develops at the apex of a non-vital tooth.

Etiology
- Cystic degeneration of Malassez epithelial rests located in the periodontal ligament.

Occurrence in children
- Relatively rare. It is more common during neonatal dentition.

Localization
- In both jaws, more often in the maxilla.

Clinical features
- The cyst is often asymptomatic, unless an acute inflammatory exacerbation occurs.
- Hard swelling close to the apex of the involved tooth.
- If the cyst becomes large, expansion of the cortical bone may occur, producing a fluctuating swelling that protrudes intraorally or extraorally (Figs. 10.**5**–10.**7**).
- Exacerbation of the cyst gives rise to a subperiosteal, submucous, and subcutaneous abscess.
- Rarely, osteomyelitis may occur.
- The thermal and electric pulp vitality tests are negative.

Radiographic features
- A well-circumscribed periapical radiolucency.

Histopathology
- The cyst is lined by a non-keratinizing stratified squamous epithelium.
- The thickness of the epithelium varies greatly.
- The lumen is filled with cellular debris and fluid.
- The cyst wall may contain an accumulation of inflammatory cells.

Differential diagnosis
- Other odontogenic cysts
- Odontogenic tumors
- Fibrous dysplasia
- Actinomycosis
- Melanotic neuroectodermal tumor of infancy

Treatment
- Conservative endodontic treatment.
- In case of failure of conservative therapy, apicectomy or surgical exploration is recommended.

Lateral Periodontal Cyst

Definition
- Lateral periodontal cyst is a rare developmental odontogenic cyst.

Etiology
- It probably arises from epithelial rests of the dental lamina in the periodontal ligament of an erupted tooth.

Occurrence in children
- Very rare. The cyst is usually discovered during adulthood.

Localization
- Often in the canine–premolar area, or between premolars of the mandible.

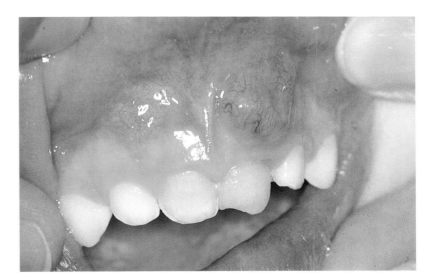

Fig. 10.**5**   Periapical cyst, intraoral swelling

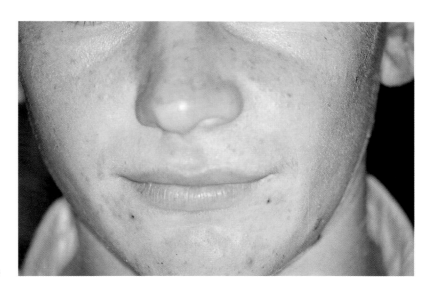

Fig. 10.**6**   Periapical cyst, extraoral swelling on the left side of the face

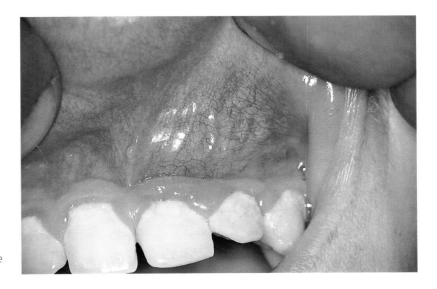

Fig. 10.**7**   Periapical cyst, extensive intraoral swelling

Clinical features

- It is usually asymptomatic, and is detected accidentally during a radiographic examination. The adjacent teeth remain vital.
- On probing, there is no communication between the dental sulcus and cyst.
- The diagnosis can be made at all ages.

Radiographic features

- It presents as a well-confined, round, radiolucent area located at the lateral surface of the teeth (Fig. 10.**8**).

Histopathology

- The cyst is lined by a thin stratified squamous epithelium. Plaque-like thickenings of the epithelial lining may be present.
- The cyst wall consists of fibrous tissue without inflammation.

Differential diagnosis

- Lateral periapical cyst
- Odontogenic keratocyst
- Gingival cyst of adults

Treatment

- Surgical removal.

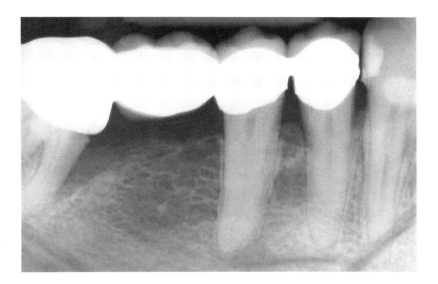

Fig. 10.**8** Lateral periodontal cyst. A well-defined, round radiolucency between the two vital premolars in a 51-year-old woman

11 Recurrent Aphthous Ulcers

Definition
- Recurrent aphthous ulcers, also known as aphthous stomatitis, are painful oral ulcerations that characteristically recur, at intervals ranging from days to months or years.

Etiology
- The exact etiology remains unknown.
- Recent data support the concept that the cell-mediated immune response plays an important role in the pathogenesis of these lesions.
- Many predisposing factors have been incriminated, such as trauma, genetics, infections, allergy, systemic diseases, hormonal disturbances, emotional stress, acquired immune deficiency syndrome (AIDS), and others.

Occurrence in children
- Common, usually after the sixth year of age.
- Girls are slightly more frequently affected than boys.
- Aphthous ulcers are one of the most common lesions of the oral mucosa, with an overall prevalence ranging from 10% to 30% in the general population.

Localization
- The non-keratinized mobile oral mucosa is most frequently affected (e.g., buccal mucosa, labial mucosa, tongue, floor of the mouth, soft palate and uvula).

Clinical features
- Based on clinical criteria, aphthous ulcers are classified as *minor, major,* and *herpetiform ulcers.*
- *Minor aphthous ulcers* are the most common in children and adults, and are clinically characterized by a shallow, round and painful ulcer 3–6 mm in diameter. The ulcer is covered by a yellow-white membrane, and is surrounded by a thin red halo (Figs. 11.**1**, 11.**2**). The lesions may be single or multiple (two to six), and they heal without scarring in 6–12 days.
- *Major aphthous ulcers* are much less common in children, and represent the more severe form of the disease. Clinically, the ulcer is deep, extremely painful, 1–2 cm in diameter, and the number varies from one to five (Figs. 11.**3,** 11.**4**). It lasts for three to six weeks or more, and may cause scarring after healing.

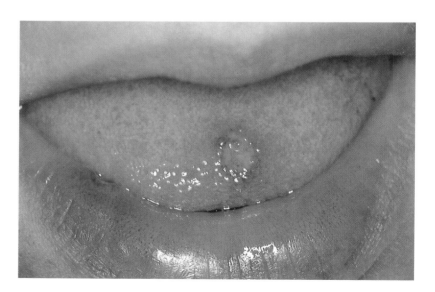

Fig. 11.**1** Minor aphthous ulcer of the tongue

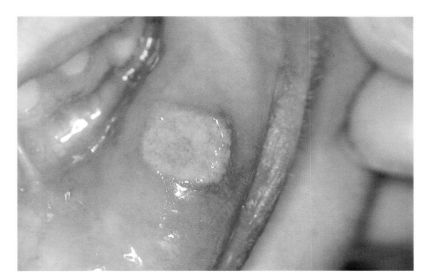

Fig. 11.**2**   Minor aphthous ulcer of the lower labial mucosa

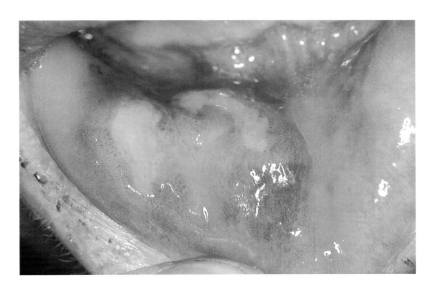

Fig. 11.**3**   Major aphthous ulcer of the lower labial mucosa

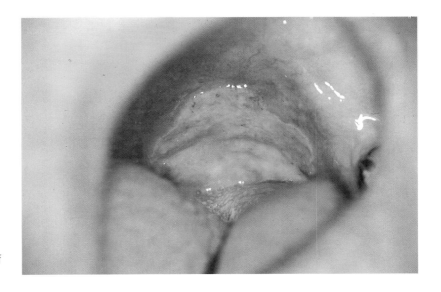

Fig. 11.**4**   Major aphthous ulcer of the soft palate

- *Herpetiform ulcers* are rare in children, and are clinically characterized by small, painful, shallow ulcers, 1–2 mm in diameter, with a tendency to occur in clusters. Characteristically, the ulcers are multiple (10–100 in number), persist for one to two weeks, and heal without scarring (Fig. 11.**5**).
- The diagnosis of all three forms of aphthous ulcer is based on clinical criteria, as there are no specific diagnostic tests.

Differential diagnosis

- Traumatic ulcer
- Herpetic stomatitis
- Herpangina
- Hand, foot and mouth disease
- Behçet's disease
- Crohn's disease
- Syphilis
- Erythema multiforme
- Cyclic neutropenia
- FAPA syndrome (Fever Aphthous ulcers Pharyngitis Adenitis)
- Sweet's syndrome

Treatment

- Topical treatment to reduce pain and shorten the course (anesthetics, e.g., 2% viscous lidocaine, benzocaine, triamcinolone 0.1% in an adhesive base–Orabase, or fluocinonide gel; intralesional injection of corticosteroids only in persistent major aphthous ulcers).
- Systemic treatment only in severe and frequently recurrent cases (corticosteroids in low dose for four to eight days, thalidomide, levamisole, pentoxifylline).

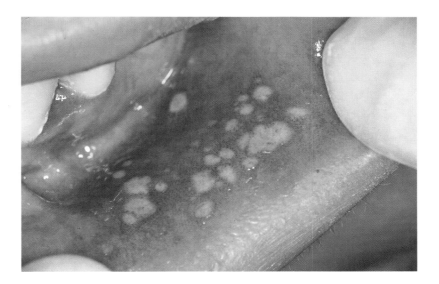

Fig. 11.**5**   Herpetiform ulcers of
the lower labial mucosa

12 Bacterial Infections

Acute Necrotizing Ulcerative Gingivitis

Definition
- Acute necrotizing ulcerative gingivitis (ANUG) is a distinctive acute gingival infection, with a characteristic clinical pattern.

Etiology
- *Bacillus fusiformis* and *Borrelia vincentii* are involved. In addition, *Prevotella intermedia* and other anaerobic bacteria may be also implicated.
- Important predisposing factors are smoking, poor oral hygiene, emotional stress, local trauma, immunosuppression and mainly human immunodeficiency virus (HIV) infection.

Occurrence in children
- Rare; more common in adolescence.

Localization
- Interdental papillae, marginal gingiva, and rarely other parts of the oral mucosa.

Clinical features
- The characteristic clinical pattern is necrosis and crater-like ulcerations.
- The lesions usually start from the tips of the interdental papillae, spreading along the free margins of the gingiva (Figs. 12.**1**, 12.**2**).
- The gingiva are fiery red, swollen, and painful.
- Spontaneous hemorrhage, intense salivation, and breath and taste disturbances are common.
- Low-grade fever, regional lymphadenopathy, malaise, and headaches may also occur.
- The lesions may occasionally spread to adjacent oral soft tissues (acute necrotizing ulcerative stomatitis), with more severe local and systemic symptoms (Fig. 12.**3**).
- The diagnosis is based on clinical criteria.

Differential diagnosis
- Primary herpetic gingivostomatitis
- Necrotizing ulcerative periodontitis
- Scurvy
- Acute leukemia
- Cyclic neutropenia
- Agranulocytosis
- Aplastic anemia
- Langerhans cell histiocytosis

Treatment
- In the acute phase, systemic antibiotics such as metronidazole, penicillin, and mouthwashes with oxygen-releasing compounds.
- Local periodontal therapy by scaling and curettage, and improvement of oral hygiene must follow the acute phase.

Periapical Abscess

Definition
- Periapical or dental abscess is an accumulation of purulent material around the apex of a non-viable tooth as a result of pulp necrosis.

Etiology
- Aerobic and anaerobic bacteria.

Occurrence in children
- Relatively common.

Localization
- Incisors and molars both in primary and secondary dentition.

Clinical features
- Tenderness or severe pain of the non-vital tooth, particularly to percussion.
- Tooth extrusion is also a common finding.
- Painful swelling of the surrounding tissues is common (Fig. 12.**4**).

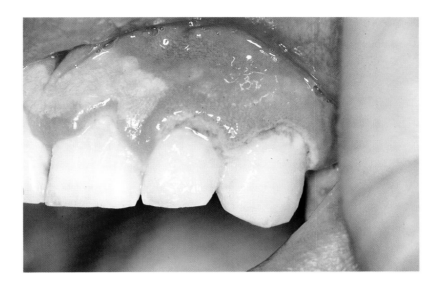

Fig. 12.**1**   Acute necrotizing ulcerative gingivitis

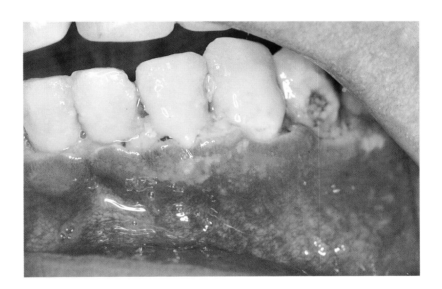

Fig. 12.**2**   Acute necrotizing ulcerative gingivitis

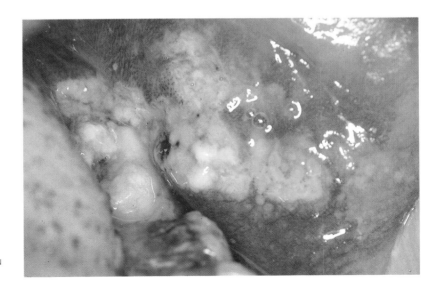

Fig. 12.**3**   Acute necrotizing ulcerative stomatitis. Extensive ulcerative lesions on the buccal mucosa and in the retromolar area

- With progression, the pus spreads along the path of least resistance, forming an intraoral or extraoral abscess or sinus tract (Figs. 12.**5**–12.**8**).
- Osteomyelitis as a result of pus extension to the medullary spaces may also occur.
- Fever, chills, headache, malaise, and lymphadenopathy are common.
- Characteristically, the thermal and electric pulp vitality tests are negative.
- The diagnosis should be made on the clinical and radiographic findings.

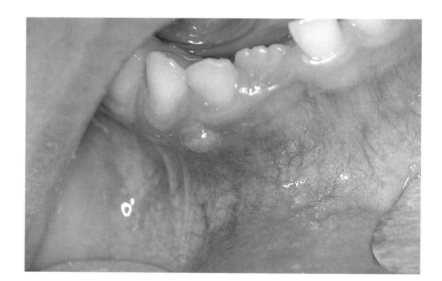

Fig. 12.**4** Periapical abscess, intraoral swelling on the buccal surface of the mandible

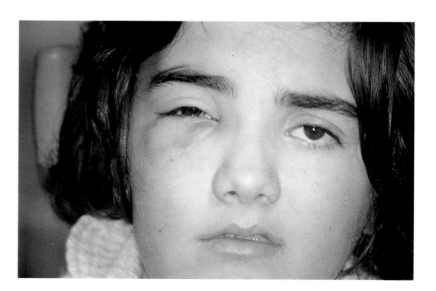

Fig. 12.**5** Periapical abscess, extraoral swelling and edema around the right eye

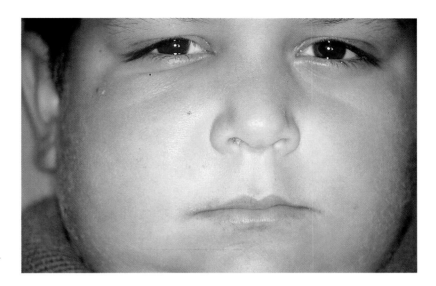

Fig. 12.**6** Periapical abscess, swelling of the right side of the face

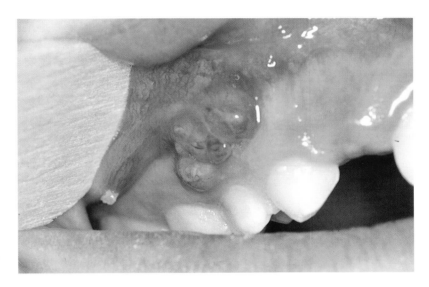

Fig. 12.**7** Periapical abscess and multiple intraoral sinus tract formation

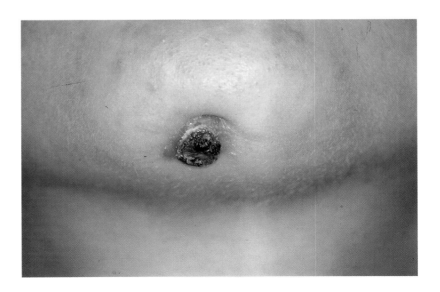

Fig. 12.**8** Periapical abscess and extraoral sinus tract on the chin

Radiographic findings	• Early lesions demonstrate thickening of the apical periodontal ligament. • Well or poorly circumscribed periapical radiolucencies, with a diameter of a few millimeters to several centimeters, are common in chronic lesions (Fig. 12.**9**).
Differential diagnosis	• Acute periodontitis and periodontal abscess • Osteomyelitis • Actinomycosis • Odontogenic cysts
Treatment	• Drainage of the abscess. • Root canal therapy, apicectomy, or extraction of the affected tooth. • Antibiotics and analgesics are usually necessary in the acute phase.

Periodontal Abscess

Definition	• Periodontal abscess is an accumulation of purulent exudate in a deep periodontal pocket.
Etiology	• Mixed aerobic and anaerobic bacterial infection.
Occurrence in children	• Rare. More common in children with diabetes mellitus.
Localization	• No specific location.
Clinical features	• Soft, edematous, usually acute swelling of the gingiva (Fig. 12.**10**). • The involved gingiva are painful, with a yellowish-red or dark red color. • Characteristically, if the swelling is pressed, pus may flow out from the periodontal pocket. • Mobility, sensitivity or pain, usually to lateral percussion, of the adjacent tooth are common. • Occasionally, regional lymphadenopathy, fever, chills and malaise may appear. • After drainage, the abscess becomes asymptomatic, but exacerbations are common. • If they are not treated, periodontal abscesses may lead to sinus tract formation (periodontal fistula). • Periodontal probing depths are exaggerated in areas of abscess formation. • The teeth are vital on thermal and electric tests, unless they have been previously treated endodontically.
Radiographic features	• Moderate or extensive bone destruction and attachment.
Differential diagnosis	• Periapical abscess and fistula • Lateral periodontal cyst • Granulomatous gingivitis • Dental papillae cyst • Pericoronitis
Treatment	• Systemic antibiotics, surgical drainage of the abscess.

Pericoronitis

Definition	• Pericoronitis is an acute or subacute gingival inflammatory reaction around a partially erupted, impacted, or erupting tooth.
Etiology	• Mechanical irritation, food debris and bacteria.
Occurrence in children	• Relatively common.
Localization	• More frequently, the mandibular first and second molars.
Clinical features	• The affected gingiva show severe painful inflammation, with edema (Fig. 12.**11**). • Foul taste, ulcerations and trismus are common (Fig. 12.**12**). • Abscess formation, low fever, and regional lymphadenopathy may occur. • The diagnosis is based on clinical criteria.
Differential diagnosis	• Herpetic gingivitis

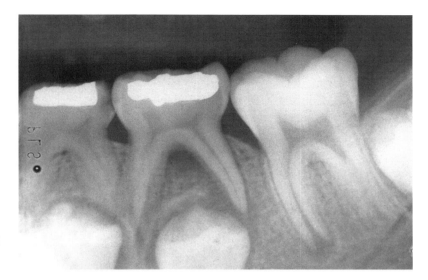

Fig. 12.**9** Periapical abscess. A poorly-defined radiolucency around the roots of the second neonatal molar

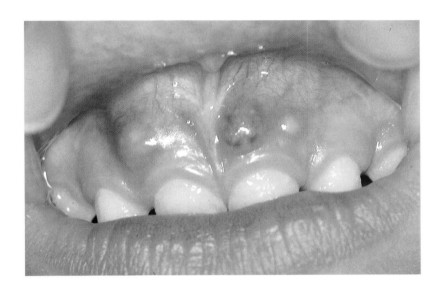

Fig. 12.**10** Multiple periodontal abscesses

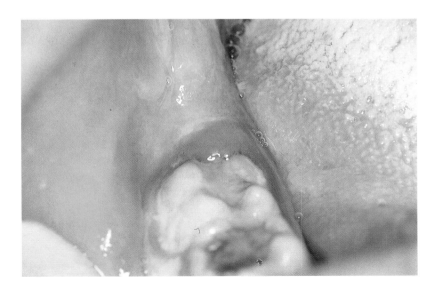

Fig. 12.**11** Pericoronitis

- Acute necrotizing ulcerative gingivitis
- Periodontal abscess
- Aphthous ulcerations

Treatment
- In the acute phase, antiseptic mouthwashes, and systemic antibiotics if general symptoms are present.
- Surgical removal of the gingival flap over the tooth, or extraction of the impacted or partially erupted tooth in severe recurrent cases.

Buccal Cellulitis

Definition
- Cellulitis is an acute and edematous inflammatory spread into the facial soft tissues.

Etiology
- Frequently, *Staphylococcus aureus*, α-hemolytic streptococci and less often Gram-negative and anaerobic microorganisms.
- *Haemophilus influenzae* type B is usually responsible for buccal cellulitis in infants.

Occurrence in children
- Relatively rare.

Localization
- Buccal and submandibular facial area.
- Facial cellulitis is usually due to the spread of dental infections.

Clinical features
- It presents as a diffuse, firm, ill-defined erythematous swelling associated with warmth and pain (Fig. 12.**13**).
- The overlying skin shows a deep purplish discoloration.
- Fever, chills, nausea, vomiting, and sweating may occur.
- The diagnosis is based on clinical criteria.

Laboratory tests
- Blood cultures
- Needle aspiration
- Biopsy

Differential diagnosis
- Erysipelas
- Acute parotitis
- Angioedema
- Leishmaniasis
- Insect bites
- Trauma

Treatment
- Systemic antibiotics.
- Occasionally, surgical drainage is recommended.

Oral Soft-Tissue Abscess

Definition
- Oral soft-tissue abscess is an acute or subacute infection of non-dental origin.

Etiology
- Usually *Staphylococcus aureus*, α-hemolytic streptococci, and rarely other microorganisms.

Occurrence in children
- Rare.

Localization
- Tongue, buccal mucosa, lips, floor of the mouth.

Clinical features
- Acute or subacute origin.
- Painful, ill-defined swelling, soft or semi-hard on palpation (Fig. 12.**14**).
- The overlying mucosa may be red or normal in color.
- Low-grade fever and regional lymphadenopathy may occur.
- On surgical or respiratory drainage, purulent material flows out.
- The diagnosis is based on clinical criteria.

Laboratory tests
- Bacterial cultures.
- Histopathological examination.

Differential diagnosis
- Soft-tissue cysts
- Actinomycosis
- Benign tumors

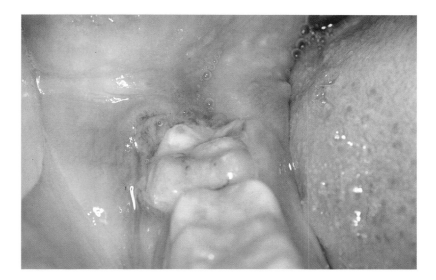

Fig. 12.**12**   Pericoronitis

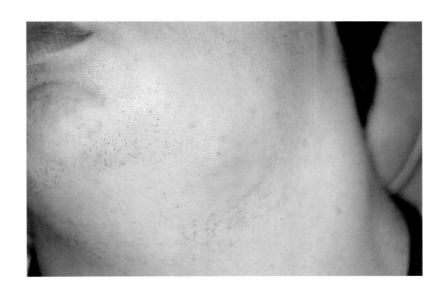

Fig. 12.**13**   Facial cellulitis due to periapical abscess

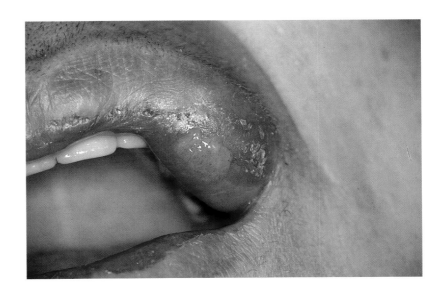

Fig. 12.**14**   Soft-tissue abscess of the upper lip

Treatment
- Antibiotics.
- Surgical drainage in persistent cases.

Acute Suppurative Sialadenitis

Definition
- Acute suppurative sialadenitis is a bacterial infectious disease of the salivary glands.

Etiology
- *Staphylococcus aureus, S. pyogenes*, and less often streptococci, pneumococci, and other microorganisms.
- Ductal obstruction by sialoliths or other causes usually help bacterial infections.

Occurrence in children
- Rare.

Localization
- Usually the parotid gland, and less often the submandibular and sublingual glands, or minor salivary glands.

Clinical features
- Painful swelling, usually unilateral in the affected gland, associated with tenderness and induration of the area (Fig. 12.**15**).
- The overlying skin may be erythematous.
- Intraorally, inflammation of the orifice of the duct is a common finding (Fig. 12.**16**). Purulent material may flow out from the duct orifice.
- Occasionally, a sialolith may be present at the orifice of the duct (Fig. 12.**17**).
- Low-grade fever, malaise, trismus may occur.
- The diagnosis is based on clinical criteria.

Laboratory tests
- Bacterial cultures
- Radiographs (occlusal, panoramic)
- Sialogram

Differential diagnosis
- Mumps
- Postoperative sialadenitis
- Sjögren's syndrome
- Mikulicz disease
- Leukemia and lymphomas
- Salivary gland tumors

Treatment
- Antibiotics.
- Surgical removal of the sialoliths.

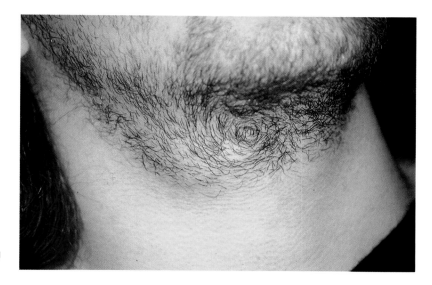

Fig. 12.**15**   Submandibular suppurative sialadenitis. Extraoral swelling of the submandibular area

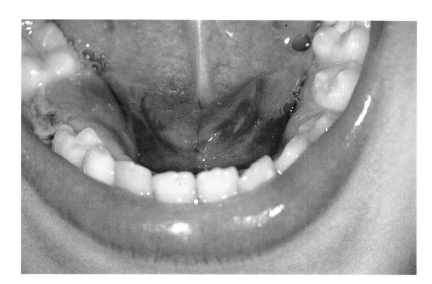

Fig. 12.**16**   Submandibular suppurative sialadenitis. Bilateral inflammation and swelling of the duct orifices

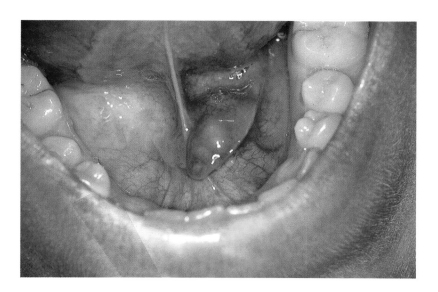

Fig. 12.**17**   Sialolith and swelling of the left orifice of the submandibular salivary duct

13 Viral Infections

Primary Herpetic Gingivostomatitis

Definition
- Primary herpetic gingivostomatitis is the most frequent acute viral infection of the oral mucosa.

Etiology
- Most frequently, herpes simplex virus type 1 (HSV-1), and rarely herpes simplex type 2 (HSV-2).

Occurrence in children
- Common.
- The incidence of primary infection with HSV-1 increases after six months of age, and peaks between the ages of two and four. New cases continue to occur in older children and adolescents.

Localization
- Gingiva, tongue, palate, lips, buccal mucosa, tonsils, posterior pharynx.

Clinical features
- Clinically, the disease is characterized by an abrupt onset accompanied by high fever, malaise, irritability, headache, and pain in the mouth, followed within one to three days by the eruptive phase.
- The affected mucosa is red and edematous, with numerous coalescing vesicles that rupture within 24 hours, leaving painful small, round, shallow ulcers that are covered by a yellowish-gray pseudomembrane and surrounded by an erythematous halo (Figs. 13.**1**, 13.**2**). The ulcers may coalesce to form larger, irregular ulcerations (Fig. 13.**3**). New elements continue to appear during the first three to five days. The ulcers gradually heal over 7–10 days without scarring.
- Bilateral painful regional lymphadenopathy is a constant feature of the disease (Fig. 13.**4**).
- Perioral lesions may occasionally occur.
- The diagnosis is usually based on clinical criteria.

Laboratory tests
- Viral culture
- Cytology smears
- Serological test (measurement of antibody titers)

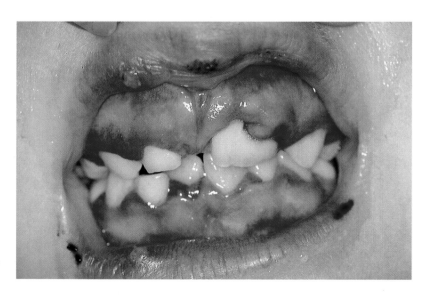

Fig. 13.**1** Primary herpetic gingivostomatitis. Enlarged and erythematous gingiva and erosions on the lips

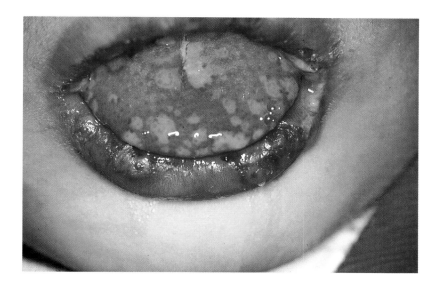

Fig. 13.**2**   Primary herpetic gingivostomatitis. Multiple shallow ulcers on the tongue and lips

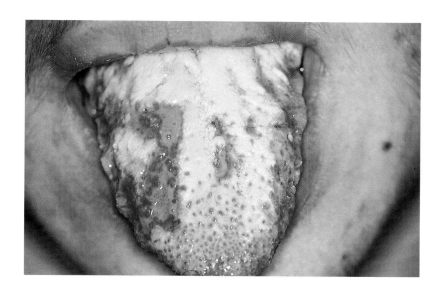

Fig. 13.**3**   Primary herpetic gingivostomatitis. Coalescing, irregular ulcers on the dorsal surface of the tongue

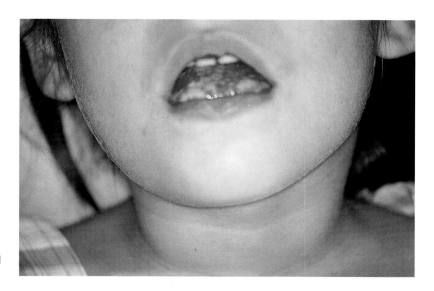

Fig. 13.**4**   Bilateral anterior cervical lymph-node enlargement

Differential diagnosis	• Herpetiform ulcers • Herpangina • Hand, foot, and mouth disease • Streptococcal stomatitis • Erythema multiforme • Infectious mononucleosis • Pemphigus
Treatment	• In most cases, the treatment is symptomatic. • In severe cases, in immunocompromised children and neonatals, systemic acyclovir is indicated.

Secondary Herpetic Infections

Definition	• Secondary or recurrent herpetic infections are the result of herpes simplex virus reactivation in pre-infected individuals.
Etiology	• HSV-1. • Predisposing factors that may precipitate virus reactivation include febrile illness, trauma, emotional stress, ultraviolet light, immunosuppression, human immunodeficiency virus (HIV) infection, leukemia.
Occurrence in children	• Rare in immunocompetent children, and common in those in whom the immune system is compromised.
Localization	• Lips, hard palate, attached gingiva.
Clinical features	• Because of acquired immunity during the primary infection, the oral complaints are usually mild (burning, itching, mild pain), and the constitutional symptoms are characteristically absent. • The oral lesions consist of a small number of discrete vesicles arranged in clusters. The vesicles rupture within about 24 hours, leaving small ulcers 1–3 mm in size, which heal spontaneously within 6–10 days (Fig. 13.**5**). The lip lesions (herpes labialis) are characteristically covered by a brownish crust (Fig. 13.**6**). • In immunocompromised children, the lesions are usually much larger, and persist for a long time (Fig. 13.**7**). • The diagnosis is based on clinical criteria.
Differential diagnosis	• Herpetiform ulcers and other forms of aphthous ulcers • Trauma • Hand, foot, and mouth disease. • Varicella
Treatment	• Symptomatic.

Herpangina

Definition	• Herpangina is an acute viral disease.
Etiology	• Usually, coxsackievirus group A (types 1–6, 8, 10, 22), and less often coxsackievirus B are responsible.
Occurrence in children	• Relatively common. The disease frequently affects children and adolescents, with a peak incidence during summer and autumn.
Localization	• Typically on the soft palate, uvula, tonsils, faucial pillars, posterior pharyngeal wall. • The tongue and buccal mucosa are rarely involved.
Clinical features	• The disease presents with sudden fever (ranging from 38–40 °C), sore throat, headache, dysphagia, and malaise, followed within 24–48 hours by diffuse erythema and vesicular eruption. • The vesicles are numerous and small, and soon rupture, leaving painful shallow ulcers that heal in 7–10 days (Figs. 13.**8,** 13.**9**). • The diagnosis is usually based on clinical criteria.
Laboratory tests	• Viral culture and serological tests may be used in atypical cases.

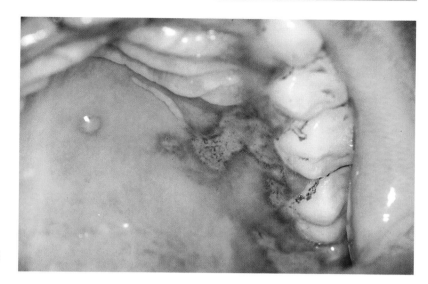

Fig. 13.**5**   Secondary herpetic infection. Multiple ulcers on the hard palate and gingiva

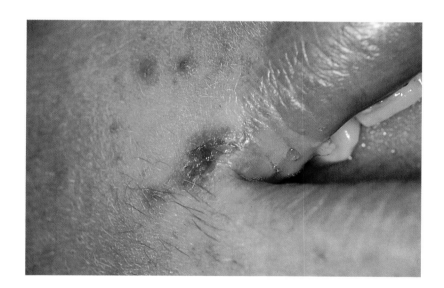

Fig. 13.**6**   Herpes labialis on the commissure

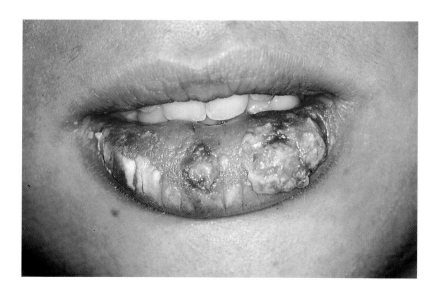

Fig. 13.**7**   Secondary herpetic infection. Severe and persistent lesions on the lower lip in an immunocompromised child

Differential diagnosis	<ul><li>Primary herpetic gingivostomatitis</li><li>Aphthous ulcers.</li><li>Lymphonodular pharyngitis</li><li>Varicella</li><li>Hand, foot, and mouth disease</li><li>Erythema multiforme</li></ul>
Treatment	• Symptomatic.

Acute Lymphonodular Pharyngitis

Definition	• Acute lymphonodular pharyngitis is an acute febrile viral disease.
Etiology	• Coxsackievirus type A_{10}.
Occurrence in children	• Relatively common.
Localization	• Soft palate, uvula, tonsillar pillars.
Clinical features	• The disease presents with fever, mild headache, anorexia and sore throat, followed within two to three days by characteristic multiple, raised, discrete, white to yellow papules surrounded by an erythematous halo (Fig. 13.**10**). • The lesions vary from 3 mm to 6 mm in diameter, and resolve within 8–10 days. • The diagnosis is usually based on clinical criteria.
Laboratory tests	• Viral culture and serological tests may be used in atypical cases.
Differential diagnosis	• Herpangina • Herpes simplex
Treatment	• Symptomatic.

Condyloma Acuminatum

Definition	• Condyloma acuminatum is a benign, viral, sexually transmitted lesion of the stratified squamous epithelium.
Etiology	• Human papillomaviruses (HPV-6, HPV-11, HPV-16, HPV-18, or others).
Occurrence in children	• Rare.
Localization	• Mainly in the anogenital area. • Rarely in the oral cavity (tongue, buccal mucosa, lip mucosa, soft palate, gingiva).
Clinical features	• The lesion presents as sessile or pedunculated well-circumscribed nodule that may proliferate and coalesce, forming cauliflower-like projections (Figs. 13.**11,** 13.**12**).

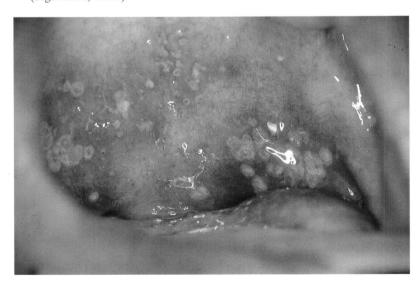

Fig. 13.**8** Herpangina. Numerous shallow ulcers on the soft palate

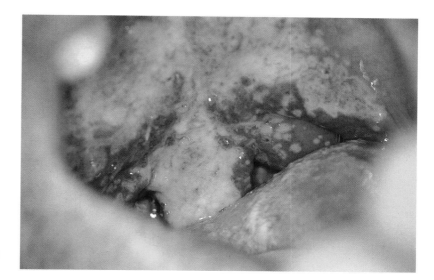

Fig. 13.**9** Herpangina. Numerous coalescing ulcers on the soft palate and uvula

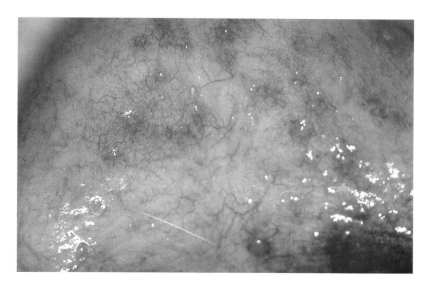

Fig. 13.**10** Acute lymphonodular pharyngitis. Multiple raised and discrete papules on the soft palate

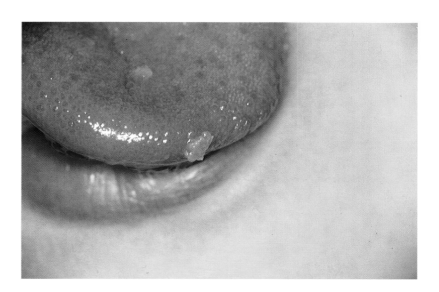

Fig. 13.**11** Condyloma acuminatum on the tip of the tongue

- Lesions may have whitish or pinkish color and are non-tender.
- They are usually multiple, but isolated lesions may be seen (Fig. 13.**13**).
- The size varies from 1 cm to 2 cm or more.
- The diagnosis is based on clinical and histopathological criteria.

Laboratory tests
- Histopathological examination reveals papillary projections of epithelium with parakeratosis, prominent acanthosis, and several koilocytes at the upper part of the epithelium. The underlying connective tissue may display a mild inflammation.

Differential diagnosis
- Verruca vulgaris
- Papilloma
- Verruciform xanthoma
- Sialadenoma papilliferum
- Focal epithelial hyperplasia
- Focal dermal hypoplasia syndrome

Treatment
- Surgical excision.

Verruca Vulgaris

Definition
- Verruca vulgaris or common wart is a benign, contagious, virus-induced lesion of the stratified squamous epithelium.

Etiology
- Human papillomaviruses (HPV-2, HPV-4, HPV-40).

Occurrence in children
- Common.

Localization
- Common on the skin fingers, hands, perioral, face.
- Uncommon in the oral mucosa (lips, commissures, tongue, palate).
- Oral lesions are due to autoinoculation of the virus by chewing or sucking the fingers.

Clinical features
- The oral lesions present as sessile or pedunculated, well-defined, rough exophytic growths, with papillary projections and a whitish color (Figs. 13.**14**–13.**16**).
- They may be single or multiple, and their size varies from 2 mm to 6 mm.
- The diagnosis is based on clinical and histopathological criteria.

Laboratory tests
- Histopathological examination reveals numerous finger-like projections of the epithelium, which is hyperkeratotic and acanthotic. The rete ridges are elongated and converge toward the center of the lesion. Koilocytes may be present on the upper part of the spinous layer. A connective-tissue core with mild chronic inflammation supports the epithelial projections.

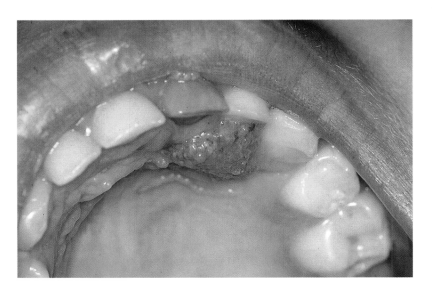

Fig. 13.**12** Condyloma acuminatum on the upper gingiva

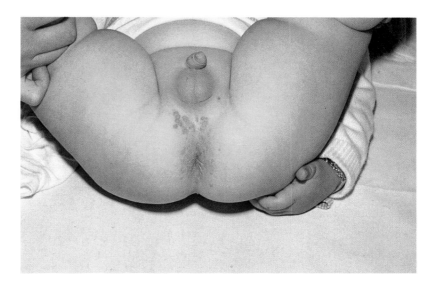

Fig. 13.**13**   Multiple condylomata acuminata in the perianal area

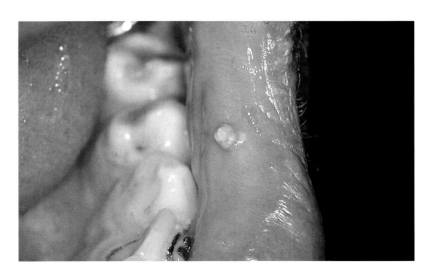

Fig. 13.**14**   Verruca vulgaris on the lip mucosa

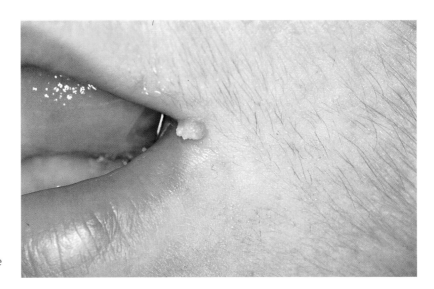

Fig. 13.**15**   Verruca vulgaris on the commissure

Differential diagnosis	● Condyloma acuminatum
	● Papilloma
	● Verruciform xanthoma
Treatment	● Surgical excision.

Focal Epithelial Hyperplasia

Definition
● Focal epithelial hyperplasia or Heck's disease is a benign, virus-induced hyperplastic lesion of the oral mucosa.

Etiology
● Human papillomaviruses (HPV-13, HPV-32).
● The disease is endemic in Eskimos, North American Indians, and South Africans, but it has also been reported in other ethnic groups.

Occurrence in children
● Common.

Localization
● Buccal mucosa, labial mucosa, tongue, gingiva, palate.

Clinical features
● The disease presents as multiple, painless, sessile, slightly elevated and well-demarcated, soft papules and nodules 1–10 mm in diameter (Figs. 13.**17,** 13.**18**).
● The lesions are whitish or have the color of the normal mucosa, with a smooth surface.
● Characteristically, the lesions tend to disappear on stretching of the oral mucosa.
● The diagnosis is based on clinical and histopathological criteria.

Laboratory tests
● Histopathological examination reveals considerable acanthosis, with broad and elongated rete ridges (Fig. 13.**19**). Parakeratosis, koilocytes, and occasionally nuclear alterations mimicking mitotic changes (mitosoid cell) may be observed. Slight inflammatory infiltration into the connective tissue may also be present.

Differential diagnosis
● Condyloma acuminatum
● Verruca vulgaris
● Multiple papillomas
● Multiple fibromas
● Focal dermal hypoplasia syndrome
● Cowden's syndrome

Treatment
● Spontaneous regression may occur after months or years.
● Surgical excision only for cosmetic purposes.

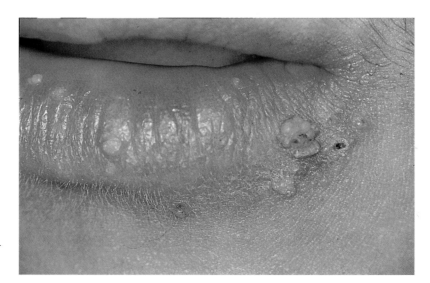

Fig. 13.**16** Verruca vulgaris. Multiple lesion on the vermilion border of the lower lip and skin

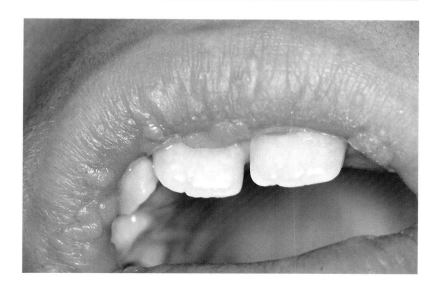

Fig. 13.**17** Focal epithelial hyperplasia. Multiple lesions on the upper lip

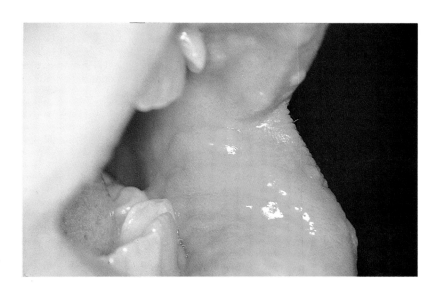

Fig. 13.**18** Focal epithelial hyperplasia. Multiple lesions on the buccal mucosa and commissure

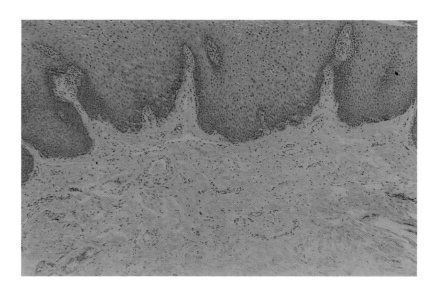

Fig. 13.**19** Focal epithelial hyperplasia. Acanthosis and broad rete ridges

14 Fungal Infections

Candidiasis

Definition

- Candidiasis, or candidosis, is the most common form of oral superficial mycosis.

Etiology

- Caused mainly by *Candida albicans,* and rarely by other *Candida* species.
- Predisposing factors for oral candidiasis include local factors (poor oral hygiene, xerostomia), iron-deficiency anemia, diabetes mellitus, malnutrition, hematologic malignancies, human immunodeficiency virus (HIV) disease, immunodeficiencies, and drugs (antibiotics, corticosteroids, and other immunosuppressives).

Occurrence in children

- Common, particularly in newborns and infants. Older children and adolescents are less commonly affected.

Localization

- Soft palate, buccal mucosa, tongue.

Clinical features

- The clinical variants of candidiasis most frequently seen in children are: pseudomembranous candidiasis, angular cheilitis, erythematous candidiasis and mucocutaneous candidiasis.
- *Pseudomembranous candidiasis,* or thrush, is the most common variant seen in children, and is usually acute. It is clinically characterized by white or whitish-yellow, slightly elevated spots or plaques, which may be removed by scraping, leaving a normal or reddish underlying mucosa (Figs. 14.**1**, 14.**2**). Xerostomia, an unpleasant taste and a mild burning sensation may occur.
- *Angular cheilitis* is relatively rare in children, and is characterized by erythema, fissured crusts with or without erosions, occasionally covered by whitish-yellow spots or plaques (Fig. 14.**3**).
- *Erythematous candidiasis* is an uncommon variant, mainly seen in HIV-infected children and in children who have received broad-spectrum antibiotic treatment. It is clinically characterized by erythematous patches or large areas, which have a predilection for the dorsum of the tongue and palate (Fig. 14.**4**). A burning sensation is common.

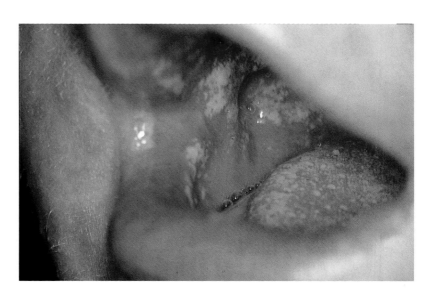

Fig. 14.**1**   Acute pseudomembranous candidiasis of the buccal mucosa and tongue

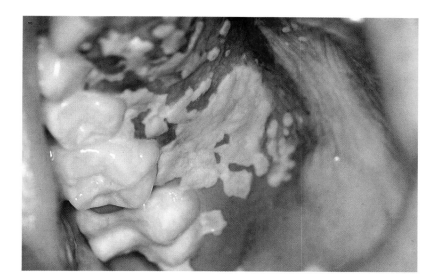

Fig. 14.**2** Acute pseudomembranous candidiasis of the palate

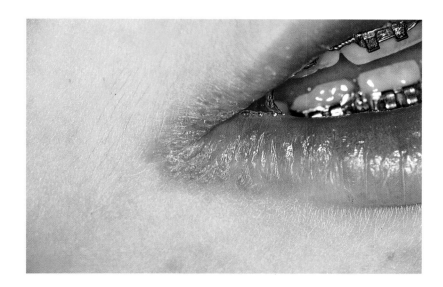

Fig. 14.**3** Angular cheilitis, associated with *Candida albicans* infection

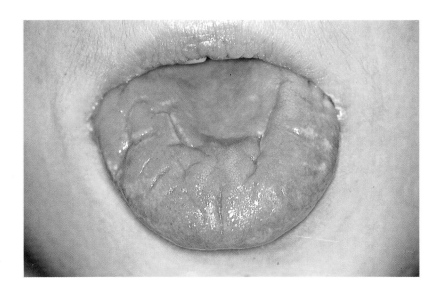

Fig. 14.**4** Erythematous candidiasis of the tongue

● *Mucocutaneous candidiasis* is a rare, chronic, and severe variant, characterized by lesions of the skin, nails and mucosae. The disease appears during childhood, and is associated with distinct immunological dysfunctions, endocrinopathies (hypoparathyroidism, hypothyroidism, hypoadrenalism, diabetes mellitus, and hypogonadism) and severe iron-deficiency anemia. Clinically, the oral lesions appear as thick and rough white plaques, usually on an erythematous base (Figs. 14.**5**–14.**7**). Characteristically, the lesions are multiple and generalized, with a predilection for the buccal mucosa, commissures, tongue, and palate, and may extend to the oropharynx and esophagus (Fig. 14.**8**). Typically, oral lesions begin between four and six years of age or later, whereas endocrinopathy follows after months or years.

● The diagnosis of all variants of candidiasis is based on clinical criteria, but can be supported by laboratory tests.

Laboratory tests

● Direct microscopic examination of oral smear.
● Culture of oral smear.
● Histopathological examination only in chronic mucocutaneous candidiasis.

Differential diagnosis

● Leukoplakia
● Hairy leukoplakia
● Lichen planus
● Plasma-cell stomatitis
● Geographic tongue
● Cinnamon contact stomatitis
● White sponge nevus
● Chemical and thermal burns
● Traumatic lesions

Treatment

● Nystatin, clotrimazole, amphotericin B for topical application.
● Ketoconazole, fluconazole, itraconazole for systemic administration.

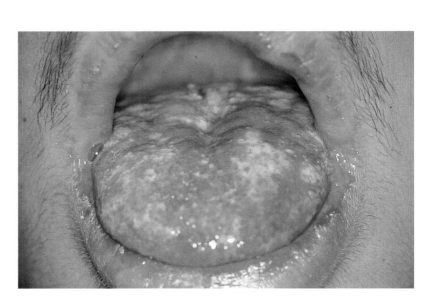

Fig. 14.**5** Chronic mucocutaneous candidiasis of the tongue

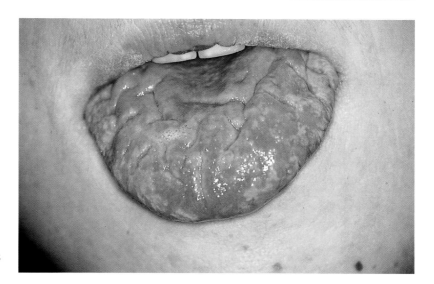

Fig. 14.**6** Chronic mucocutaneous candidiasis of the tongue

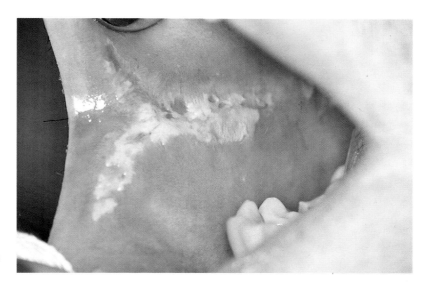

Fig. 14.**7** Chronic mucocutaneous candidiasis of the buccal mucosa

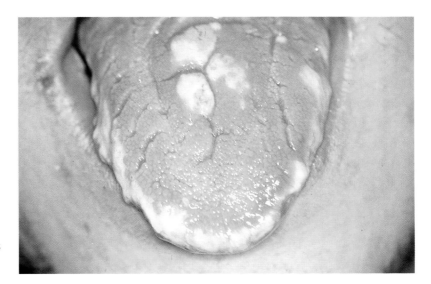

Fig. 14.**8** Chronic mucocutaneous candidiasis of the tongue (same patient as in Fig. 14.**7**)

Part II
Systemic Diseases

15 Genetic Disorders

Hypophosphatasia

Definition
- Hypophosphatasia is an inherited enzyme deficiency disorder, characterized by decreased serum and tissue alkaline phosphatase production and activity.

Etiology
- Genetic. It is inherited as an autosomal recessive trait. An autosomal dominant form has also been reported.

Occurrence
- Rare; one in 100 000 births.

Localization
- Periodontium, skeleton, skull, eyes.

Clinical forms
- Neonatal, infantile, childhood and adult forms.
- The childhood form mainly affects the periodontium, and usually occurs during the second to third year of life.

Clinical features
- Delayed teeth eruption, premature exfoliation of deciduous and permanent teeth without inflammatory response are typical findings.
- Early exfoliation mainly affects the anterior teeth, and may be the only clinical sign of the disease (Fig. 15.**1**).
- Radiographically, alveolar destruction and enlargement of pulp chambers and root canals may be seen (Fig. 15.**2**).
- Craniosynostosis, intracranial hypertension, growth retardation.
- Skeletal abnormalities, ocular defects.
- The diagnosis is based on clinical criteria and laboratory tests.

Laboratory tests
- Low serum alkaline phosphatase concentrations.
- Increased phosphoethanolamine in both blood and urine.
- Low serum levels of Vitamin B_6 and pyridoxal phosphate.
- Radiographic examination of the skull and skeleton.

Differential diagnosis
- Acatalasia
- Osteogenesis imperfecta
- Papillon–Lefèvre syndrome
- Other congenital forms of osteochondrodysplasia

Treatment
- Phosphorus, vitamin D and parathormone have been used, with poor results.
- Prosthetic substitution of missing teeth.

Papillon–Lefèvre Syndrome

Definition
- Papillon–Lefèvre syndrome is a genetic disorder characterized by periodontal and skin manifestations.

Etiology
- Genetic. It is inherited as an autosomal recessive trait.
- Periodontal lesions are caused by multiple leukocyte dysfunctions, and presumably by a specific bacterial infection, such as *Actinobacillus actinomycetemcomitans*.

Occurrence
- Rare. The prevalence is about one to four per million live births.
- Onset usually during the first three years of life.

Localization
- Periodontium, skin.

Clinical features
- Eruption of the deciduous teeth proceeds normally.
- Reddish and hyperplastic gingivae, deep periodontal pockets.
- Advanced periodontitis, with severe bone destruction of the jaws, mobility, migration, and exfoliation of all primary teeth by the fourth to fifth year (Fig. 15.**3**).

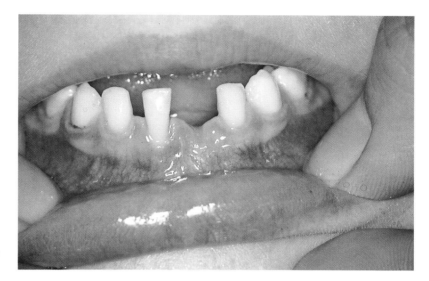

Fig. 15.**1**   Hypophosphatasia, early exfoliation of deciduous tooth

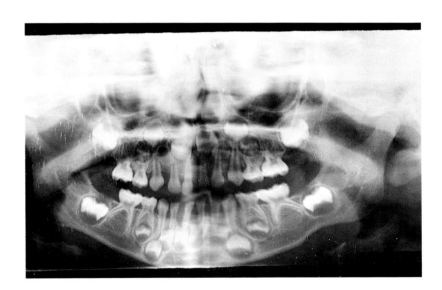

Fig. 15.**2**   Hypophosphatasia, extensive bone loss

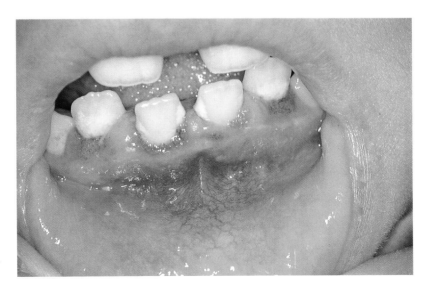

Fig. 15.**3**   Papillon–Lefèvre syndrome. Severe periodontitis and migration of primary teeth

- Normal eruption of permanent teeth and recurrence of periodontal destruction resulting in loss of all permanent teeth by 14 years of age (Fig. 15.**4**).
- The teeth are involved almost in the same order in which they erupt.
- When teeth are absent, the alveolar mucosa is normal.
- Marked halitosis is common.
- Hyperkeratosis of palms and soles, which become diffusely red and scaly (Figs. 15.**5**, 15.**6**).
- Hyperkeratosis and psoriasis-like scaly redness in other skin areas (elbows, knees, dorsal fingers and feet, external malleoli).
- Worsening of the skin lesions during winter.
- Diagnosis is based on clinical criteria.

Laboratory features

- Panoramic radiography shows remarkable alveolar bone destruction (Fig. 15.**7**).
- Histopathological examination is not specific.

Differential diagnosis

- Acatalasia
- Hypophosphatasia
- Juvenile periodontitis
- Congenital neutropenia
- Cyclic neutropenia
- Glycogen storage disease type Ib
- Langerhans cell histiocytosis
- Focal palmoplantar and oral mucosa hyperkeratosis syndrome
- Psoriasis
- Hypohidrotic ectodermal dysplasia

Treatment

- Intensive oral hygiene, periodontal treatment. However, the prognosis is poor, and complete prostheses are necessary.
- Symptomatic therapy for the cutaneous lesions and retinoid acid products.

Focal Palmoplantar and Oral Mucosa Hyperkeratosis Syndrome

Definition

- Focal palmoplantar and oral mucosa hyperkeratosis syndrome, or hyperkeratosis palmoplantaris and attached gingival hyperkeratosis, is an unusual genetic disorder characterized by dermal and oral mucosa hyperkeratosis.

Etiology

- Genetic. It is inherited as an autosomal dominant trait.

Occurrence

- Very rare. The lesions appear in early childhood, and increase in severity with age.

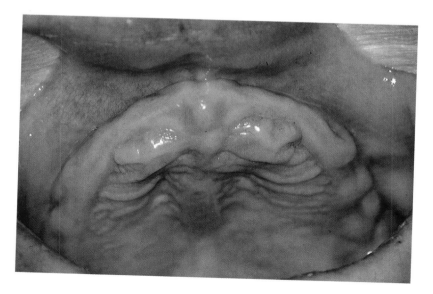

Fig. 15.**4** Papillon–Lefèvre syndrome. Premature loss of permanent teeth in an 18-year-old boy

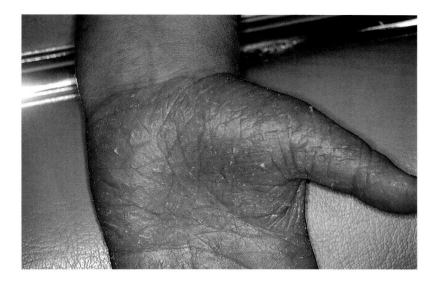

Fig. 15.**5** Papillon–Lefèvre syndrome. Red and scaly palm

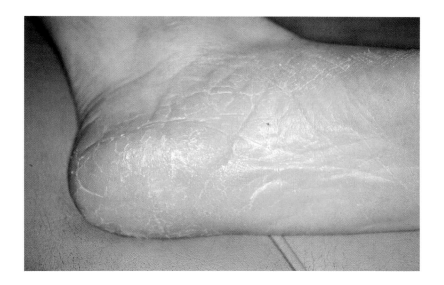

Fig. 15.**6** Papillon–Lefèvre syndrome. Hyperkeratosis of the sole

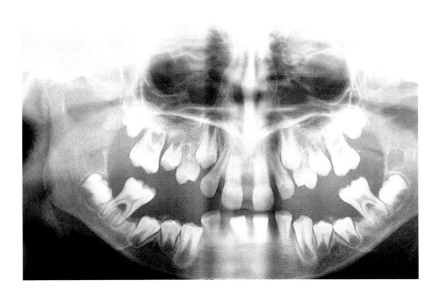

Fig. 15.**7** Papillon–Lefèvre syndrome. Severe alveolar bone destruction

Localization
- Oral mucosa (mainly attached gingiva and other areas subject to mechanical pressure or friction, such as the hard palate, the retromolar pad mucosa, alveolar mucosa, lateral border or dorsum of the tongue, and buccal mucosa along the occlusal line).
- Skin, mainly over the weight-bearing and pressure-related areas, such as the soles (toe pads, heels, metatarsal heads) and palms.
- Nails.

Clinical features
- The oral mucosa hyperkeratosis clinically manifests as a non-removable, painless white plaque (Fig. 15.**8**).
- In the skin, focal hyperkeratotic lesions of various degrees, which may be painful (Fig. 15.**9**).
- The severity of the hyperkeratotic lesions increases with age and varies among patients, even in the same family.
- Hyperhidrosis, follicular keratosis of the face, hyperkeratosis, and thickening of the nails may rarely occur (Fig. 15.**10**).
- Diagnosis is based on clinical criteria.

Laboratory tests
- Not helpful.

Differential diagnosis
- Papillon–Lefèvre syndrome
- Congenital pachyonychia
- Congenital dyskeratosis
- White sponge nevus

Treatment
- Not available. Partial improvement using aromatic retinoids.

Hypohidrotic Ectodermal Dysplasia

Definition
- Hypohidrotic ectodermal dysplasia is a genetic disorder characterized by defects in tissues derived from the ectoderm.

Etiology
- Genetic. It is inherited as an X-linked recessive trait, and therefore primarily affects males.

Occurrence
- Rare (approximately one in 100 000 births).

Localization
- Oral cavity, skin and skin appendages, skull, eyes, pharynx and larynx.

Clinical features
- The disorder becomes apparent usually during the first year of life, with fever of unknown origin, particularly during summer, and retarded eruption or absence of the deciduous teeth.
- Hypodontia and rarely anodontia of deciduous and permanent teeth (Fig. 15.**11**).
- Conical shape of the teeth appears frequently.
- Defective alveolar process is common, but jaw development is normal.
- Xerostomia may rarely occur as a result of salivary gland hypoplasia.

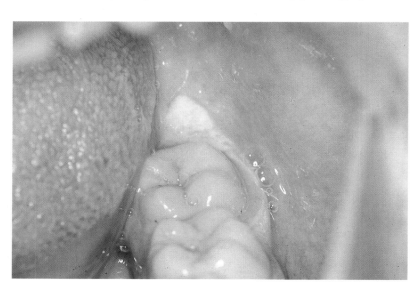

Fig. 15.**8** Focal palmoplantar and oral mucosa hyperkeratosis syndrome. Hyperkeratotic white plaque on the retromolar pad mucosa

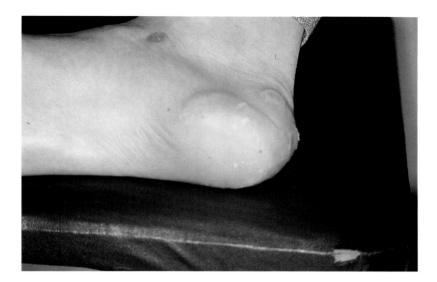

Fig. 15.**9**   Focal palmoplantar and oral mucosa hyperkeratosis syndrome. Focal hyperkeratosis of the sole

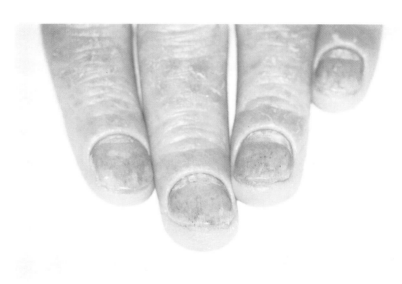

Fig. 15.**10**   Focal palmoplantar and oral mucosa hyperkeratosis syndrome. Hyperkeratosis and thickening of the nails

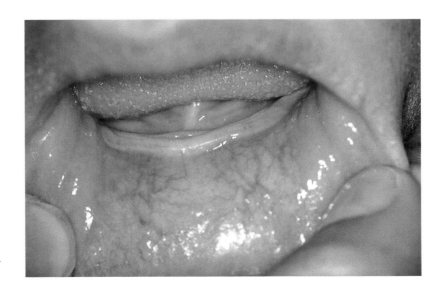

Fig. 15.**11**   Hypohidrotic ectodermal dysplasia. Anodontia

- Decreased sweating and, rarely, complete anhidrosis due to severely reduced number of sweat glands.
- The skin is dry, thin, and sparse. The scalp hair is often blond, short and fine. The nails are usually normal.
- Characteristic facies (frontal bossing, saddle nose, large lips and ears) (Fig. 15.**12**).
- Reduction of nasopharyngeal secretions. The pharyngeal and laryngeal mucosae may be atrophic, resulting in an abnormal voice.
- Eye lesions (reduction of lacrimal secretions, corneal defects, absence of eyebrows).
- Respiratory infections may rarely occur during infancy.

Laboratory tests
- Dental radiographs.
- Demonstration of reduced sweating using several tests.

Differential diagnosis
- Idiopathic hypodontia
- Incontinentia pigmenti
- Cleidocranial dysplasia
- Ellis–van Creveld syndrome
- Focal dermal hypoplasia syndrome
- Papillon–Lefèvre syndrome

Treatment
- There is no specific treatment. Full or partial dentures should be constructed as early as possible.

Focal Dermal Hypoplasia Syndrome

Definition
- Focal dermal hypoplasia syndrome, or Goltz–Gorlin syndrome, is a genetic disorder characterized by multisystemic manifestations.

Etiology
- Genetic. It has an X-linked dominant mode of inheritance. It is fatal in male hemizygotes.
- Over 95% of the cases are sporadic, and the condition rarely occurs in males.

Occurrence
- Rare.

Localization
- Oral cavity (tongue, buccal mucosa, palate, gingiva, lips), skin, facies, eyes, musculoskeletal system, central nervous system (CNS).

Clinical features
- Oral lesions include multiple papillomas, hypodontia or oligodontia, small or large teeth, enamel dysplasia, and malocclusion (Figs. 15.**13**, 15.**14**). Orofacial clefts may rarely occur.
- Skin lesions include thin skin with linear irregular pigmentation, atrophy, and telangiectasia present at birth (Fig. 15.**15**). Localized deposits of sub-

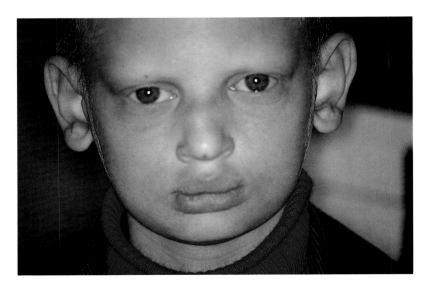

Fig. 15.**12** Hypohidrotic ectodermal dysplasia. Characteristic facies

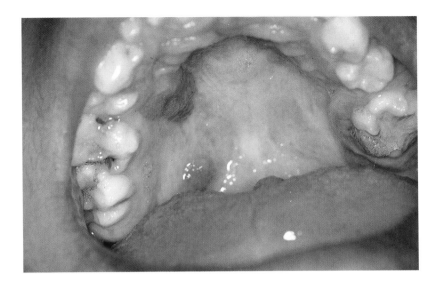

Fig. 15.**13**   Focal dermal hypoplasia syndrome. Multiple papillomas on the palate

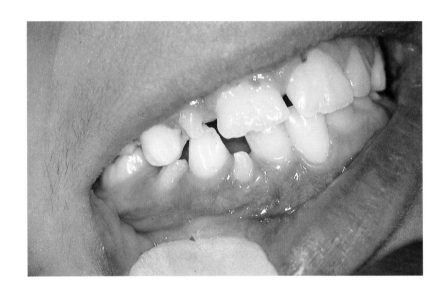

Fig. 15.**14**   Focal dermal hypoplasia syndrome. Dental defects (small and large teeth, malocclusion)

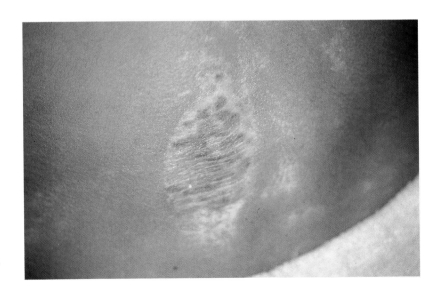

Fig. 15.**15**   Focal dermal hypoplasia syndrome. Atrophic and hyperpigmented plaque on the skin

cutaneous fat that present as soft reddish-yellow nodules are a common finding. Dystrophic nails and sparse hair may also be observed (Fig. 15.**16**).

- Musculoskeletal anomalies such as syndactyly, brachydactyly, and oligodactyly are common. Clinodactyly and polydactyly are less common.
- Asymmetry of the extremities, scoliosis, midclavicular aplasia, microcephaly are seen.
- Eye anomalies (coloboma of iris, strabismus, optic atrophy, microphthalmia), mental handicap, and genitourinary anomalies may occur.
- The diagnosis is mainly made on the basis of clinical criteria.

Laboratory tests
- Biopsy and histopathological examination of oral and skin lesions.

Differential diagnosis
- Incontinentia pigmenti
- Rothmund–Thomson syndrome
- Focal epithelial hyperplasia
- Multiple papillomas and condylomata acuminata for the oral lesions

Treatment
- Not available. Surgical excision of oral papillomas.

White Sponge Nevus

Definition
- White sponge nevus, or Cannon's disease, is a relatively uncommon genetic disorder.

Etiology
- Genetic. It is inherited as an autosomal dominant trait.

Occurrence
- Relatively rare.

Localization
- Most frequently, the buccal mucosa, tongue, floor of the mouth.
- Less commonly, other mucosae, such as the vaginal, rectal, nasal, and esophageal mucosae may be affected.

Clinical features
- Clinically, the lesions appear as white, thickened, with multiple furrows, diffuse plaques with a spongy texture (Figs. 15.**17**, 15.**18**).
- The lesions are benign, asymptomatic, and usually symmetrical.
- Lesions may appear at birth, or more commonly during childhood. The disease is progressive until early adulthood, remaining stable thereafter.
- The diagnosis is made mainly on the basis of the history and the clinical features.

Histopathology
- Histopathological examination shows parakeratosis and marked acanthosis.
- On the upper part of the spinous layer, the cells are vacuolated with small pyknotic nuclei, without evidence of atypia.

Differential diagnosis
- Leukoedema
- Hereditary benign intraepithelial dyskeratosis
- Leukoplakia

Treatment
- Not available.

Neurofibromatosis

Definition
- Neurofibromatosis is a group of conditions including at least nine hereditary forms. The most common form is the classic neurofibromatosis, type I, or von Recklinghausen's disease, which accounts for about 90% of cases.

Etiology
- Genetic. Genetic disorder inherited as an autosomal dominant trait. However, new mutations are common and represent 50% of all cases.

Occurrence
- Relatively common. The classic form occurs in approximately one in every 3000 births.

Localization
- Oral mucosa, skin, central nervous system, eyes, skeletal system, endocrine systems.

Clinical features
- Oral lesions occur in about of 60–70% of cases, and are characterized by multiple or isolated nodular neurofibromas, which vary in size (Fig. 15.**19**). Tumors usually involve the tongue, although other oral mucosa areas may

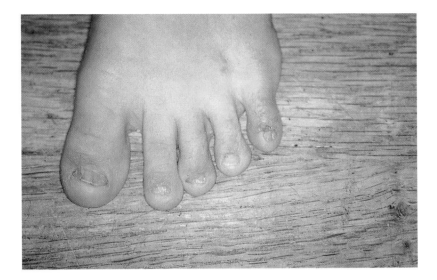

Fig. 15.**16** Focal dermal hypoplasia syndrome. Nail dystrophy

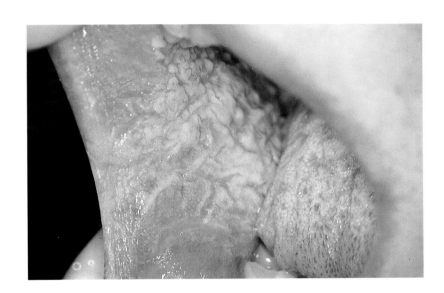

Fig. 15.**17** White sponge nevus.
White and thickened plaques on
the buccal mucosa

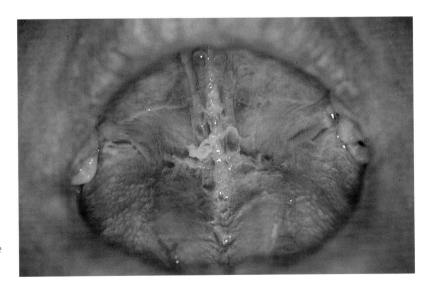

Fig. 15.**18** White sponge nevus.
White and thickened lesions on the
ventral surface of the tongue and
floor of the mouth

be affected. Enlargement of fungiform papillae is common, and macroglossia is less common. Lesions on the maxilla and the mandible are relatively uncommon.

- Skin lesions are the cardinal features of the disease, and are characterized by multiple neurofibromas (varying from a few to hundreds or thousands of tumors), and café-au-lait spots (Fig. 15.**20**). The presence of four or more café-au-lait skin spots larger than 1.5 cm in diameter has been considered as a strong diagnostic criterion for neurofibromatosis. Axillary freckling is an additional important diagnostic sign, occurring in about 50% of cases.
- Other abnormalities, including CNS tumors, mental deficiency, seizures, scoliosis, kyphosis, macrocephaly, and eye and endocrine disorders may be less commonly seen.
- Malignant transformation of the neurofibromas into neurofibrosarcomas may occur in 3–12% of cases.

Laboratory tests
- Histopathological examination.
- Computed tomography (CT).
- Panoramic radiography.

Differential diagnosis
- Multiple endocrine neoplasia type III syndrome
- Klippel–Trenaunay–Weber syndrome
- LEOPARD syndrome

Treatment
- There is no specific therapy, and treatment is supportive.
- Surgical excision of the tumors.

Tuberous Sclerosis

Definition
- Tuberous sclerosis, or Bourneville–Pringle syndrome, is a rare disorder mainly characterized by angiofibromas, mental retardation, and seizures.

Etiology
- Genetic. It is transmitted as an autosomal dominant trait, with variable expressivity.

Occurrence
- Rare. The prevalence varies from one in 100 000 to one in 170 000 in the general population.
- The lesions usually present between three to six years of age.

Localization
- Oral cavity, skin, central nervous system, eyes, skeletal system.

Clinical features
- Oral lesions present as multiple fibrous nodules, a few millimeters to 1 cm in diameter, with whitish or normal color. Approximately 11% of the patients have such lesions, which are predominantly seen on the anterior gingiva (Fig. 15.**21**), although other parts of the oral mucosa may be involved. Enamel pits are common. A high-arched palate, cleft lip and palate and macroglossia, with loss of the filiform papillae of the tongue may rarely be seen (Fig. 15.**22**).

Fig. 15.**19** Neurofibromatosis. Neurofibroma on the tongue

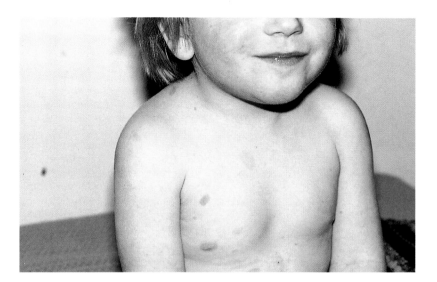

Fig. 15.**20**   Neurofibromatosis.
Café-au-lait spots on the skin

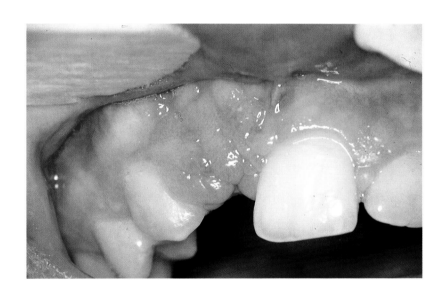

Fig. 15.**21**   Tuberous sclerosis.
Multiple nodules on the gingiva
and alveolar mucosa

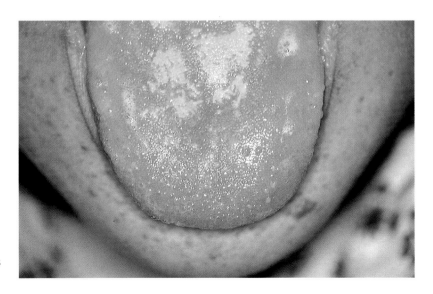

Fig. 15.**22**   Tuberous sclerosis. Loss
of filiform papillae of the tongue

- The most characteristic and common skin lesions are facial angiofibromas, which present as numerous small nodules, red to pink in color, occurring primarily in the nasolabial fold and cheeks (Fig. 15.**23**). Hypomelanotic areas (ash-leaf muscles) and raised connective-tissue plaques (Shagreen patches) are early and common signs. Periungual or subungual fibromas and nail dystrophy may also occur (Fig. 15.**24**).
- Central nervous system manifestations occur approximately in 90% of the patients and present as seizures, mental retardation, and hamartomatous tumors.
- Cardiac rhabdomyoma, multiple retinal hamartomas, renal angiomyolipomas, polycystic kidneys, and cystic lesions on the lungs may also occur.
- The diagnosis of the disease is based on the presence of one of the primary diagnostic criteria (facial angiofibromas, ungual fibromas, CNS hamartomas), or on the presence of two secondary criteria (infantile seizures, ash-leaf muscles, Shagreen patches, cardiac rhabdomyomas, renal angiomyolipomas or cysts, retinal hamartoma).

Laboratory tests

- Histopathological examination of the skin and the oral angiofibromas.
- Electroencephalography, brain CT scan.

Differential diagnosis

- Neurofibromatosis
- Cowden's syndrome
- Focal dermal hypoplasia syndrome
- Multiple fibromas
- Lipoid proteinosis

Treatment

- Symptomatic when required.

Gardner's Syndrome

Definition

- Gardner's syndrome is a disorder classified among the group of familial colorectal polyposis syndromes.

Etiology

- Genetic. It is transmitted as an autosomal dominant trait.

Occurrence

- Rare.

Localization

- Gastrointestinal tract, bone, skin, oral cavity.

Clinical features

- The oral manifestations include multiple osteomas of the jaws and, occasionally, exostoses, supernumerary and impacted teeth, multiple odontomas, and fibrous soft-tissue tumors (Fig. 15.**25**).
- Skin lesions consist of epidermoid cysts, fibromas and increased pigmentation (Fig. 15.**26**).

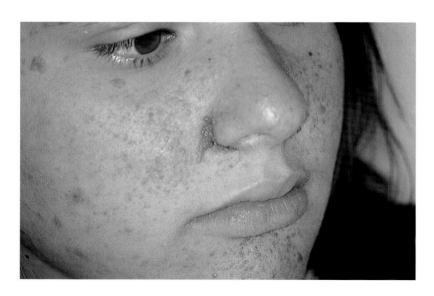

Fig. 15.**23** Tuberous sclerosis. Typical facial angiofibromas

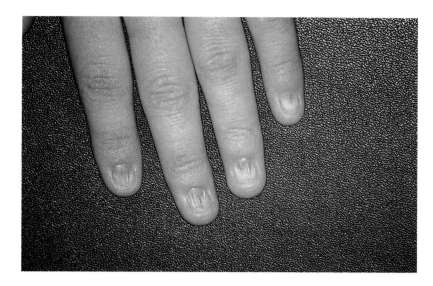

Fig. 15.**24**   Tuberous sclerosis. Nail dystrophy

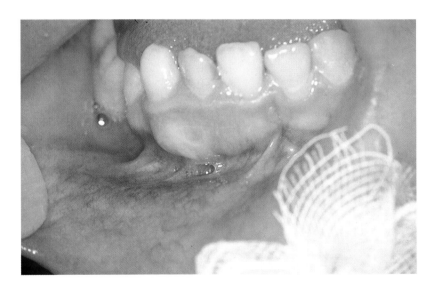

Fig. 15.**25**   Gardner's syndrome. Multiple exostoses of the mandible

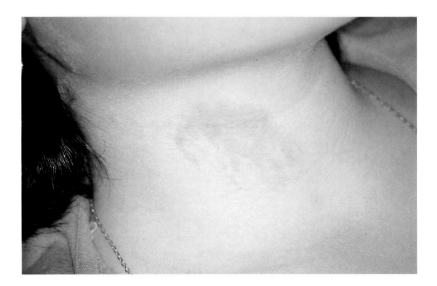

Fig. 15.**26**   Gardner's syndrome. Increased skin pigmentation

- Bone lesions include multiple osteomas, mainly in the calvaria, facial bones, and occasionally exostoses.
- Gastrointestinal manifestations are multiple polyps, mainly in the colon and rectum, with a marked tendency to malignant transformation.
- Ocular lesions and various neoplasias of the central nervous system may rarely occur.

Laboratory features
- Radiographic investigation of the jaws, skull and intestinal tract (Fig. 15.**27**).
- Histopathological examination of the tumors.

Differential diagnosis
- Peutz–Jeghers syndrome
- Cowden's syndrome
- Other multiple tumor intestinal syndromes

Treatment
- Symptomatic. Surgical removal of jaw osteomas and epidermoid cysts is recommended.

Incontinentia Pigmenti

Definition
- Incontinentia pigmenti, or Bloch–Sulzberger syndrome, is an inherited multisystemic disorder.

Etiology
- Genetic. It is transmitted with an X-linked dominant mode of inheritance.

Occurrence
- Rare. The disease begins at birth, or during the first month of life.

Localization
- Skin, teeth, eyes, central nervous system.

Clinical features
- Teeth anomalies, occur in about 90% of the cases and are characterized by oligodontia, delayed tooth eruption, enamel disorders, and peg-shaped or conical teeth (Fig. 15.**28**). Both the deciduous and permanent teeth are affected.
- Skin lesions are the main clinical features of the disease, and are classified intro three stages. The *first stage* is characterized by vesicular lesions of the extremities and the trunk in a linear pattern, and resolves in about two to four months. The *second stage* is characterized by hyperkeratotic verrucous lesions on the limbs, digits and joints; these lesions usually begin during the first month of age, and resolve spontaneously by six months of age. The *third stage* is characterized by macular brownish hyperpigmentation in a reticular pattern, or in whorls or patches (Fig. 15.**29**). This stage usually begins between the third and sixth months of life. Atrophy of the skin, depigmentation, alopecia and nail dystrophy may also be rarely seen.
- Eye lesions occur in about 30% of cases, and include strabismus, cataracts, optic atrophy, and retinal abnormalities.
- CNS lesions occur in about 30–40% of cases, and include mental retardation, seizures, microcephaly, eye muscle paralysis, and other motor disorders.

Laboratory tests
- Histopathological examination of skin lesions.

Differential diagnosis
- Epidermolysis bullosa
- Hypomelanosis of Ito
- Focal dermal hypoplasia syndrome
- Hypohidrotic ectodermal dysplasia
- Ellis–van Creveld syndrome
- Congenital syphilis

Treatment
- Symptomatic.

Hypomelanosis of Ito

Definition
- Hypomelanosis of Ito, or incontinentia pigmenti achromians, is a heterogeneous and clinically variable disorder, with cutaneous involvement resembling a negative image of that of incontinentia pigmenti.

Etiology
- Genetic. The disease is probably sporadic; mosaicism of different types of aneuploidy is frequently present, and most commonly involves chromosome X.

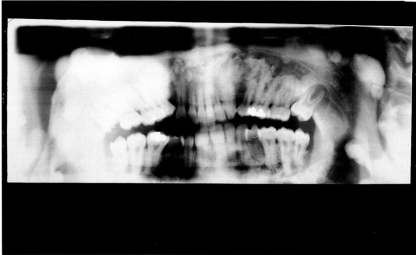

Fig. 15.**27**   Gardner's syndrome. Multiple osteomas of the mandible

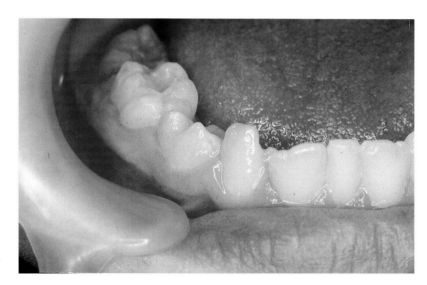

Fig. 15.**28**   Incontinentia pigmenti. Peg-shaped teeth

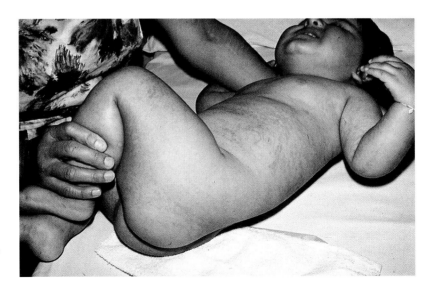

Fig. 15.**29**   Incontinentia pigmenti. Linear and whorl hyperpigmentation on the skin

Occurrence	• Rare.
Localization	• Skin, teeth, central nervous system, eyes, skeleton.
Clinical features	• Tooth anomalies are relatively uncommon, and include conical anterior teeth with pitted, yellow-brown crowns (Fig. 15.**30**). Talon cusps, multiple caries of the anterior teeth, and irregularly formed dentin may also occur.
• Skin lesions are common, and are characterized by unilateral or bilateral macular hypopigmented whorls, streaks, and patches, typically distributed along Blaschko lines, which are described as the "negative pattern" of the hyperpigmented lesions of incontinentia pigmenti (Fig. 15.**31**). Nail and hair anomalies may also be seen.
• Seizures, delay in psychomotor development, mental retardation, hypotonia, limb asymmetry, scoliosis, short stature, ocular abnormalities, and precocious puberty may occur (Fig. 15.**32**).
Laboratory tests	• Histopathological examination of the skin lesions
• Radiographs of the skeleton
• CT scan
• Electroencephalogram
Differential diagnosis	• Incontinentia pigmenti
• McCune–Albright syndrome
• Naegeli syndrome
Treatment	• Symptomatic.

Ehlers–Danlos Syndrome

Definition	• Ehlers–Danlos syndrome includes a heterogeneous group of inherited defects of collagen biosynthesis.
Etiology	• Genetic. The syndrome includes several genetic disorders inherited as autosomal dominant, autosomal recessive, or X-linked recessive traits.
• On the basis of clinical, genetic, and biochemical criteria, at least 11 types of the syndrome are recognized. Types I and II are the most common, and both are inherited as autosomal dominant traits.
Occurrence	• Rare.
Localization	• Oral cavity, skin, joints.
Clinical features	• Oral manifestations include thin and fragile oral mucosa. Easy bruising and bleeding on minor trauma are a common finding. Periodontal disease, gingival bleeding, and delayed wound healing are relatively common. Approximately 50% of the patients have the ability to touch their nose with the tip of the tongue, compared with 10% of normal people (Fig. 15.**33**).

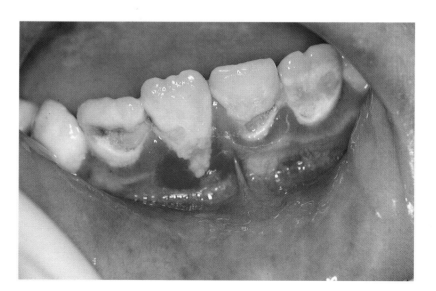

Fig. 15.**30** Hypomelanosis of Ito. Multiple caries of the anterior teeth, with pitted, yellow-brown crowns

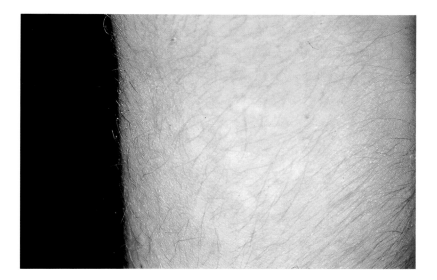

Fig. 15.**31**   Hypomelanosis of Ito. Hypopigmented whorls and small patches on the skin

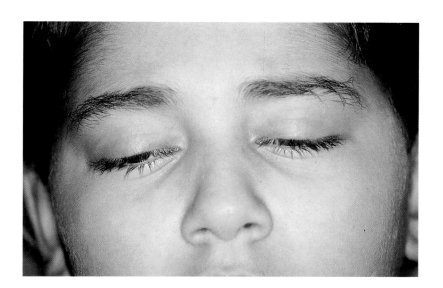

Fig. 15.**32**   Hypomelanosis of Ito. Photophobia and blepharoptosis

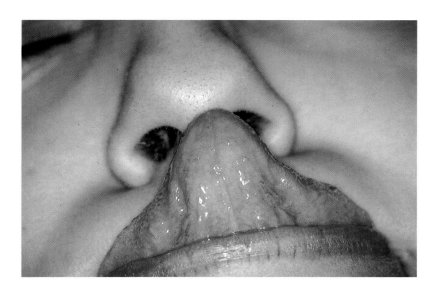

Fig. 15.**33**   Ehlers–Danlos syndrome. Ability to touch the tip of the nose with the tongue tip

Dental anomalies such as enamel, dentine, and cementum defects, as well as an increased tendency to develop multiple pulp stones and temporomandibular joint hypermobility, may occur (Fig. 15.**34**).
- Skin manifestations include hyperextensibility and skin fragility, frequent bruising, abnormal healing (papyraceous scarring), especially over the elbows, knees, chin, and pseudotumors (Fig. 15.**35**).
- Joint hypermobility, kyphoscoliosis, and cardiovascular and ocular abnormalities may occur (Fig. 15.**36**).

Laboratory tests
- There are no specific tests.

Differential diagnosis
- Cutis laxa
- Marfan's syndrome and Marfanoid hypermobility syndrome

Treatment
- Symptomatic.

Orofaciodigital Syndrome Type I

Definition
- Orofaciodigital syndrome type I is the most common genetic disorder in the group of orofaciodigital syndromes.

Etiology
- Genetic. The condition is inherited as an X-linked dominant trait, limited to females and fatal in males.

Occurrence
- Rare. The incidence of the syndrome is probably about one in 50 000 live births.

Localization
- Oral cavity, digits, facies, skin.

Clinical features
- Oral manifestations are common, and include multiple, large hyperplastic fibrous bands traversing the mucobuccal fold, hypertrophy and shortening of the frenulum of the lips and tongue, and multilobed or bifid tongue with multiple hamartomas (Figs. 15.**37, 15.38**). Lips and palate clefts, supernumerary teeth, malposition of the maxillary canine teeth, missing mandibular lateral incisors, and hypoplastic mandible with a short ramus are common findings.
- Digital malformations include polydactyly, brachydactyly, clinodactyly, and syndactyly (Figs. 15.**39, 15.40**).
- The facial anomalies include frontal bossing, euryopia, ocular hypertelorism, short upper lip, broad nasal root, and asymmetry of the nostrils (Fig. 15.**41**).
- Skin manifestations include xeroderma, alopecia, milia, sparse hair, and dermatoglyphic abnormalities.

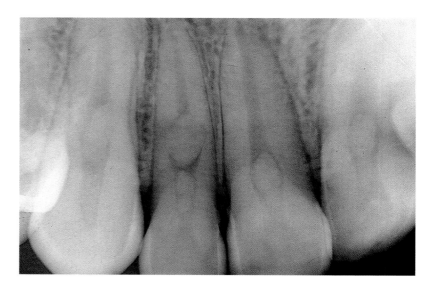

Fig. 15.**34** Ehlers–Danlos syndrome. Multiple pulp stones

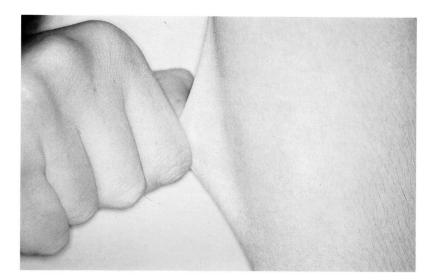

Fig. 15.**35**   Ehlers–Danlos syndrome. Hyperelastic skin

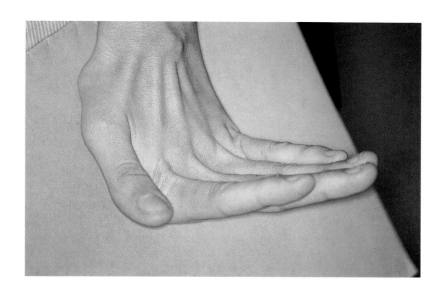

Fig. 15.**36**   Ehlers–Danlos syndrome. Joint hypermobility

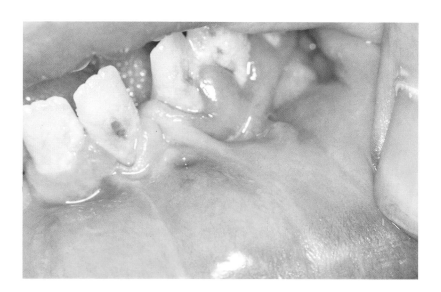

Fig. 15.**37**   Orofaciodigital syndrome, type I. Hyperplastic fibrous bands traversing the mucolabial fold

- Mild mental retardation and bilateral polycystic kidneys are less common findings.

Laboratory tests
- No specific tests.

Differential diagnosis
- Orofaciodigital syndrome type II (Mohr's syndrome)
- Chondroectodermal dysplasia
- Oculodentodigital syndrome

Treatment
- Symptomatic.

Sturge–Weber Angiomatosis

Definition
- Sturge–Weber angiomatosis, or encephalotrigeminal angiomatosis, is a sporadic congenital hamartomatous vascular proliferation, mainly involving areas along the trigeminal nerve distribution.

Etiology
- Not clear, but it is thought to be caused by the persistence of a vascular plexus around the cephalic portion of the neural tube and under the ectoderm, destined to become facial skin.

Occurrence
- Rare. The disorder is usually apparent at birth.

Localization
- Facial skin, oral mucosa, central nervous system, eyes.

Clinical features
- The principal clinical features are hemangiomas of the leptomeninges, the skin, face, and oral mucosa, calcifications of the brain, ocular disorders, epilepsy and mild mental retardation.
- Facial hemangioma is the most characteristic and constant finding, and is evident at birth. Clinically, it appears bright red or purple in color, and it is confined roughly to the area supplied by the trigeminal nerve, usually unilateral (Fig. 15.**42**).
- Oral hemangioma is also unilateral, and may involve the upper gingiva and alveolar ridges, the buccal mucosa, the tongue and the lips. The lesions have a bright red or purple color and are usually flat, but may also have a raised irregular surface that causes tissue enlargement (Fig. 15.**43**). Delayed teeth eruption, early eruption, and dental ectopia are common findings.

Laboratory tests
- Histopathological examination shows multiple dilated blood vessels with excessive dilatation.

Differential diagnosis
- Isolated disseminated hemangiomas
- Klippel–Trenaunay–Weber syndrome

Treatment
- Treatment depends on the severity and location of the lesions.
- Laser therapy usually improves the lesions.

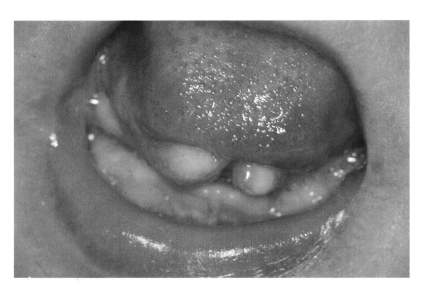

Fig. 15.**38** Orofaciodigital syndrome, type I. Two sublingual hamartomas

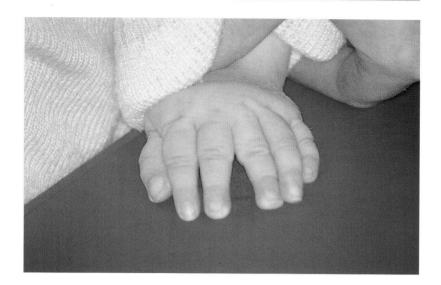

Fig. 15.**39** Orofaciodigital syndrome, type I. Hexadactyly and clinodactyly

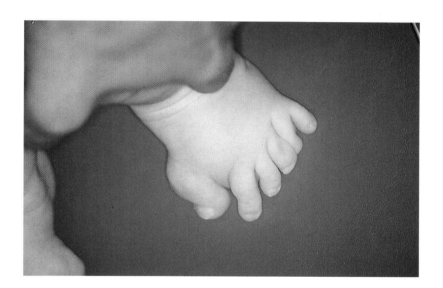

Fig. 15.**40** Orofaciodigital syndrome, type I. Hexadactyly and clinodactyly

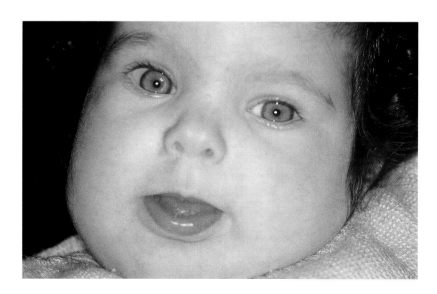

Fig. 15.**41** Orofaciodigital syndrome, type I. Frontal bossing and ocular hypertelorism

Chondroectodermal Dysplasia

Definition
- Chondroectodermal dysplasia, or Ellis–van Creveld syndrome, is a genetic disorder of the osteochondrodysplasia group of defects.

Etiology
- It is inherited as an autosomal recessive trait.

Occurrence
- Rare. The prevalence has been estimated at seven per million births.

Localization
- The skeleton, oral cavity, hair and nails, heart, eyes, central nervous system.

Clinical features
- The most constant oral finding is fusion of the middle portion of the upper or the lower lip to the gingiva, resulting in the disappearance of the mucolabial fold (Fig. 15.**44**). Congenitally missing teeth, small teeth with conical crowns, and natal teeth are also present.
- Bilateral polydactyly, and plump, shortened extremities are common.
- Skeletal anomalies, mainly chondrodysplasia of the long bones.
- The hair is thin and sparse, and the fingernails are dystrophic.
- Congenital heart defects, genital anomalies are frequent.

Laboratory tests
- Radiographic examination

Differential diagnosis
- Orofaciodigital syndrome
- Other chondrodysplasia syndromes
- Acrofacial dysostosis of Weyers

Treatment
- Symptomatic.

Congenital Osteopetrosis

Definition
- Congenital osteopetrosis, or severe infantile osteopetrosis, is a rare hereditary disorder characterized by failure of the primary spongiosa resorption by osteoclasts, resulting in increased osseous density in which cortical and cancellous bone are indistinguishable. Osteopetrosis has been classified into two forms, *congenital* and *adult*.

Etiology
- Genetic. The congenital form is inherited as an autosomal recessive trait.
- The adult form is inherited as an autosomal dominant trait.

Occurrence
- Rare. It may be recognized in utero, at birth, or within the first few months of life.

Localization
- Nearly all bones, including the jaws.

Clinical features
- Increased density of the bones. The involved bones are expanded, splayed, and dense. Characteristically, the skull is thickened and dense, mainly the cranial base and the calvaria (Fig. 15.**45**). A broad face, snub nose, frontal bossing, and hypertelorism may be seen.

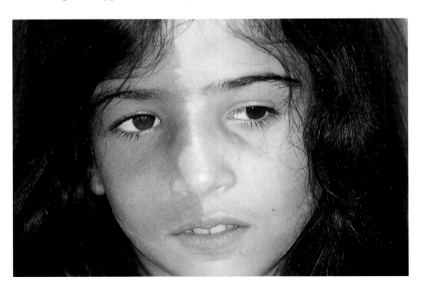

Fig. 15.**42** Sturge–Weber angiomatosis. Unilateral facial hemangioma

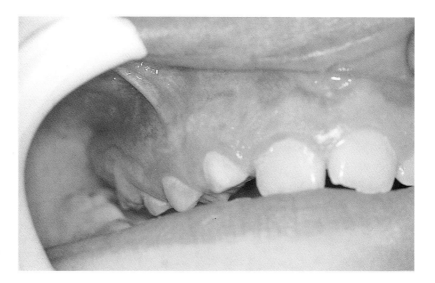

Fig. 15.**43**   Sturge–Weber angiomatosis. Unilateral hemangioma of the gingiva and alveolar mucosa

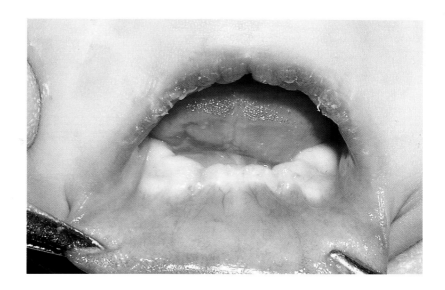

Fig. 15.**44**   Chondroectodermal dysplasia. Fusion of the middle portion of the lower lip to the gingiva and disappearance of the mucolabial fold

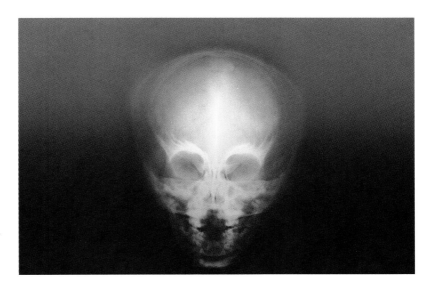

Fig. 15.**45**   Congenital osteopetrosis. The skull is thickened and dense, mainly the cranial base and the calvaria

- Defective vision and nystagmus are common.
- Delayed tooth eruption, embedded teeth, expanded jaws, and ankylosis of the cementum to the bone may occur. Jaw osteomyelitis, leading to intraoral and extraoral fistulas, is a common complication (Fig. 15.**46**).
- Anemia, hepatomegaly, splenomegaly, blindness, deafness, facial paralysis, and pathological bone fractures are common signs and complications.

Laboratory tests
- Radiographic examination
- Histopathological examination

Differential diagnosis
- Other forms of osteopetrosis

Treatment
- Symptomatic or supportive.

Down's Syndrome

Definition
- Down's syndrome, or trisomy 21, is a chromosomal disorder with variable clinical manifestations. Most patients show full trisomy 21, but there are a few cases of trisomy 21 mosaic, normal, and translocation.

Occurrence
- Common. The overall prevalence rate is approximately one per 800 live births. The risk increases with increasing maternal age, reaching one in 50 for mothers over 45 years of age.

Localization
- Great distribution in different tissues and organs.

Clinical features
- The most frequent oral lesions are macroglossia, fissured and geographic tongue, high-arched palate, cleft palate, periodontal disease, delayed tooth eruption, and hypoplastic teeth (Fig. 15.**47**).
- Mental retardation, hypotonia, mongoloid slanting of the eyes, short ears, and flat face with a broad nose bridge are common findings (Fig. 15.**48**).
- Follicular hyperkeratosis, persistent facial flushing, alopecia areata, and dry skin are common.
- Polydactyly, syndactyly, clinodactyly, hyperextensibility of joints, other skeletal abnormalities, small penis and scrotum, cryptorchidism, congenital heart anomalies, dermatoglyphic abnormalities, and hormonal disturbances are common clinical features.
- There is an increased risk for leukemia, and respiratory diseases are common complications.

Laboratory tests
- Chromosomal analysis is necessary. Prenatal diagnosis has become widely available.

Differential diagnosis
- Hypothyroidism

Treatment
- Supportive.

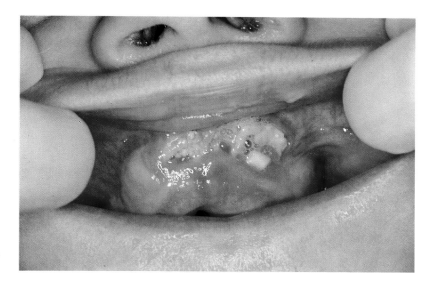

Fig. 15.**46**   Congenital osteopetrosis. Osteomyelitis of the maxilla

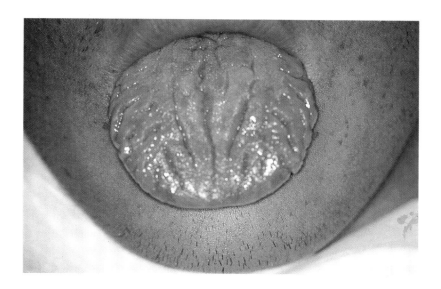

Fig. 15.**47**   Down's syndrome, macroglossia and fissured tongue

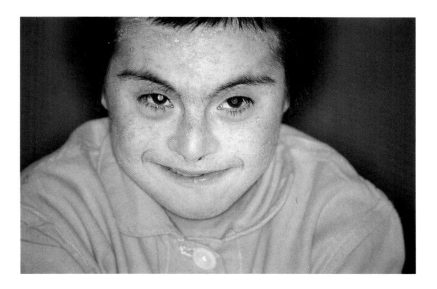

Fig. 15.**48**   Down's syndrome, characteristic facies

16 Skin Diseases

Pemphigus Vulgaris

Definition

- Pemphigus is a chronic autoimmune bullous disease involving the mucous membranes and the skin.

Etiology

- The exact etiology remains unknown.

Classification

- Pemphigus is classified into four main forms: *vulgaris, vegetans, foliaceus,* and *erythematosus.*
- Drug-induced pemphigus and paraneoplastic pemphigus are also two unique varieties of the pemphigus group.
- Pemphigus vulgaris is the most common form of pemphigus, representing about 95% of cases both in children and adults.

Occurrence in children

- Very rare (less than approximately 0.5% of cases).
- The mean age of onset is usually in the fifth decade.

Localization

- Soft palate, uvula, buccal mucosa, gingiva, floor of the mouth, lips.
- Skin involvement is common, and less common sites are the conjunctival, nasal and genital mucosae.

Clinical features

- In children, the oral lesions precede the onset of skin lesions by weeks or months in 90% of cases.
- Bullae that rapidly rupture, leaving painful, persistent erosions without a tendency for healing (Figs. 16.**1,** 16.**2**).
- The lesions may be localized for a long time, and gradually become generalized if left untreated.
- Detachment of clinically healthy epithelium by rubbing is a common sign of pemphigus (Nikolsky's sign).
- Pain, discomfort during mastication, dysphagia, increased salivation, and halitosis, are common.
- Lesions may also develop on other mucosal surfaces (Fig. 16.**3**).
- Skin bullae and erosions are also common during the course of the disease (Fig. 16.**4**).
- The clinical diagnosis should always be confirmed by laboratory tests.

Laboratory tests

- Histopathologically, the lesions show intraepithelial bulla formation, acantholysis, and villous projections of the corium (Fig. 16.**5**).

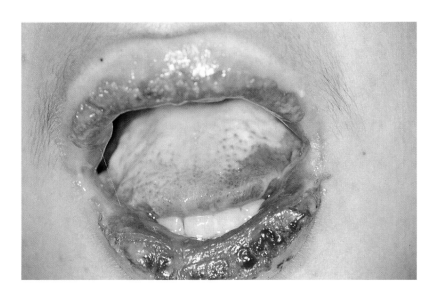

Fig. 16.**1** Pemphigus vulgaris. Severe erosions on the lips in a young girl

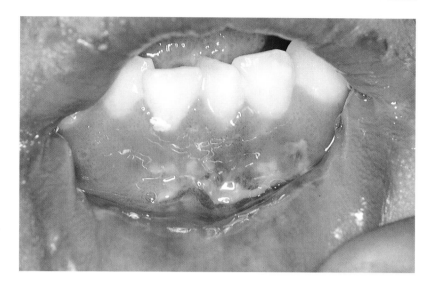

Fig. 16.**2** Pemphigus vulgaris. Erythema and erosions on the gingiva and alveolar mucosa in a six-year-old girl

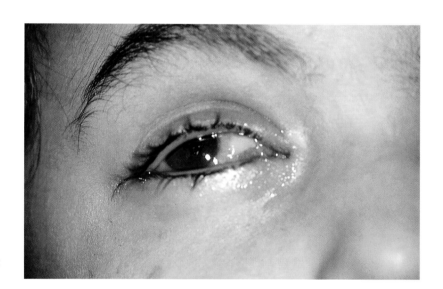

Fig. 16.**3** Pemphigus vulgaris. Severe conjunctivitis (same patient as in Fig. 16.**2**)

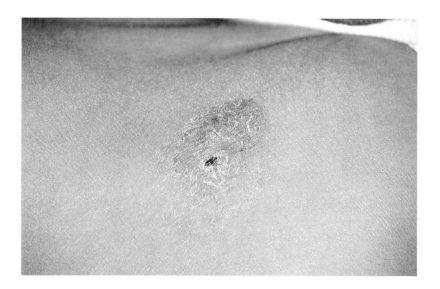

Fig. 16.**4** Pemphigus vulgaris. Flaccid bulla on the skin (same patient as in Fig. 16.**2**)

- Direct immunofluorescence: IgG and C_3 deposition in the intercellular substance areas of the epithelium (Fig. 16.**6**).
- Indirect immunofluorescence: Circulating intercellular IgG antibodies can be demonstrated in over of 80% of patients with active disease.
- Cytological smears show Tzanck cells.

Differential diagnosis

- Cicatricial pemphigoid
- Juvenile bullous pemphigoid
- Childhood linear IgA disease
- Childhood dermatitis herpetiformis
- Epidermolysis bullosa
- Primary herpetic gingivostomatitis
- Erythema multiforme
- Aphthous ulcers

Treatment

- Systemic steroids.
- Immunosuppressive drugs (adjuvant therapy) such as azathioprine, cyclophosphamide, cyclosporine.
- Topical steroids.

Cicatricial Pemphigoid

Definition

- Cicatricial pemphigoid, or benign mucous membrane pemphigoid, is a chronic autoimmune disease of elderly patients that primarily affects the mucous membranes, and rarely the skin.

Etiology

- The exact etiology remains unknown.

Occurrence in children

- Very rare.

Localization

- Often on the oral mucosa (gingiva, buccal, soft palate, tongue, lips).
- Less often, other mucosae (eyes, genitalia, lips).
- Skin lesions are uncommon.

Clinical features

- The oral lesions are a constant finding, and are usually localized.
- Erythema and hemorrhagic bullae that rupture within one to three days, leaving clean, relatively painless erosions.
- The lesions usually recur and persist for a long time, leading occasionally to scar formation.
- Desquamative gingivitis may be the only manifestation of the disease (Fig. 16.**7**).
- Inflammation, bullae, and erosions may rarely also occur on other mucosal surfaces and the skin.
- Usually, the lesions regress after two to four years.
- The clinical diagnosis should be confirmed by laboratory tests.

Laboratory tests

- Histopathologically, the condition is characterized by subepithelial bulla formation, with little inflammation (Fig. 16.**8**).

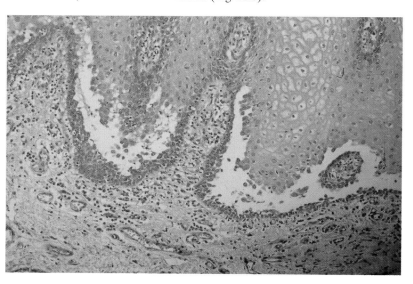

Fig. 16.**5** Pemphigus vulgaris. Acantholysis and intraepithelial clefts

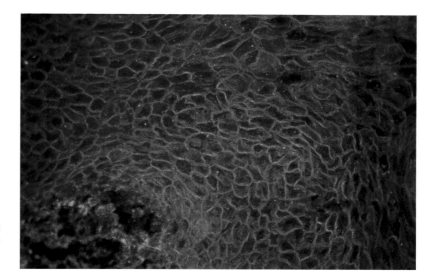

Fig. 16.**6**   Pemphigus vulgaris. IgG deposition in the intercellular areas between the epithelial cells (direct immunofluorescence)

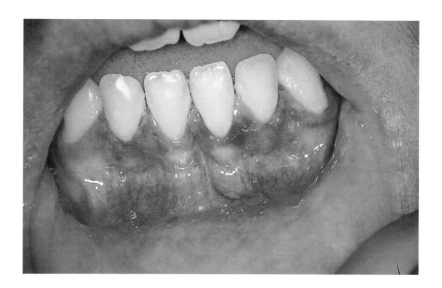

Fig. 16.**7**   Cicatricial pemphigoid. Desquamative gingivitis in a 13-year-old boy

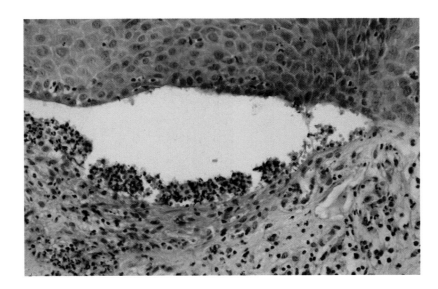

Fig. 16.**8**   Cicatricial pemphigoid. Subepithelial clefting with mild chronic inflammation in the connective tissue

- Direct immunofluorescence, usually linear deposition of IgG and complement along the basement membrane zone are found (Fig. 16.**9**).
- Indirect immunofluorescence, circulating IgG and IgA antibodies are rarely found (about 10% of cases).

Differential diagnosis

- Pemphigus vulgaris
- Juvenile bullous pemphigoid
- Childhood linear IgA disease
- Childhood dermatitis herpetiformis
- Epidermolysis bullosa
- Lichen planus
- Herpetic gingivostomatitis

Treatment

- Topical steroids in mild cases, and systemic steroids in severe cases.
- Dapsone, cyclosporine, and azathioprine may also be used.

Juvenile Bullous Pemphigoid

Definition

- Juvenile bullous pemphigoid is a chronic autoimmune mucocutaneous recurrent bullous disease of children.

Etiology

- The etiology remains unknown.
- The same pathogenetic factors as in bullous pemphigoid of adults are implicated.

Occurrence in children

- Very rare. Usually over the age of five.

Localization

- The disease affects mainly the skin (arms and legs, genital area, groin, abdomen, palms and soles).
- The oral mucosa (palate, gingiva, buccal mucosa, tongue) is rarely affected.

Clinical features

- The oral lesions appear as bullae which rupture in one to three days, leaving painful erosions that show no tendency to spread (Fig. 16.**10**).
- Oral lesions are usually mild and transient.
- The skin lesions are usually generalized, and begin as edematous erythema soon after isolated tense bullae, or develop in clusters (Figs. 16.**11**, 16.**12**). Most bullae rupture in about four to eight days, leaving erosions which have no tendency to spread and heal relatively rapidly.
- Nikolsky's sign is negative.
- The disease lasts about three to four years. Recurrences are not rare, but are less severe than the initial attack.

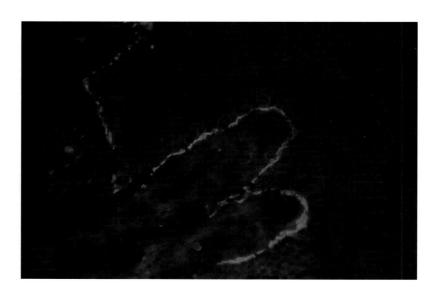

Fig. 16.**9** Cicatricial pemphigoid. IgG deposition in a linear pattern along the basement membrane zone of the epithelium (direct immunofluorescence)

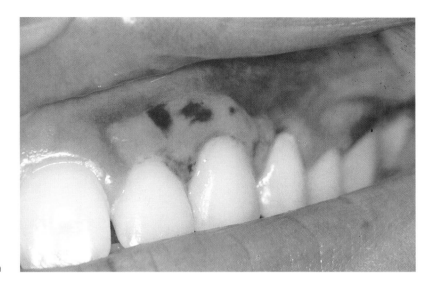

Fig. 16.**10**   Juvenile bullous pemphigoid. Intact hemorrhagic bullae on the gingiva and alveolar mucosa

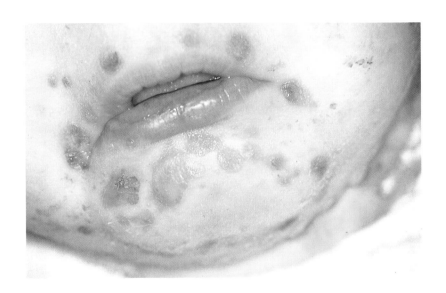

Fig. 16.**11**   Juvenile bullous pemphigoid. Multiple perioral skin lesions

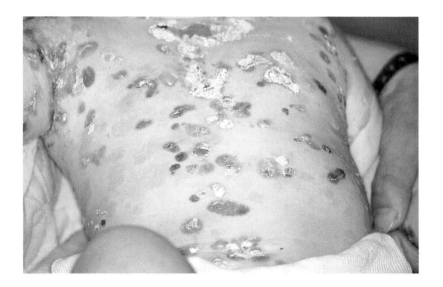

Fig. 16.**12**   Juvenile bullous pemphigoid. Generalized skin lesions

Laboratory tests

- Histopathologically, the condition is characterized by subepithelial bulla formation with eosinophils in the corium and in the bulla cavity (Fig. 16.**13**).
- Direct immunofluorescence often shows IgG and/or C_3, and less often IgA, IgM, and fibrin deposits in a linear pattern along the basement membrane zone (Fig. 16.**14**).
- On indirect immunofluorescence, circulating IgG antibodies are present in approximately 80% of cases.

Differential diagnosis

- Pemphigus vulgaris
- Cicatricial pemphigoid
- Childhood linear IgA disease
- Childhood dermatitis herpetiformis
- Epidermolysis bullosa

Treatment

- Systemic steroids is the treatment of choice.
- Sulfones.
- Immunosuppressive drugs as adjuvant therapy.
- Topical steroids.

Juvenile Dermatitis Herpetiformis

Definition

- Juvenile dermatitis herpetiformis, or Duhring–Brocq disease, is a rare chronic, recurrent pruritic vesicular skin disease, similar to the adult type, affecting children.

Etiology

- The etiology remains unknown.
- There is a strong association with specific HLA antigens, such as: HLA-B_8, HLA-DR_3, HLA-DW_3, HLA-DQW_2.
- In addition, several immunological mechanisms may be involved in the pathogenesis.
- Gluten hypersensitivity plays an important role in the pathogenesis of childhood dermatitis herpetiformis.

Occurrence in children

- Rare, usually over the age of five.

Localization

- Common on the skin (symmetrical distribution on the extensor aspects of the elbows and knees, shoulders, buttocks, posterior neck, and scalp).
- Rare (5–10%) on the oral mucosa (tongue, buccal mucosa, palate, gingiva, lips).

Clinical features

- Clinically, the disease presents with a few itching erythematous papules or plaques on the skin, followed by intensely burning papules, vesicles, and less often bullae in groups, in a herpes-like pattern (Fig. 16.**15**).
- The lesions are symmetrically distributed, and are usually generalized.
- The oral lesions usually follow the skin eruption, and very rarely may precede them. They appear as maculopapular lesions or vesicles that rupture, leaving painful erosions (Fig. 16.**16**).

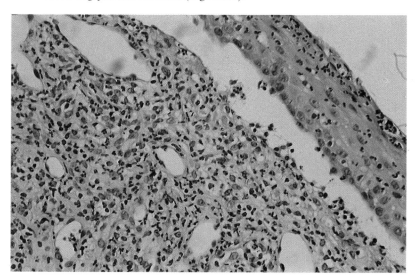

Fig. 16.**13** Juvenile bullous pemphigoid. Subepithelial cleft with mild inflammation in the upper corium and eosinophils within the cleft

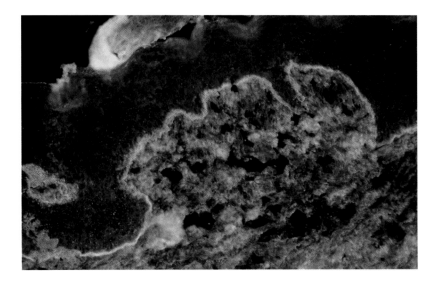

Fig. 16.**14** Juvenile bullous pemphigoid. IgG deposition in a linear pattern along the basement membrane zone of the skin (direct immunofluorescence)

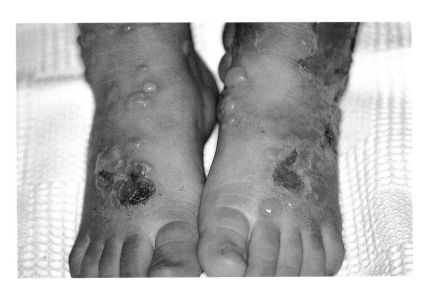

Fig. 16.**15** Juvenile dermatitis herpetiformis. Clusters of bullae on the skin

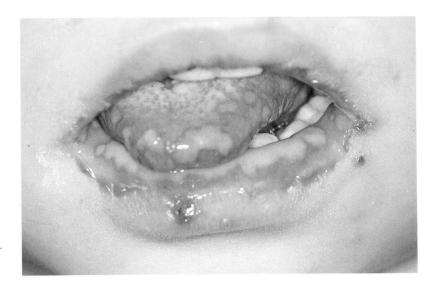

Fig. 16.**16** Juvenile dermatitis herpetiformis. Severe erosions on the lips and tongue

- In the celiac type, permanent dental enamel defects are found in almost half of the patients with dermatitis herpetiformis.
- There is an association between dermatitis herpetiformis and various thyroid disorders. In addition, gluten-sensitive enteropathy is commonly associated with juvenile dermatitis herpetiformis.

Laboratory tests

- Histopathologically, the lesions show subepithelial clefts, with microabscesses of neutrophils and eosinophils in the corium papillae (Fig. 16.**17**).
- On direct immunofluorescence, granular or fibrillar IgA deposits in the dermal papillae and along the dermoepidermal junction (Fig. 16.**18**).
- On indirect immunofluorescence, circulating IgA antiendomysial antibodies are found in approximately 70–80% of patients.

Differential diagnosis

- Herpetic gingivostomatitis
- Juvenile bullous pemphigoid
- Childhood linear IgA disease
- Cicatricial pemphigoid
- Pemphigus vulgaris
- Aphthous ulcers
- Erythema multiforme

Treatment

- Gluten-free diet.
- Sulfones or sulfapyridines.
- Tetracycline and nicotinamide may also be used in some cases.

Childhood Linear IgA Disease

Definition

- Childhood linear IgA disease is an autoimmune vesiculobullous mucocutaneous disorder characteristically seen in children.

Etiology

- Remains unknown.
- An autoimmune mechanism analogous to that of linear IgA disease of adulthood seems to play a role in the pathogenesis.

Occurrence in children

- Rare. The onset is usually before the age of five years.

Localization

- Common on the skin, in a symmetrical distribution (perioral, genital, buttocks, arms).
- The oral mucosa is affected in about 30–50% of patients.
- Rarely, other mucosae may be affected (ocular, nasal, larynx).

Clinical features

- The skin lesions usually have an abrupt onset, and are characterized by pruritus and vesicles, either alone or at the periphery of annular erythema, distributed in a symmetrical pattern (Figs. 16.**19**–16.**21**).
- The lesions tend to occur in clusters, and heal with postinflammatory discoloration.

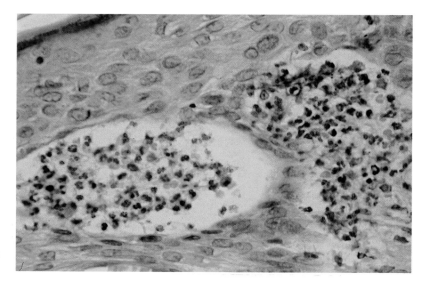

Fig. 16.**17** Juvenile dermatitis herpetiformis. Microabscesses of neutrophils and eosinophils into the dermal papillae of the skin

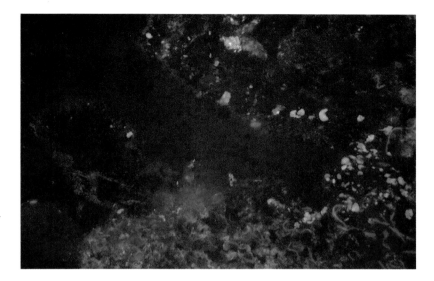

Fig. 16.**18**   Juvenile dermatitis her-petiformis. IgA deposition in a granular pattern along the dermo-epidermal junction and dermal papillae

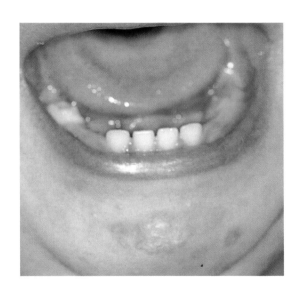

Fig. 16.**19**   Linear IgA disease. Vesicles on the perioral skin

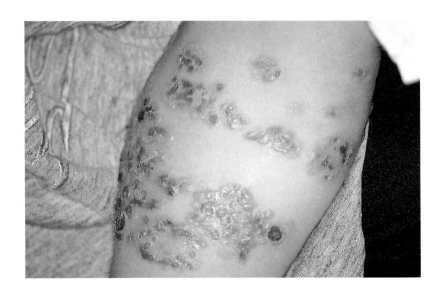

Fig. 16.**20**   Linear IgA disease. Clusters of vesicles on the skin

- The oral lesions usually appear after the skin manifestations, and are characterized by vesicles that soon rupture, leaving painful erosions (Fig. 16.**22**).
- The disease usually resolves during puberty.

Laboratory tests

- Histopathologically, the lesion shows subepidermal vesicles, eosinophilic spongiosis within the epidermis, and eosinophilic infiltration of the upper corium.
- Direct immunofluorescence reveals a homogeneous deposition of IgA in a linear pattern along the dermoepidermal junction (Fig. 16.**23**). Rarely, IgG, IgM or C_3 deposition may occur in a similar distribution.
- On indirect immunofluorescence, circulating IgA anti-basement membrane antibodies are found in about 80% of patients.

Differential diagnosis

- Juvenile bullous pemphigoid
- Childhood dermatitis herpetiformis
- Pemphigus vulgaris
- Cicatricial pemphigoid
- Erythema multiforme
- Varicella
- Impetigo

Treatment

- Dapsone and sulfapyridine are the drugs of choice.
- Systemic steroids may also be used.

Hereditary Epidermolysis Bullosa

Definition

- Hereditary epidermolysis bullosa is a rare, chronic, mechanobullous group of genetic disorders affecting mainly the skin, and less frequently the oral and other mucosae.

Etiology

- The etiology and the exact pathogenesis remain unknown.

Classification

- On the basis of the anatomical level of blister formation, the clinical features (e.g., scarring or non-scarring), the pattern of inheritance, and the expression of specific basement membrane features, the disease is classified into three major types, and numerous subtypes. The major types are:

Type I. The intraepidermal form, characterized by a non-scarring pattern and transmitted as an autosomal and X-linked trait.

Type II. The junctional form, characterized by skin atrophy and transmitted as an autosomal recessive trait.

Type III. The dermal form, characterized by skin atrophy and scarring and transmitted as an autosomal dominant or recessive trait.

Occurrence in children

- Exclusively in infants and children.

Localization

- Skin (hands, feet, fingers, toes, ankles, knees, elbows, trunk, scalp, nails) particularly in areas of friction and pressure.
- Mainly oral mucosa (tongue, palate, buccal mucosa, gingiva, lips).
- Other mucosal surfaces (eyes, larynx, esophagus, genitals) are less often affected.

Clinical features

- Skin manifestations are common in all types of the disease, and are characterized by bulla formation, erosions or ulcerations, scarring, deformities, milia, pigmentation or depigmentation, claw hand and enclosure of the hand in a glove-like sac, nail dystrophy (Figs. 16.**24**–16.**28**).
- Oral and dental manifestations are common in some varieties of types II and III, and rare in type I.
- Common oral manifestations are bullae formations that rupture, leaving painful erosions or ulcerations. Depending on the disease type, repeated blistering with scar formation may lead to diminished oral opening, epithelial atrophy, ankyloglossia, elimination of tongue movement, elimination of vestibular and buccal sulci, perioral stricture, periodontal destruction, milia nodules (Figs. 16.**29**–16.**32**).

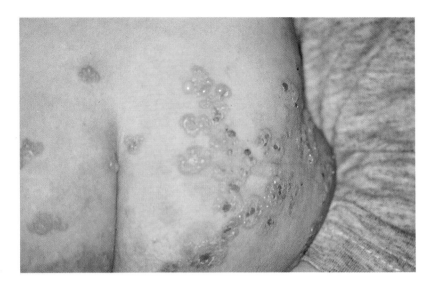

Fig. 16.**21**   Linear IgA disease. Clusters of vesicles on the buttocks

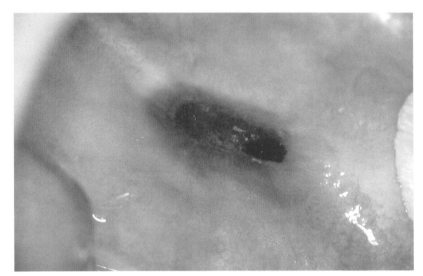

Fig. 16.**22**   Linear IgA disease. Erosion on the buccal mucosa

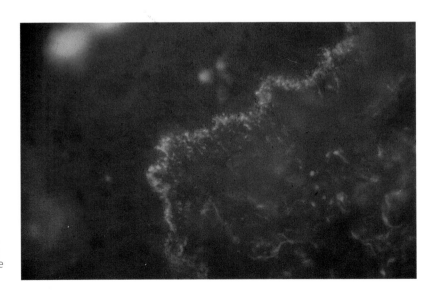

Fig. 16.**23**   Linear IgA disease. IgA deposition in a linear pattern along the dermoepidermal junction of the skin

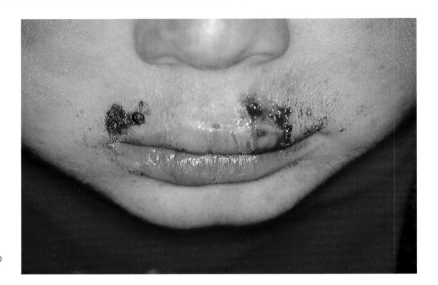

Fig. 16.**24**   Epidermolysis bullosa, type I. Mild lesions on the upper lip and adjacent skin

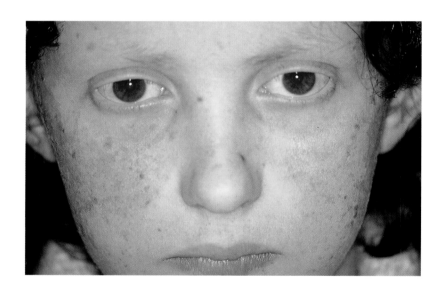

Fig. 16.**25**   Epidermolysis bullosa, type III. Milia and dryness of the skin

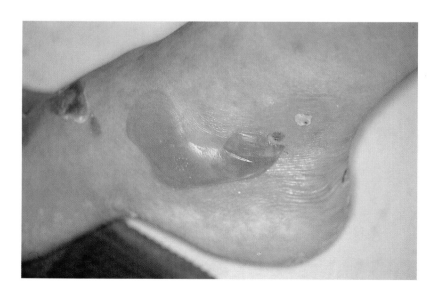

Fig. 16.**26**   Epidermolysis bullosa, type III. Intact bulla and atrophy of the skin

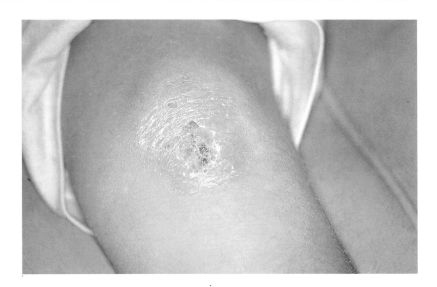

Fig. 16.**27**   Epidermolysis bullosa, type III. Scarring of the skin of the knee

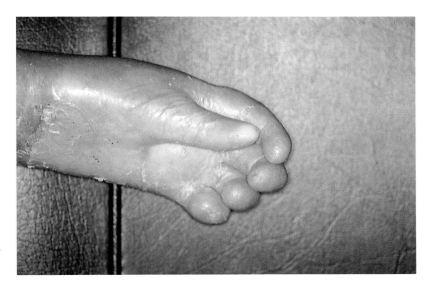

Fig. 16.**28**   Epidermolysis bullosa, type III. Scarring, loss of fingernails, and enclosure of the hand in a glove-like sac

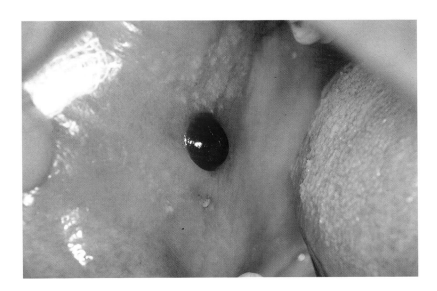

Fig. 16.**29**   Epidermolysis bullosa, type I. Hemorrhagic bulla on the buccal mucosa

- Teeth are rarely affected (hypoplasia and pitted enamel) in scarring epidermolysis bullosa, with dermolytic blisters, and in atrophicans generalisata gravis (Fig. 16.**33**).
- The severity of the oral and skin manifestations depends on the type of the disease.
- Rarely, leukoplakia and squamous-cell carcinoma may develop on the oral lesions of type III disease.

Laboratory tests

- Histopathological examination reveals: a) in the intraepidermal forms, split-through in the epidermal basal cells; b) in the junctional forms, split-through in the basement membrane region; and c) in the dermal forms, split-through in the upper dermis.
- Electron microscopic examination is essential for an accurate diagnosis of the different forms of the disease.
- Immunofluorescence tests for localization of type IV collagen, laminin, lamina densa antigen-1, and bullous pemphigoid antigen in the different levels of cleavage of bullae is useful to differentiate the forms of the disease.

Differential diagnosis

- Pemphigus vulgaris
- Cicatricial pemphigoid
- Juvenile bullous pemphigoid
- Childhood dermatitis herpetiformis
- Childhood linear IgA disease

Treatment

- First of all, patients must avoid trauma.
- Symptomatic treatment of the lesions.
- Topical or systemic steroids, or both.

Erythema Multiforme

Definition

- Erythema multiforme in an acute, self-limited, and often recurrent inflammatory disease characterized mainly by skin manifestations, and less often by mucosal manifestations.

Etiology

- Many factors have been implicated in the etiology of erythema multiforme, including herpesvirus, *Mycoplasma pneumoniae* infection, drugs, and others. However, in over 50% of cases a cause cannot be found.
- The disease is currently considered to have an immunological pathogenesis.

Occurrence in children

- Common, more often in adolescents.
- The disease is rare under the age of three.

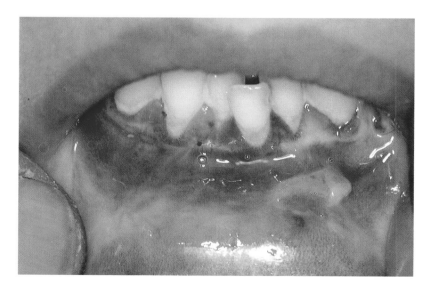

Fig. 16.**30** Epidermolysis bullosa, type III. Erosions and scarring on the labial mucosa and gingiva

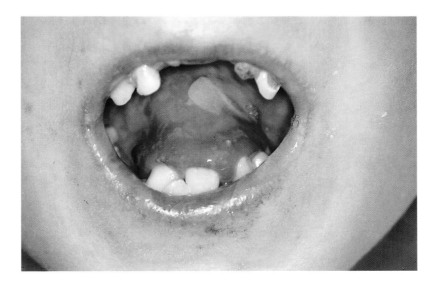

Fig. 16.**31**   Epidermolysis bullosa, type III. Erosions, scarring, and microstomia

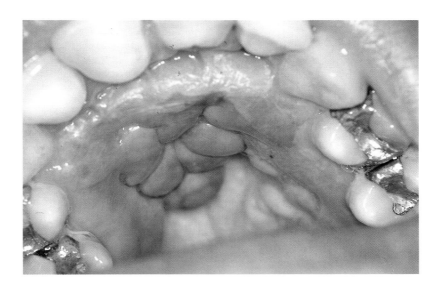

Fig. 16.**32**   Epidermolysis bullosa, type III. Multiple lobulated hyperplastic nodules on the middle of hard palate

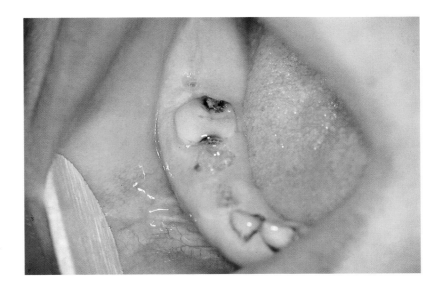

Fig. 16.**33**   Epidermolysis bullosa, type III. Hypoplastic and pitted enamel and dental caries

Localization

- The oral mucosa is affected in about 20–30% of cases (lips, soft palate, tongue, buccal mucosa, gingiva), usually in association with skin manifestations. Rarely, the oral lesions are the only manifestations of the disease.
- The skin is very often affected in a symmetrical pattern (palms and soles, backs of the hands and feet, extensor aspect of the forearms and legs, neck, trunk).
- Other mucosae (conjunctiva, genital) may also be affected.

Clinical features

- Often, the disease begins with modest prodromal symptoms, malaise, low fever, arthralgias, or burning and itching at the sites where the eruption will occur.
- The disease usually has a sudden onset, and the skin lesions start as round red maculopapules. The lesions grow centrifugally, reaching a diameter of 1–3 cm in 24–48 hours. Over the following days, a peripheral ring of lighter color forms around the lesion, and the center becomes cyanotic or purpuric, forming the characteristic target or "iris" lesions (Figs. 16.**34**, 16.**35**). Rarely, purpuric plaques and bullous elements may develop in association with target lesions.
- The oral lesions appear as small vesicles, which soon rupture, leaving extensive erosions covered by pseudomembranes (Figs. 16.**36**, 16.**37**).
- The disease recurs in 20–30% of cases.
- Diagnosis is primarily based on clinical criteria.

Histopathology

- The most important histopathological alterations are found in the upper corium and the lowest layers of the epithelium.
- The corium lesions are characterized by vasodilation of the blood vessels, swelling of the endothelial cells and perivascular mononuclear cells, and polymorphonuclear leukocyte infiltration.
- The epithelial lesions are characterized by hydropic degeneration of the lower layers of the cells and necrotic degeneration of a number of epidermal cells.

Differential diagnosis

- Stevens–Johnson syndrome
- Primary herpetic gingivostomatitis
- Recurrent aphthous ulcers
- Pemphigus vulgaris
- Cicatricial pemphigoid
- Bullous pemphigoid

Treatment

- Systemic steroids.
- Oral acyclovir prevents herpes-associated recurrent erythema multiforme in some cases.

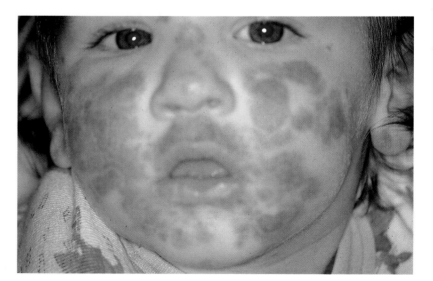

Fig. 16.**34** Erythema multiforme. Skin lesions on the face

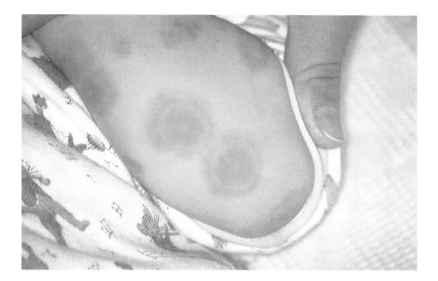

Fig. 16.**35**   Erythema multiforme. Characteristic target-like (iris-like) lesions on the skin

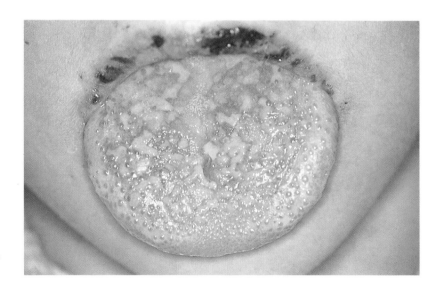

Fig. 16.**36**   Erythema multiforme. Erosions on the tongue and upper lip

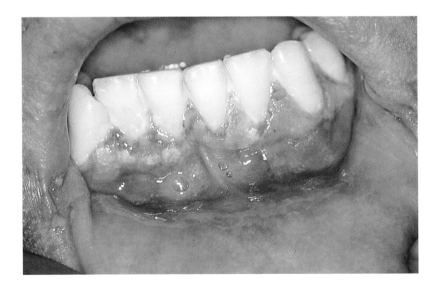

Fig. 16.**37**   Erythema multiforme. Erosions on the gingiva

Stevens–Johnson Syndrome

Definition
- Stevens–Johnson syndrome, or erythema multiforme major, is the more severe mucocutaneous variety of erythema multiforme, with prominent involvement of mucous membranes.

Etiology
- As in erythema multiforme, but drugs are the most common cause.

Occurrence in children
- Common; more frequent in boys.

Localization
- Mainly mucous membranes (oral, ocular, nares, pharynx, larynx, esophagus, genitalia, urethral meatus, anorectal junction), and less often the skin (mainly the trunk or widespread).

Clinical features
- In almost all cases, serious prodromal symptoms (in particular high fever, general discomfort, malaise, diarrhea, vomiting, muscular pains, arthralgias, pharyngitis) precede the mucocutaneous eruptions by several days. The early symptoms are followed by a rapid, sudden mucosal and skin involvement.
- The oral manifestations are the most common signs (95–100%), and present as erythematous and edematous lesions very soon developing into blisters that rapidly rupture, leaving widespread, painful erosions covered by yellowish-white pseudomembranes or hemorrhagic crusts, especially on the lips (Fig. 16.**38**).
- More rarely, severe inflammation, blisters, and erosions occur in other mucosal surfaces (Figs. 16.**39**, 16.**40**).
- The skin lesions may be similar to those seen in erythema multiforme, but are further characterized by asymmetry, involvement of non-typical skin regions, and a longer duration. The severity of the skin lesions may vary from minor to extremely severe.
- The diagnosis is usually based on clinical criteria.

Histopathology
- As in erythema multiforme.

Differential diagnosis
- Erythema multiforme
- Toxic epidermal necrolysis
- Pemphigus vulgaris
- Bullous pemphigoid
- Behçet's syndrome
- Kawasaki's disease
- Staphylococcal scalded skin syndrome.

Treatment
- Systemic steroids.
- Secondary infection is treated with oral antibiotics.

Toxic Epidermal Necrolysis

Definition
- Toxic epidermal necrolysis, or Lyell's disease, is a severe exfoliative disease of the skin and mucous membranes with a high rate of mortality.

Etiology
- Drug-induced reaction (antibiotics, anticonvulsants, non-steroidal anti-inflammatory agents).
- Infections may also be responsible, but less often.

Occurrence in children
- Rare.
- The "staphylococcal scalded skin syndrome," which has a similar clinical presentation to toxic epidermal necrolysis, appears almost exclusively in children under the age of five years.

Localization
- The whole skin.
- Mucous membranes (oral, oropharynx, ocular, genitalia, anus).

Clinical features
- The disease usually begins rapidly, with non-specific symptoms and signs such as cough, fever, sore throat, burning eyes, malaise etc, that precede the skin and mucosal manifestations by one to three days.
- The skin lesions usually appear as macules with darker purpuric centers, or as an extensive scarlatiniform eruption. In one to two days, the typical manifestations develop, characterized by a sheet-like loss of epidermis

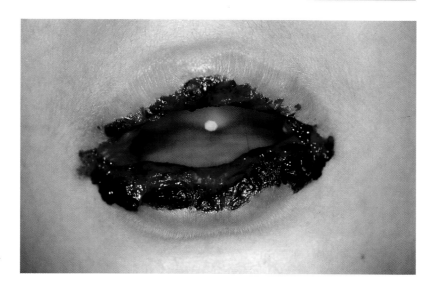

Fig. 16.**38**   Stevens–Johnson syndrome. Erosions covered by hemorrhagic crusting on the lips

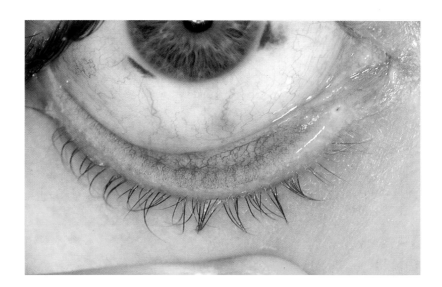

Fig. 16.**39**   Stevens–Johnson syndrome. Conjunctivitis

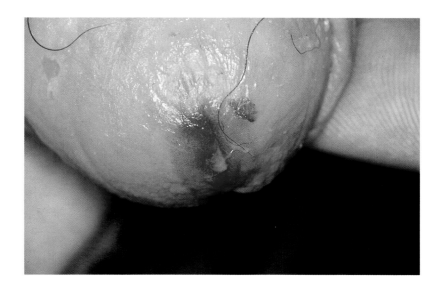

Fig. 16.**40**   Stevens–Johnson syndrome. Erythema and a small erosion on the glans penis

(Fig. 16.**41**). The epidermis is raised by flaccid blisters which spread on pressure.

- Nikolsky's sign is positive.
- The oral lesions appear early and are characterized by severe inflammation, blistering, and painful, widespread erosions, primarily on the lips (Fig. 16.**42**).
- Similar lesions may appear on other mucous membranes.
- The prognosis in children appears to be much better compared to that in adults.

Histopathology

- Histopathologically, the lesions show necrosis of the whole epidermis, detached from a little-altered dermis.

Differential diagnosis

- Stevens–Johnson syndrome
- Staphylococcal scalded skin syndrome
- Pemphigus vulgaris
- Kawasaki disease

Treatment

- Management of the patients must be undertaken as soon as possible in burn units or intensive-care units.
- The use of systemic steroids is still controversial.

Lichen Planus

Definition

- Lichen planus is a relatively common chronic inflammatory cutaneous and mucous membrane disease.

Etiology

- Unknown. It is probably of multifactorial origin.
- Recent evidence supports the concept that this is an immunologically mediated disease. Cell-mediated immunity appears to play a major role in the pathogenesis.

Occurrence in children

- Very rare.

Localization

- In children, usually the skin (legs, arms, trunk, nails).
- Very rarely, the oral mucosa is involved (lips, tongue, buccal mucosa, gingiva).

Clinical features

- The two main forms of oral lichen planus—reticular and erosive—are more often seen in children.
- The early oral lesions are usually single, discrete, whitish papules that tend to coalesce into interlacing white lines (Wickham's striae), or form an annular pattern (Fig. 16.**43**). These lesions may remain asymptomatic for a long time.
- Painful erosions and atrophy of the epithelium may be seen, usually in association with papules (Fig. 16.**44**).

Fig. 16.**41** Staphylococcal scalded skin syndrome. Severe skin lesion in an infant

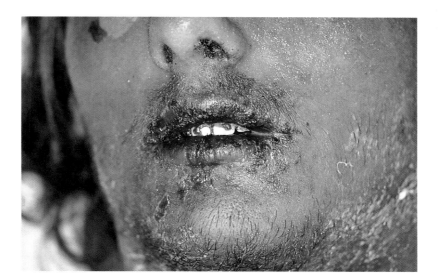

Fig. 16.**42** Toxic epidermal necrolysis. Erosions covered by hemorrhagic crusting on the lips and perioral skin

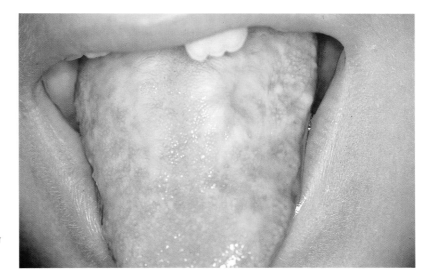

Fig. 16.**43** Lichen planus. Reticular and atrophic lesions on the dorsal surface of the tongue

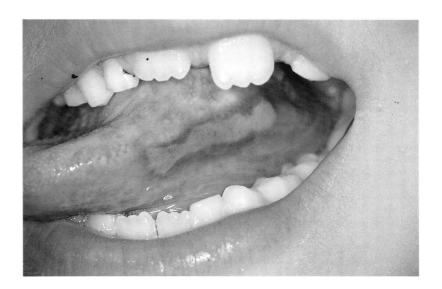

Fig. 16.**44** Lichen planus. Linear erosion along the lateral border of the tongue

- The chronicity, recurrence, and bilateral involvement are characteristic of oral lichen planus.
- The skin lesions present as pruritic, purple polygonal papules. Nail involvement is not unusual (Fig. 16.**45**).
- The diagnosis is usually based on clinical criteria, particularly in the reticular form of the disease.

Laboratory tests

- Histopathologically, the lesions are characterized by varying degrees of hyperkeratosis, parakeratosis, and acanthosis. Hydropic degeneration of the basal cell layer and colloid bodies are a constant findings. A band-like accumulation of T-lymphocytes along the epidermal–dermal junction is always present.
- Direct immunofluorescence shows ovoid globular deposits of IgG, IgM, IgA, and complement. Basement membrane zone deposits of fibrin and fibrinogen are present in a linear pattern (Fig. 16.**46**). However, these findings are not specific.

Differential diagnosis

- Lichen planus reaction due to drugs or to dental materials
- Mechanical chronic friction
- Graft-versus-host disease
- Leukoplakia
- Cicatricial pemphigoid
- Candidiasis
- Geographic tongue

Treatment

- Topical application of steroids in an adhesive base (Orabase).
- Intralesional steroids, particularly for erosive lichen planus.
- Topical cyclosporine mouthwash.
- Systemic steroids in severe painful lesions.

Familial Acanthosis Nigricans

Definition

- Familial or juvenile acanthosis nigricans is a rare benign mucocutaneous disease, characterized by papillary lesions and dark discoloration.

Etiology

- Inherited as an irregular autosomal dominant trait.

Occurrence in children

- This form of acanthosis nigricans occurs exclusively in children. The disease may begin during childhood, or more often at puberty, during which it becomes more severe.

Localization

- Oral mucosa (tongue, lips, gingiva, palate).
- Skin (axillae, neck, groins, umbilicus, perianal area, genitalia).

Clinical features

- The oral mucosa is affected in about 10–25% of cases, with as multiple, small, finely papillary lesions of normal color appearing (Fig. 16.**47**).
- Gingival enlargement may occur (Fig. 16.**48**).

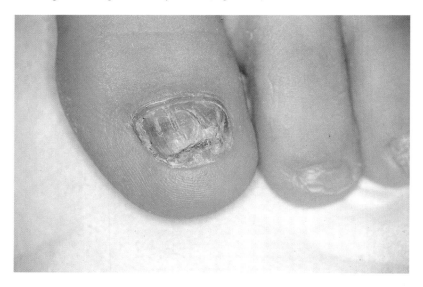

Fig. 16.**45** Lichen planus. Nail dystrophy

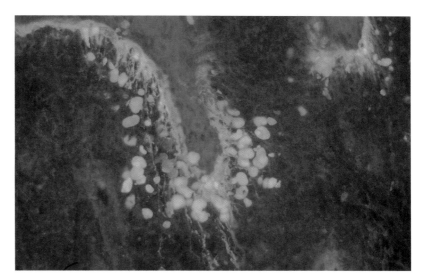

Fig. 16.**46** Lichen planus. Fibrin deposition in a globular pattern along the basement membrane and the upper corium (direct immuno-fluorescence)

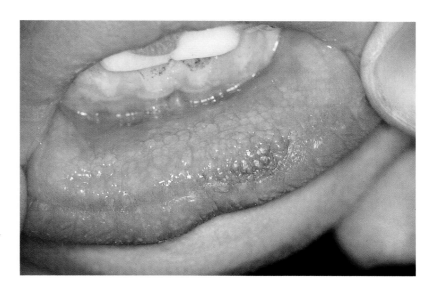

Fig. 16.**47** Familial acanthosis nigricans. Multiple coalescent small papillary lesions on the labial mucosa

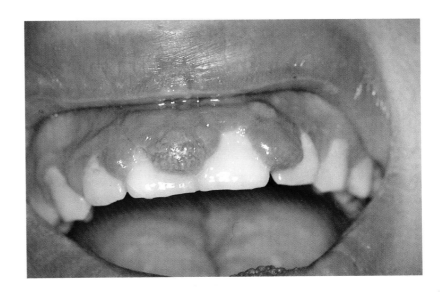

Fig. 16.**48** Familial acanthosis nigricans. Gingival enlargement

- The dorsum of the tongue may show hypertrophy and elongation of the papillae, resulting in a shaggy appearance.
- In contrast to the skin lesions, the oral lesions are usually not pigmented.
- The skin is usually thick, with small papillary lesions (tags) and dark pigmentation (Fig. 16.**49**).
- The diagnosis is usually based on clinical criteria.

Histopathology

- The histopathological features are not specific, and are characterized by hyperorthokeratosis, acanthosis, and papillomatosis. Increased melanin deposition usually occurs in the skin lesions, and rarely in the oral lesions.

Differential diagnosis

- Hairy tongue
- Multiple verrucae vulgaris or papillomas
- Pseudoacanthosis nigricans
- Acanthosis nigricans is associated with some congenital syndromes.
- Malignant acanthosis nigricans
- Cowden's syndrome

Treatment

- There is no satisfactory therapy.
- Keratolytic drugs may occasionally improve the lesions.
- Surgical reconstruction in cases of severe aesthetic problems.

Kawasaki's Syndrome

Definition

- Kawasaki's syndrome, or mucocutaneous lymph-node syndrome, is an acute multisystem inflammatory febrile illness of young children.

Etiology

- The etiology remains unknown.

Occurrence in children

- It is a relatively rare disease that predominantly appears during childhood.
- The peak incidence is between one and two years of age, and 80–90% of the affected children are under five years of age.

Localization

- Skin, oral mucosa, eyes, lymph nodes, cardiovascular system.

Clinical features

- The cardinal signs of the syndrome are the following:
- Fever (usually ranging from 38.5 °C to 40 °C), lasting five days or longer.
- Erythema, edema and fissuring of the lips, diffuse erythema, and prominent papillae of the tongue (strawberry tongue) (Fig. 16.**50**). Bright erythema of the palate and the oropharynx may also be seen.
- Polymorphous erythematous non-vesicular skin exanthem.
- Intense reddening and indurative edema of the hands and feet, followed by membranous desquamation, usually of the fingertips and toe tips and rarely of other skin areas (Figs. 16.**51**–16.**53**).

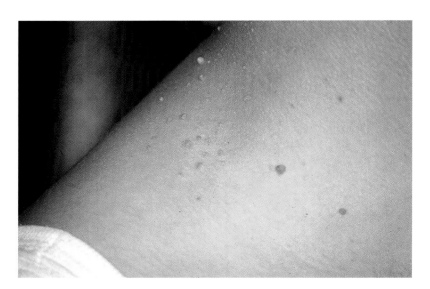

Fig. 16.**49** Familial acanthosis nigricans. Skin tags

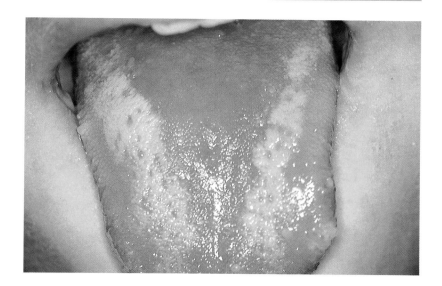

Fig. 16.**50**   Kawasaki's syndrome. Loss of filiform papillae of the tongue and erythema

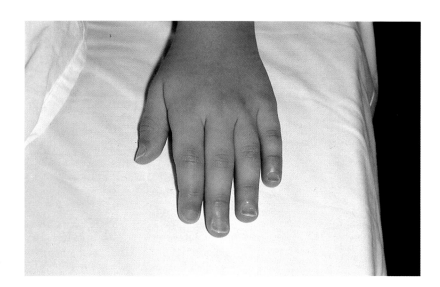

Fig. 16.**51**   Kawasaki's syndrome. Erythema and edema of the hand

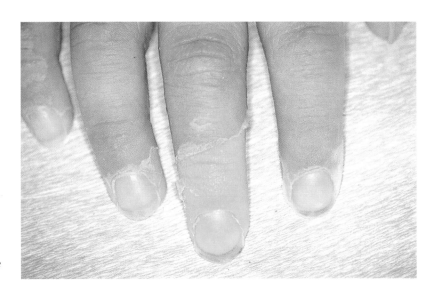

Fig. 16.**52**   Kawasaki's syndrome. Characteristic desquamation of the fingertips skin

- Bilateral conjunctival infection, and occasionally mild anterior uveitis (Fig. 16.**54**).
- Acute, non-purulent swelling of a single or multiple anterior cervical lymph nodes.
- Musculoskeletal disorders, abdominal symptoms, neurological involvement, coronary artery dilation, and aneurysms, myocarditis, and urinary tract involvement may be less commonly associated features.
- The diagnosis is made clinically when five of the above principal signs are present.

Laboratory tests

- Laboratory tests are non-specific. The most characteristic abnormal values are: marked leukocytosis, thrombocytosis, elevated erythrocyte sedimentation rate (ESR), sterile pyuria and proteinuria, and elevated serum immunoglobulins.

Differential diagnosis

- Scarlet fever
- Erythema multiforme
- Staphylococcal scalded skin syndrome
- Rubella
- Reiter's syndrome
- Drug reaction

Treatment

- Hospitalization during the acute phase and supportive care.
- Aspirin and intravenous gamma globulin are the mainstay of treatment.

Vitiligo

Definition

- Vitiligo is an acquired melanocytopenic disorder, characterized histologically by the absence of epidermal melanocytes.

Etiology

- Unknown. However, an autoimmune mechanism is involved in the pathogenesis.

Occurrence in children

- Approximately 50% of cases begin before age 20.
- Childhood vitiligo is a distinct subset of the disease.

Localization

- Skin (dorsal aspect of the hands, neck, face, and periorificial regions).
- Lips (rarely).
- The oral mucosa is not affected.

Clinical features

- Appears as white, asymptomatic macules, varying in size from several millimeters to several centimeters in diameter, which are surrounded by a zone of normal or hyperpigmented skin (Fig. 16.**55**).
- The lesions progressively increase in size, forming various irregular patterns.

Treatment

- Topical psoralens and UVA light.
- Topical steroids.

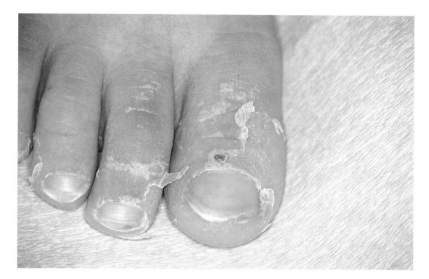

Fig. 16.**53**   Kawasaki's syndrome. Characteristic desquamation of the toe tips skin

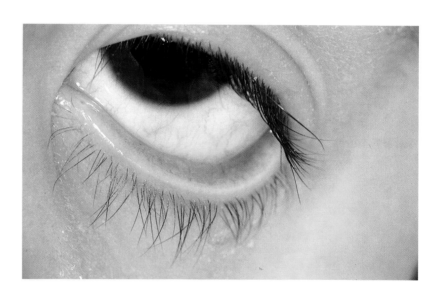

Fig. 16.**54**   Kawasaki's syndrome. Conjunctivitis

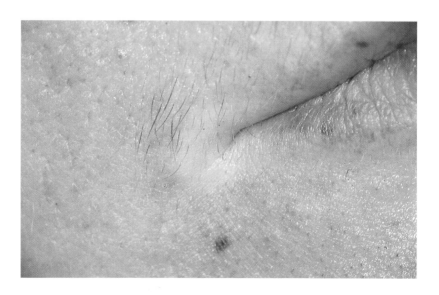

Fig. 16.**55**   Vitiligo. Hypopigmented skin patch around the angle of the mouth

17 Autoimmune Diseases

Lupus Erythematosus

Definition

- Lupus erythematosus is a chronic inflammatory autoimmune disease with a variable spectrum of clinical forms, in which mucocutaneous manifestations may occur with or without systemic manifestations.

Etiology

- Unknown etiology. However, a genetically determined autoimmune mechanism is implicated in the pathogenesis of the disease.

Classification

- Two major forms of lupus erythematosus are recognized: *discoid* and *systemic*. An additional form, subacute cutaneous lupus erythematosus, is also recognized.

Occurrence in children

- The discoid form is rare (less than 2% of patients develop the disease before 10 years of age).
- The systemic form is relatively common in children, particularly girls over eight years of age.
- Neonatal lupus erythematosus appears in the first month of life, and is due to maternal passage of different lupus erythematosus antibodies.

Localization

- The discoid form most commonly affects the face, but lesions may occur on any body surface. The oral mucosa is involved in 15–25% of cases (buccal mucosa, lower lip, gingiva, palate, tongue), usually in association with skin lesions.
- The systemic form affects the skin and many organ systems. The oral mucosa is involved in 30–45% of cases.

Clinical features

- *Discoid lupus erythematosus* is usually confined to the skin, and the lesions are characterized by scaling, flat or slightly elevated erythematous papules, and plaques with prominent follicular hyperkeratosis. The lesions are sharply demarcated from the surrounding healthy skin, and gradually progress to scarring and depigmentation. Usually, the lesions on the face form the characteristic "butterfly" erythema (Fig. 17.**1**). The oral lesions are characterized by a well-defined central atrophic red plaque surrounded by a sharp elevated border of irradiating whitish striae (Fig. 17.**2**). Erosions, white plaques, atrophy, and telangiectasias of the oral mucosae may be seen.
- *Systemic lupus erythematosus* (SLE) is a multisystemic disease characterized by 11 clinical and laboratory diagnostic criteria. If any four or more of these criteria are present, the diagnosis of systemic lupus erythematosus is made. The criteria are: malar rash, discoid rash, photosensitivity, oral ulcers, arthritis, serositis, renal, neurological, hematological, and immunological disorders, and antinuclear antibody.
  The oral manifestations of SLE include localized or extensive painful erosions or ulcers, petechiae, edema, hemorrhages, and xerostomia (Figs. 17.**3**, 17.**4**).

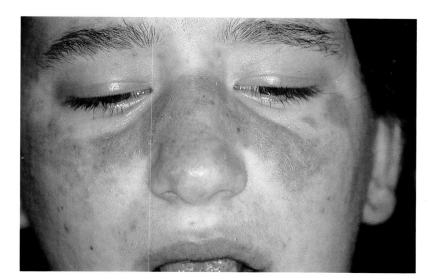

Fig. 17.**1**   Discoid lupus erythematosus. Typical "butterfly" erythema on the face

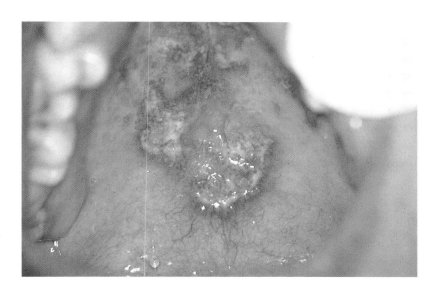

Fig. 17.**2**   Discoid lupus erythematosus. Atrophic red plaque with irradiating whitish striae on the palate

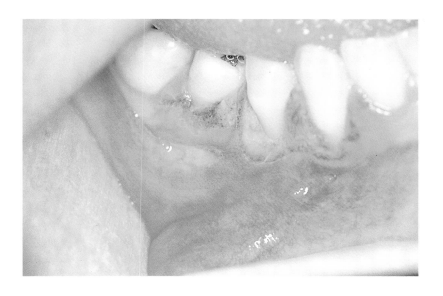

Fig. 17.**3**   Systemic lupus erythematosus. Erosions on the gingiva and alveolar mucosa

The skin manifestations may be localized or widespread, similar to those seen in discoid lupus erythematosus, or even more severe (Figs. 17.**5**, 17.**6**).

Laboratory tests

- Histopathological examination demonstrates perivascular lymphocytic infiltration, vascular dilation, and edema in the upper connective tissue, hydropic degeneration of the basal-cell layer, and atrophy of the epithelium.
- Direct immunofluorescence shows granular or linear thick bands of IgG or IgM, IgA and C_3 deposition at the basal membrane zone of the epithelium and in the dermal vessels walls (Fig. 17.**7**).
- Serological and other findings in the systemic form, such as antinuclear antibodies (anti-ANA), anti-native deoxyribonucleic acid (anti-nDNA), anti-Sjögren's syndrome A antibody (anti–SS-A, anti-Ro), anti-Sjögren's syndrome B antibody (anti–SS-B, anti-La), anti-nuclear ribonucleoprotein (anti-nRNP), erythrocyte sedimentation rate (ESR).

Differential diagnosis

- Lichen planus
- Cicatricial pemphigoid, bullous pemphigoid, linear IgA disease, pemphigus
- Erythema multiforme and Stevens–Johnson syndrome

Treatment

- Topical steroids, intralesional steroids, antimalarials, dapsone, systemic steroids, isotretinoin, azathioprine and other immunosuppressive drugs.

Systemic Sclerosis

Definition

- Systemic sclerosis is a relatively rare chronic multisystemic inflammatory connective-tissue disorder, with a wide spectrum of manifestations.

Etiology

- The etiology remains unknown, although an autoimmune pathogenesis has been suggested.

Classification

- There are two forms, *systemic* and *localized*. The localized form is restricted to the skin in an asymmetric manner.

Occurrence in children

- Rare.

Localization

- Skin, oral mucosa, synovium, digital arteries, and several internal organs (esophagus, intestinal tract, heart, lungs, kidney, skeletal muscles).

Clinical features

- The oral features include thin and pale oral mucosa, short and hard lingual frenulum, gingival regression, atrophy of the tongue papillae, loss of tissue elasticity, microglossia. The lips are pale, thin, and sclerotic. Microstomia,

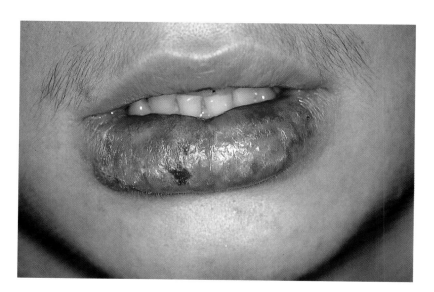

Fig. 17.**4** Systemic lupus erythematosus. Edema and erosions on the lower lip

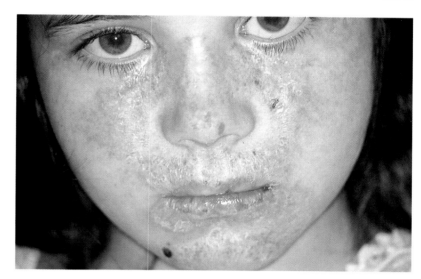

Fig. 17.**5** Systemic lupus erythematosus. Severe scarring of the skin of the face

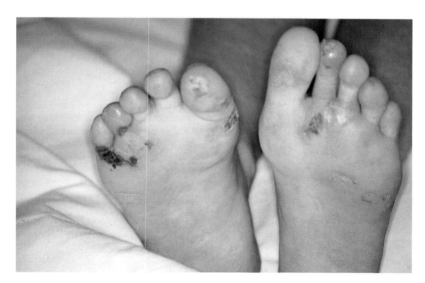

Fig. 17.**6** Systemic lupus erythematosus. Edema and necrotic ulcers on the soles

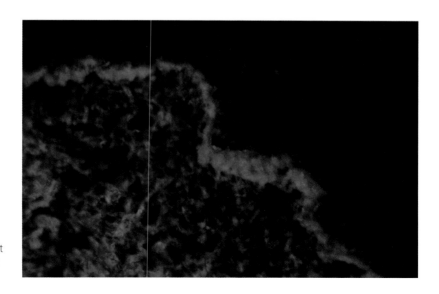

Fig. 17.**7** Systemic lupus erythematosus. Granular thick band of IgG deposition along the basement membrane zone of the epithelium (direct immunofluorescence)

limitation of mouth opening (Fig. 17.**8**), xerostomia, inelastic esophagus, dysphagia, difficulty in swallowing, diffuse widening of the periodontal ligament on dental radiographs (10–20%). A characteristic clinical feature is the perioral radial folds (Fig. 17.**9**).

- Three stages of the skin lesions are recognized: *edematous, sclerotic,* and *atrophic.* Initially, the skin is edematous, and as the disease progresses, it becomes thin, hard, and inelastic, with a pale color. Facial skin involvement results in characteristic facies (mask-like facies) with smooth, taut skin, small, sharp nose, narrow oral aperture and thin lips.
- Skin necrosis, ulcers, and telangiectasia may gradually appear.
- Raynaud's phenomenon is a common disorder in patients with systemic sclerosis, and represents an episodic vasoconstriction of the digital arteries and arterioles that is precipitated by cold or stress.
- Involvement of the gastrointestinal tract, joints, heart, lungs, kidney, etc., is frequent and leads to organ failure.
- CREST syndrome (calcinosis cutis, Raynaud's phenomenon, esophageal dysmotility, sclerodactyly, telangiectasia) is a clinical variant of systemic sclerosis.

Laboratory tests

- Skin biopsy and histopathological examination, which reveals diffuse deposition of dense collagen.
- Specific circulating antibodies are useful in establishing the diagnosis: anti-DNA antibodies, centromere antibodies, Scl-70 antibodies, anti-Sjögren's syndrome A antibody (anti–SS-A, anti-Ro), anti-Sjögren's syndrome B antibody (anti–SS-B, anti-La).

Differential diagnosis

- Epidermolysis bullosa
- Lipoid proteinosis
- Atrophic lichen planus
- Cicatricial pemphigoid

Treatment

- Corticosteroids, antimalarials, D-penicillamine, colchicine, azathioprine and other immunosuppressives, calcium-channel blockers, and potassium para-aminobenzoate have been used, with limited success.
- There is no specific management for the oral lesions.

Dermatomyositis

Definition

- Dermatomyositis is a relatively rare multisystemic disease, characterized by an inflammatory reaction of the striated muscles and secondarily of the skin.

Etiology

- The etiology remains unclear, although an autoimmune pathogenic mechanism has been proposed.

Occurrence in children

- Rare.

Localization

- Striated muscles, skin and oral mucosa.

Clinical features

- Juvenile dermatomyositis is characterized by a non-suppurative myositis that causes symmetric weakness, rash, and vasculitis.
- Muscle weakness, myalgias, fever, and fatigue are early and common symptoms and signs.
- Muscle atrophy, residual proximal weakness, calcinosis of the subcutaneous tissues, arthritis, joint contractures, and Raynaud's phenomenon may be late manifestations.
- The skin lesions appear in about 40–50% of patients, and present as skin edema and a characteristic periorbital violaceous discoloration. An additional characteristic sign is the appearance of violaceous flat-topped papules, 0.2–1.0 cm in size, usually along the sides of the fingers and over the knuckles (Gottron's sign). Periungual erythema, telangiectasia, poikiloderma, violaceous scaling patches, and scalp scaling may also occur.
- The oral lesions are rare and non-specific, and may present as erythema, painful erosions, telangiectasias, and tongue edema.
- The incidence of an underlying malignancy in children is low, in contrast to the adults.

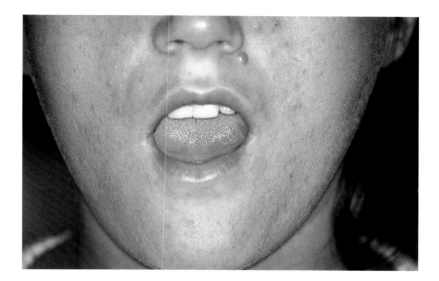

Fig. 17.**8**   Systemic sclerosis. Microstomia

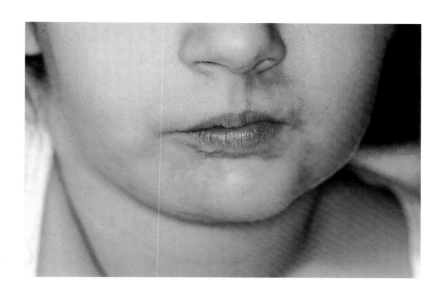

Fig. 17.**9**   Systemic sclerosis. Perioral radial folds

Laboratory tests	• Histopathological examination of the muscles.
	• Serum measurement of certain enzymes (creatine kinase, phosphokinase, transaminases, aldolase) and urinary creatine.
	• Antinuclear antibodies are usually present. Anti–SS-A (anti-Ro), anti–SS-B (anti-La), Sm, nRNP, J0–1, may also be present, but are of limited diagnostic value.
Differential diagnosis	• Systemic lupus erythematosus
	• Stomatitis medicamentosa
	• Erythema multiforme
Treatment	• Corticosteroids, immunosuppressive, drugs, antimalarials, plasmapheresis.
	• Non-steroidal anti-inflammatory drugs.
	• Physical therapy.

Mixed Connective-Tissue Disease

Definition	• Mixed connective-tissue disease is a multisystemic disorder characterized by a combination of clinical manifestations and laboratory findings seen in lupus erythematosus, scleroderma, dermatomyositis, rheumatoid arthritis, and Sjögren's syndrome. A high serum titer of antibodies against ribonucleoprotein antigens is a characteristic finding, and occurs in all such patients.
Etiology	• The cause and pathogenesis are unknown.
	• Probably autoimmune.
Occurrence in children	• Very rare.
	• The disease is more common in women over 35 years.
Localization	• Skin, oral mucosa, skeletal, muscles, lymph nodes and many other organs.
Clinical features	• Oral lesions are rare and are characterized by a non-specific erythema, edema, erosions and xerostomia (Fig. 17.**10**).
	• Swollen hands and tapered fingers, polyarthritis, myositis, esophageal motility, pulmonary involvement, Raynaud's phenomenon, and lymphadenopathy are the most common signs and symptoms.
	• Alopecia, skin lesions suggestive of lupus erythematosus, scleroderma, and dermatomyositis may occur.
Laboratory tests	• High titers of anti-ribonucleoprotein antibodies (anti-RNP). Antinuclear antibodies (ANAs) may also be found on direct immunofluorescence of normal skin.
Differential diagnosis	• Other connective-tissue diseases
	• Juvenile rheumatoid arthritis
Treatment	• Corticosteroids.
	• Immunosuppressive drugs.

Sjögren's Syndrome

Definition	• Sjögren's syndrome is a chronic autoimmune exocrinopathy.
Etiology	• The exact cause remains unknown. Genetic factors, viral infection, and autoimmunity are involved in the pathogenesis.
Classification	• Two forms of the syndrome are recognized: *primary,* and *secondary* if it coexists with other connective-tissue diseases.
Occurrence in children	• Rare.
	• More than 90% of patients are women over 40 years of age.
Localization	• Salivary, lacrimal, and other exocrine glands.
Clinical features	• The oral mucosa is reddish, dry, smooth, and shiny. The tongue is smooth, with furrowing (Fig. 17.**11**). Dysphagia, cheilitis, candidiasis, and multiple dental caries are common (Fig. 17.**12**).

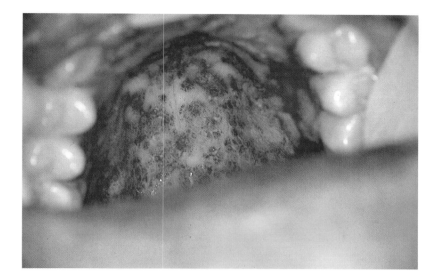

Fig. 17.**10** Mixed connective-
tissue disease. Severe erythema,
edema, and erosions on the palat

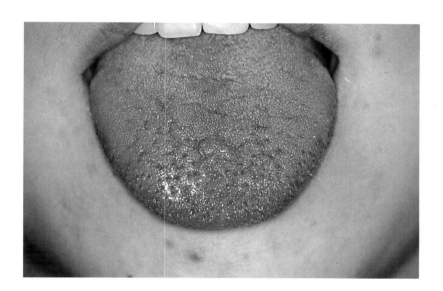

Fig. 17.**11** Sjögren's syndrome.
Dry tongue

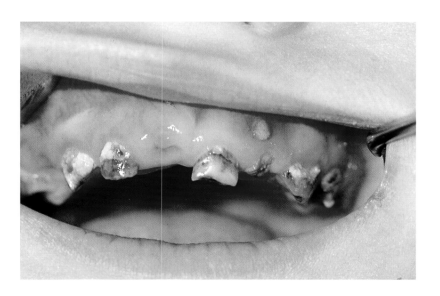

Fig. 17.**12** Sjögren's syndrome.
Multiple dental caries

- Recurrent enlargement of the parotid and other major and/or minor salivary glands (Fig. 17.**13**).
- The ocular manifestations include a burning sensation, keratoconjunctivitis sicca, enlargement of lacrimal glands, and more severe lesions as the disease progresses.
- Recurrent infections of the respiratory system may often develop.
- In secondary Sjögren's syndrome, the clinical manifestations depend on the accompanying diseases, e.g., rheumatoid arthritis, lupus erythematosus, systemic scleroderma, dermatomyositis, human immunodeficiency virus (HIV) infection, thyroiditis, vasculitides, and/or cryoglobulinemia.

Laboratory tests

- Quantitative measurement of saliva and tears, scintigraphy, sialography.
- Biopsy and histopathological examination of the minor salivary glands of the lower lip is very useful.
- Serum immunological evaluation for anti–SS-A (anti-Ro), anti–SS-B (anti-La), anti-DNA, and other non-specific antibodies.

Differential diagnosis

- Graft-versus-host disease
- Pernicious anemia
- Systemic scleroderma
- HIV infection
- Xerostomia due to drugs or other causes

Treatment

- Corticosteroids, immunosuppressive and antimalarial drugs.
- Sialagogue drugs (pilocarpine) may stimulate salivary flow.
- Saliva and tear substitutes.
- Scrupulous oral hygiene and fluoride applications.

Graft-Versus-Host-Disease

Definition

- Graft-versus-host disease (GVHD) is a multisystemic immunological phenomenon caused by an immune reaction between the transplanted T-lymphocytes and the patient's normal tissues.

Etiology

- It occurs in patients who receive allogeneic bone-marrow transplants to treat life-threatening hematological diseases such as leukemia, aplastic anemia, or even myelodysplastic syndrome.

Occurrence in children

- Common in transplant patients (20–50%).

Localization

- Skin, oral mucosa (buccal mucosa, tongue, eyes, lips), gastrointestinal tract, liver, lungs and other organs.

Clinical features

- *Acute GVHD.* The signs and symptoms are usually observed during the second week after bone-marrow transplantation, and include diarrhea, nausea, skin, gastrointestinal tract and oral mucosa manifestations.
- *Chronic GVHD* develops 100 days after bone-marrow transplantation from an HLA-matched donor. It is characterized by fatigue and lesions on the skin and in the gastrointestinal tract, oral cavity, liver, eyes, and lungs.
- Oral lesions develop more commonly in the chronic form of the disease, and are characterized by a diffuse erythema, lichenoid reactions, and painful ulcerations with an irregular surface (Fig. 17.**14**). A burning sensation and atrophy of the oral mucosa are common.
- Xerostomia is a common symptom, due to salivary gland involvement.
- Oral opportunistic infections are also common (herpes, candidiasis).

Laboratory findings

- Biopsy of the oral mucosa and the minor salivary glands of the lower lip. The histopathological features resemble those seen in lichen planus and Sjögren's syndrome.
- Increased salivary sodium concentrations.

Differential diagnosis

- Lichen planus, lupus erythematosus
- Langerhans cell histiocytosis, leukemia
- Sjögren's syndrome, scleroderma
- Oral lesions due to drugs
- Acrodermatitis enteropathica

Treatment

- Corticosteroids, immunosuppressive drugs, thalidomide.

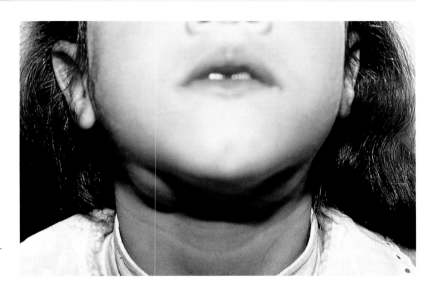

Fig. 17.**13** Sjögren's syndrome. Bilateral submandibular gland swelling

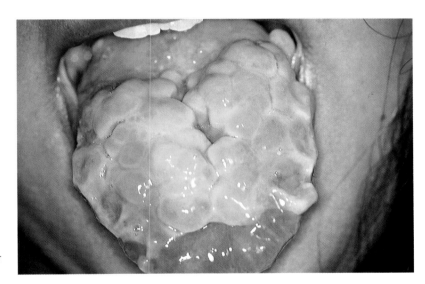

Fig. 17.**14** Graft-versus-host disease. Severe ulcers with an irregular surface on the tongue

Behcet's Syndrome

Definition
- Behçet's syndrome is a chronic inflammatory multisystemic disease.

Etiology
- Unknown. Genetic, immunological factors, and viral infection may be involved in the pathogenesis of the disease.
- The disorder is more common in some ethnic groups (Japanese, Turkish, Greek and other Mediterranean countries).

Occurrence in children
- Rare. It usually develops in children over 15 years old.
- Neonatal Behçet's syndrome has been described in infants born from mothers with the disease.
- Males are more frequently affected than females (5 : 1 or more).

Localization
- Oral mucosa, eyes, genitalia, skin.
- Gastrointestinal tract, cardiovascular system, joints.
- The lungs and central nervous system are rarely involved.

Clinical features
- Oral involvement, with lesions similar to aphthous ulcerations (minor, major, herpetiform ulcers or atypical), which recur more than two or three times a year, is a constant finding (Figs. 17.**15**, 17.**16**).
- Conjunctivitis, iritis, iridocyclitis with hypopyon, uveitis. All these lesions may eventually lead to vision loss (Fig. 17.**17**).
- Genital round ulcerations on the scrotum or penis and in the vulva or vagina and balanitis (Figs. 17.**18**, 17.**19**).

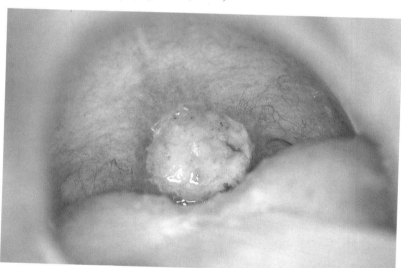

Fig. 17.**15** Behçet's syndrome. Minor aphthous ulcer on the soft palate

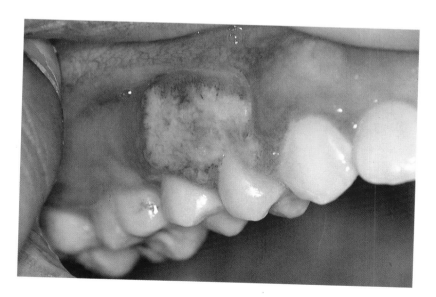

Fig. 17.**16** Behçet's syndrome. Major aphthous ulcer on the gingiva

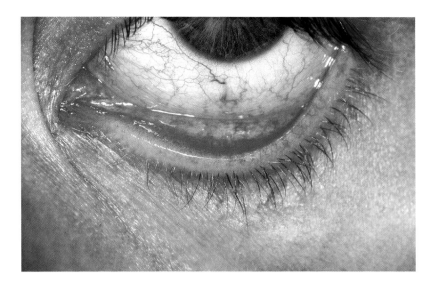

Fig. 17.**17**   Behçet's syndrome.
Conjunctivitis

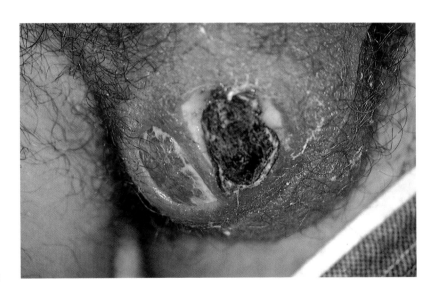

Fig. 17.**18**   Behçet's syndrome.
Major round ulcers on the scrotum

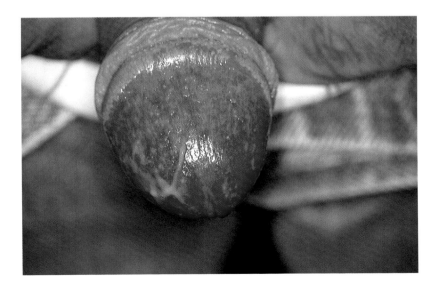

Fig. 17.**19**   Behçet's syndrome.
Severe balanitis

- Cutaneous involvement includes folliculitis, nodular erythema, papules, vesicles, pustules, and necrotic lesions.
- Positive pathergy test in 60–70% of the cases.
- Involvement of other organs and systems is common (vascular, neurologic, skeletal, intestinal).
- Malaise and fever may accompany the other manifestations.
- The diagnosis is based on clinical criteria.

Laboratory tests
- There is no diagnostic laboratory test.

Differential diagnosis
- Aphthous ulcers
- Reiter's syndrome
- Erythema multiforme
- Stevens–Johnson syndrome
- Pemphigus and pemphigoid
- Crohn's disease
- HIV infection

Treatment
- Corticosteroids, cyclosporine and other immunosuppressive drugs, colchicine, thalidomide.

Reiter's Syndrome

Definition
- Reiter's syndrome is a multisystemic disease that usually develops in genetically susceptible individuals after an episode of dysentery or a sexually transmitted infection.

Etiology
- The etiology and pathogenesis of the disease remain unknown, although it has been suggested that the tissue destruction is mediated by an immunological mechanism. Infectious agents (*Mycoplasma, Chlamydia, Yersinia, Salmonella,* etc.) and genetic factors (increased frequency of HLA-27) seem to play an important role in the pathogenesis of the disease.

Occurrence in children
- Relatively rare. It usually affects boys over 15 years of age.

Localization
- Oral mucosa (tongue, buccal mucosa, gingiva, palate, upper and lower lips), genitals, skin, eyes, skeletal and cardiovascular system.

Clinical features
- A characteristic sign is the arthritis that affects the joints of the upper and lower extremities, and may lead to deformation. Six to seven joints are usually symmetrically involved.
- Non-gonococcal urethritis, prostatitis, cervicitis.
- Non-bacterial conjunctivitis, which is usually bilateral, iritis, choroiditis (Fig. 17.**20**).
- Mucocutaneous lesions, such as macular, vesicular, or pustular lesions, keratoderma blennorrhagicum, psoriasiform lesions, cyclic balanitis, nail disturbances, pustule formation under the nails (Figs. 17.**21,** 17.**22**).

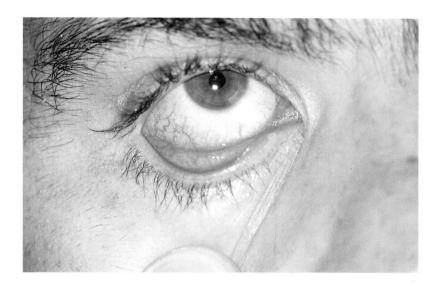

Fig. 17.**20**   Reiter's syndrome.
Conjunctivitis

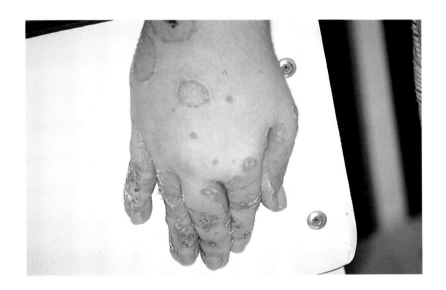

Fig. 17.**21**   Reiter's syndrome.
Psoriasiform skin lesions and joint
involvement, leading to deformation

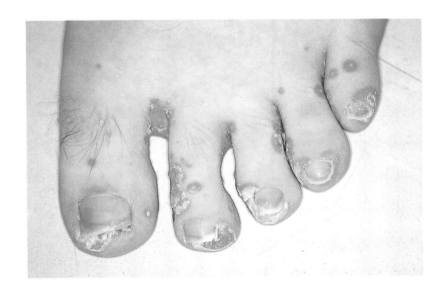

Fig. 17.**22**   Reiter's syndrome.
Psoriasiform skin lesions and nail
pustule formation under the nails

- Oral lesions develop in 20–40% of cases, and are characterized by erythematous areas surrounded by a thin, whitish margin, erosions, and loss of the filiform papillae (Fig. 17.**23**).
- In children, the disease is usually less severe than in adults.

Laboratory tests

- Blood and serologic tests, HLA antigens, synovial fluid analysis, radiographs of the affected joints, biopsy of skin lesions.
- The laboratory tests are non-pathognomonic.

Differential diagnosis

- Behçet's syndrome
- Erythema multiforme and Stevens–Johnson syndrome
- Geographic tongue and geographic stomatitis

Treatment

- Bed rest.
- Non-steroidal anti-inflammatory drugs, salicylates, methotrexate.
- The use of antibiotics and corticosteroids remains unclear.

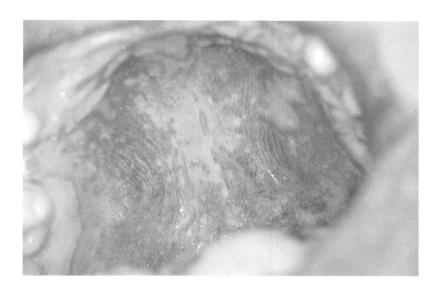

Fig. 17.**23** Reiter's syndrome.
Severe erythema and whitish lines
and plaques on the palate

18 Gastrointestinal Diseases

Crohn's Disease

Definition
- Crohn's disease is a chronic inflammatory granulomatous disease that affects the gastrointestinal tract from the mouth to the anus.

Etiology
- Unknown. Probably, the pathogenesis of the disease is immunologically mediated.

Occurrence in children
- Common. It affects children over 10 and those younger than 20 (30% of cases).

Localization
- Gastrointestinal tract.
- The oral mucosa is involved in 10–20% of cases (lips, buccal mucosa, gingiva, mucolabial and mucobuccal folds, palate).
- Skin, eyes, joints may rarely be affected.

Clinical features
- Oral lesions present as granulomatous lip swelling, angular cheilitis, diffuse or nodular swelling resulting in a cobblestone appearance of the mucosa, mucosal tags, soft-tissue swellings, and granulomatous ulcers (Figs. 18.**1**, 18.**2**). Aphthous-like ulcerations, pyostomatitis vegetans, metallic dysgeusia, and persistent lymphadenopathy are common. The oral lesions usually regress when intestinal symptoms are in remission.
- Gastrointestinal signs and symptoms include abdominal pain, diarrhea, vomiting, rectal bleeding, and loss of appetite. Weight loss, low-grade fever, decreased growth, and fatigue may occur.
- Extra-abdominal manifestations include arthritis, spondylitis, and uveitis.

Laboratory findings
- Histopathological examination reveals a granulomatous inflammation with epithelioid cells, Langhans giant cells, and lymphocytes, with no evidence of caseous necrosis.
- Increased sedimentation rate.
- Low levels of hemoglobulin and protein.

Differential diagnosis
- Granulomatous cheilitis and Melkersson–Rosenthal syndrome
- Sarcoidosis, tuberculosis
- Behçet's syndrome
- Ulcerative colitis

Treatment
- Appropriate diet.
- Corticosteroids.
- Sulfasalazine, azath oprine, cyclosporine, metronidazole.

Peutz–Jeghers Syndrome

Definition
- Peutz–Jeghers syndrome is a genetic disorder characterized by mucocutaneous pigmentation and hamartomas of the intestine.

Etiology
- It is inherited as an autosomal dominant trait.

Occurrence in children
- Rare.

Localization
- The lips (vermilion zone), perioral area, gingiva, buccal mucosa, tongue, palate.
- Skin of the face, mainly around the nose and eyes, and rarely on the hands and feet.
- The small bowel is the most frequently involved portion of the intestinal tract.

Clinical features
- Several characteristic small asymptomatic flat, irregularly oval, pigmented macules, usually 1–10 mm in diameter, are the cutaneous and oral mucosal markers of the syndrome (Figs. 18.**3**, 18.**4**). These lesions are often apparent in early childhood.

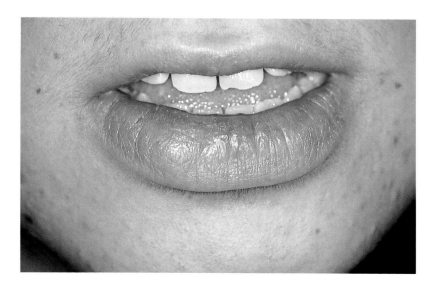

Fig. 18.**1**   Crohn's disease. Swelling of the lower lip

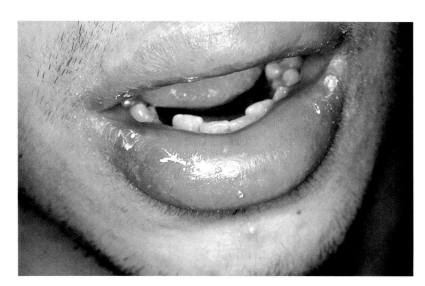

Fig. 18.**2**   Crohn's disease. Erythema and swelling of the lower lip

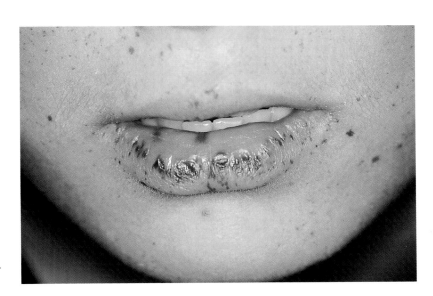

Fig. 18.**3**   Peutz–Jeghers syndrome. Typical flat pigmented macules on the lower lip

- Intestinal polyps, which may cause abdominal pain, hemorrhage, constipation, and intussusception.
- The polyps themselves do not appear to be premalignant.

Laboratory findings
- Histopathological examination of the mucocutaneous macules reveals increased melanin pigmentation.
- Endoscopy.

Differential diagnosis
- Multiple freckles and ephelides
- Gardner's syndrome
- Albright's syndrome
- Cronkhite–Canada syndrome
- Addison's disease

Treatment
- Surgical intervention when the polyps cause severe symptoms.
- Oral and skin lesions require no treatment.

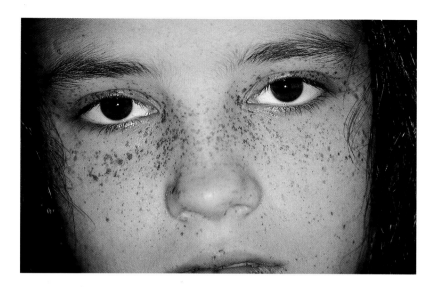

Fig. 18.**4**   Peutz–Jeghers syndrome. Typical pigmented macules of the skin of the face

19 Hematological Diseases

Thalassemia

Definition
- Thalassemia represents a heterogenous group of genetically inherited disorders with a variable degree of severity in hemoglobin synthesis.
- The most common form is β-thalassemia, which is classified as heterozygous (thalassemia minor) and homozygous (thalassemia major).

Etiology
- Inherited defects resulting in abnormal hemoglobins.
- Disturbance in the hemoglobin molecule (reduced synthesis of the alpha-globin or beta-globin chains of the hemoglobin molecule).
- When two defective genes for the beta-globin molecule are inherited, the child is affected with thalassemia major.

Occurrence in children
- Exclusively in children.
- Thalassemia major becomes symptomatic usually during the first year of life.

Localization
- Skin, skeletal, bone marrow, liver, spleen, heart, endocrine glands.
- Oral cavity.
- Salivary gland involvement is relatively rare.

Clinical features
- Bone marrow hyperplasia; the bones become thin.
- Massive expansion of the face marrow and skull bones produces a characteristic facies.
- Marked painless enlargement of the maxilla and the mandible.
- The teeth are displaced, with occlusion problems (Figs. 19.**1**, 19.**2**).
- The oral mucosa is pale, and there is loss of tongue papillae and glossodynia.
- Parotid and other salivary gland enlargement may rarely occur.
- Skin pallor, malaise, weakness.
- Spleen and liver enlargement, endocrine disturbances, cardiac failure.
- The above disturbances are observed in the major form of the disease, and depend on whether or not the child is maintained on a blood transfusion program.

Laboratory tests
- Specialized hematological tests, including electrophoresis of hemoglobin and genetic typing.

Differential diagnosis
- Iron-deficiency anemia

Treatment
- Blood transfusions, chelation therapy, hormonal replacement therapy, general supportive measures.

Iron-Deficiency Anemia

Definition
- Iron-deficiency anemia is the most common hematological disease of infancy and childhood.

Etiology
- It is due to lack of sufficient iron for hemoglobin synthesis.

Occurrence in children
- Relatively common.

Clinical features
- Pallor of the oral mucosa.
- Atrophy of the lingual papillae and burning sensation on the tongue.
- Bilateral angular cheilitis and candidiasis (Figs. 19.**3**, 19.**4**).
- Skin pallor and koilonychia.
- Irritability, loss of appetite, fatigue, headache, tachycardia.
- Rarely, neurological disturbances and spleen enlargement.
- The signs and symptoms depend on the severity and duration of the disease.

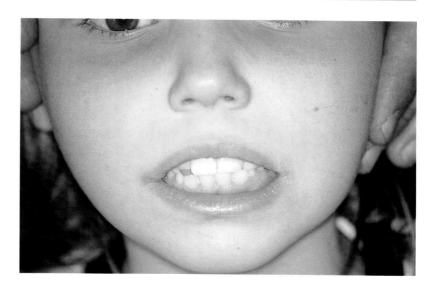

Fig. 19.**1**   Thalassemia major. Protrusion of the upper anterior tooth and malocclusion

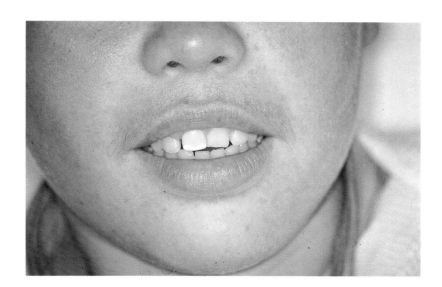

Fig. 19.**2**   Thalassemia major. Malocclusion

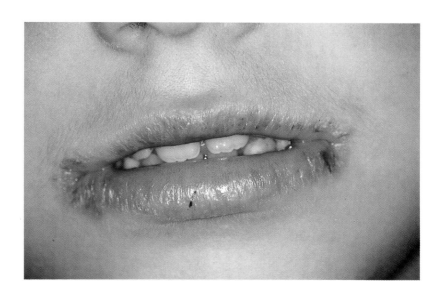

Fig. 19.**3**   Iron-deficiency anemia. Bilateral angular cheilitis

Laboratory tests	• Hemoglobin, ferritin and iron determination. • Complete blood count.
Differential diagnosis	• Other types of anemia • Atrophic lichen planus
Treatment	• Iron supplementation and proper diet.

Pernicious Anemia

Definition	• Pernicious anemia is a form of megaloblastic anemia.
Etiology	• It is due to vitamin B_{12} deficiency, usually caused by a gastric mucosal defect that reduces intrinsic factor synthesis. • In contrast to adults, in children the stomach is histopathologically normal and secretes normal amounts of acid.
Occurrence in children	• Rare. Occasionally between the first and tenth years.
Clinical features	• A burning sensation on the tongue and taste disturbances are common early symptoms. • Smooth, red, shiny and painful tongue, rarely with erosions. • Anorexia, weakness, fatigue, irritability, gastrointestinal and neurological disturbances (ataxia, paresthesias, hyporeflexia).
Laboratory tests	• Hematological evaluation of the vitamin B_{12} level. • Schilling test. • Biopsy and histopathological examination of the gastric mucosa.
Differential diagnosis	• Other types of anemia • Pellagra • Malnutrition disorders
Treatment	• Vitamin B_{12} replacement.

Congenital Neutropenia

Definition	• Congenital neutropenia is a hematological disorder characterized by severe and constant decrease of neutrophils in the peripheral blood, and is associated with an increased susceptibility of the patients to bacterial infections.
Etiology	• The etiology is unknown. The disease is probably inherited by an autosomal recessive trait.
Occurrence in children	• Rare. The neutropenia is present at birth.
Clinical features	• Oral lesions are a common finding, and may be the initial sign of the disease. • Recurrent ulcerations, which may lead to scar formation (Fig. 19.**5**). • Bacterial infections are common, while candidiasis and viral infections are less common. • Periodontal disease leading to bone destruction, tooth mobility, and occasionally tooth loss (Fig. 19.**6**). • Recurrent infections of the skin (particularly when neutrophil counts drop below 500/mm³), otitis media, and respiratory tract and urinary system infections are common. • The signs and symptoms usually improve with age.
Laboratory tests	• Complete blood count. • Radiographic examination of the jaws usually shows severe alveolar bone loss.
Differential diagnosis	• Cyclic neutropenia • Agranulocytosis • Aplastic anemia • Leukemia • Glycogen storage disease type Ib

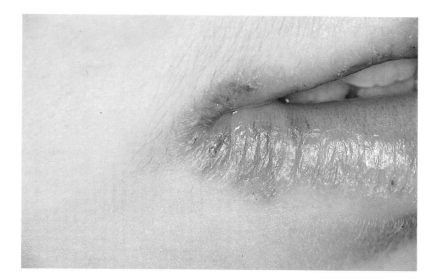

Fig. 19.**4**   Iron-deficiency anemia. Persistent angular cheilitis, associated with *Candida* infection

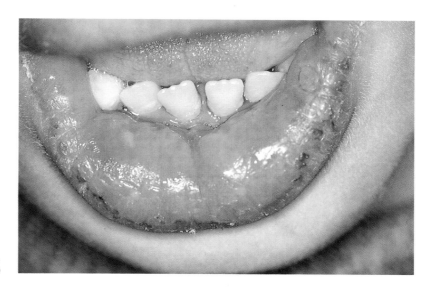

Fig. 19.**5**   Congenital neutropenia. Ulcers and scarring on the lower lip

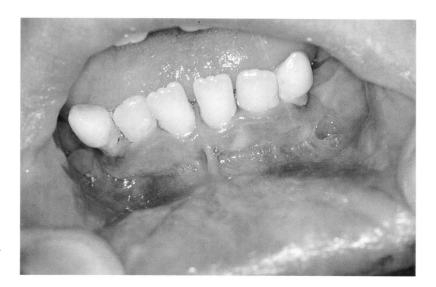

Fig. 19.**6**   Congenital neutropenia. Periodontitis, teeth migration, and scarring of the labial mucosa

Treatment
- Good oral hygiene.
- Periodontal treatment.
- Appropriate antibiotic therapy, granulocyte colony-stimulating factor (G-CSF).
- Bone-marrow transplantation may also offer some hope of cure.

Cyclic Neutropenia

Definition
- Cyclic neutropenia is a hematological disorder characterized by regular periodic reduction of the neutrophil population in the affected patient.

Etiology
- The etiology remains unknown, although an autosomal dominant trait has been described in some cases.

Occurrence in children
- Rare. It usually begins after 10 years of age.

Clinical features
- The symptoms and signs of cyclic neutropenia occur in a cyclic pattern of three weeks' duration and persist for 5–10 days, after which the neutrophil counts gradually return to normal.
- Painful oral ulcerations covered by a whitish membrane and surrounded by slight erythema are the most constant findings (Fig. 19.**7**). The lips, tongue, buccal mucosa, and gingiva are the areas most commonly affected.
- Gingivitis is also common, but bacterial infection is relatively rare (Fig. 19.**8**).
- Low-grade fever, malaise, headache, arthralgia, cervical adenitis, otitis media, and skin infections may occur during an episode of profound neutropenia.

Laboratory tests
- Repeated complete blood count.

Differential diagnosis
- Aphthous ulcers
- Herpetic stomatitis
- Congenital neutropenia
- Agranulocytosis
- Leukemia
- Primary and secondary syphilis

Treatment
- Symptomatic and topical antiseptics for the oral lesions.
- Corticosteroids and occasionally splenectomy in severe cases.
- Granulocyte-colony stimulating factor (G-CSF) may also be effective.

Agranulocytosis

Definition
- Agranulocytosis is a serious hematological disorder that occurs as a result of a severe reduction or even absence of neutrophils or all granulocytes in the blood or bone marrow.

Etiology
- Drugs are the most common cause of the disease. Idiopathic cases or cases induced by infection may occur less frequently.

Occurrence in children
- Rare.

Clinical features
- The oral manifestations are early, and consist of necrotic ulcers covered by gray-white or dark, dirty pseudomembranes with a characteristically absent red halo (Figs. 19.**9**, 19.**10**). The gingiva, tongue, buccal mucosa, palate, tonsils are the most common sites affected.
- Sialorrhea, dysphagia, and difficulty in swallowing are common symptoms.
- The onset is sudden and is characterized by fever, chills, headache, malaise, and sweats.
- Pharyngeal, pulmonary, and gastrointestinal infections are common.

Laboratory tests
- Complete blood count and bone-marrow aspiration.

Differential diagnosis
- Necrotizing ulcerative gingivitis and stomatitis
- Congenital neutropenia
- Cyclic neutropenia
- Infectious mononucleosis
- Acute leukemia

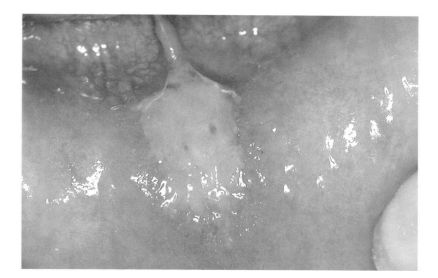

Fig. 19.**7** Cyclic neutropenia. Irregular superficial ulcer on the labial mucosa

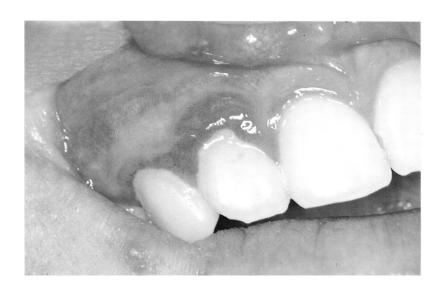

Fig. 19.**8** Cyclic neutropenia. Localized gingivitis

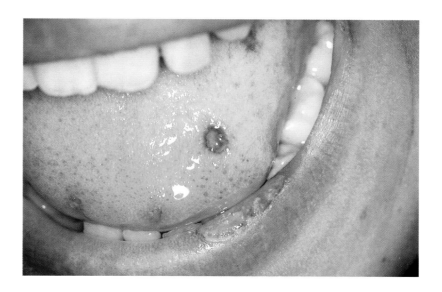

Fig. 19.**9** Agranulocytosis. Necrotic ulcers on the tongue and lower lip

Treatment

- Antibiotics, corticosteroids in low doses.
- Discontinuation of the responsible drug as soon as possible.
- Granulocyte macrophage–colony stimulating factor (GM-CSF) may be useful.

Aplastic Anemia

Definition

- Aplastic anemia is a life-threatening hematological disorder in which acellular or markedly hypocellular bone marrow results in pancytopenia.

Etiology

- Idiopathic cases have been described, but drugs, chemicals, infections, radiation, metabolic and immunological abnormalities are mainly associated with the disease.
- A congenital type, inherited as an autosomal recessive trait (Fanconi's anemia), may develop in childhood.

Occurrence in children

- Rare.

Clinical features

- The onset of the disease is usually insidious, and the presenting symptoms include headache, fever, progressive weakness, fatigue, and mild hemorrhage.
- Slight pallor, petechiae, or ecchymoses of the skin, mucous membranes, and eyes are early diagnostic signs.
- Lymph-node enlargement and hepatosplenomegaly are notably absent.
- The oral manifestations are related to the degree of neutropenia and thrombocytopenia. Gingival bleeding is a common early sign (Fig. 19.**11**). Necrotic ulcers may develop on the lips, buccal mucosa, palate, and gingiva (Fig. 19.**12**). Pallor of the oral mucosa, petechiae, and ecchymoses may be seen.
- The course of the disease is determined by the severity of the aplasia.

Laboratory tests

- Complete blood count.
- Bone-marrow biopsy.

Differential diagnosis

- Agranulocytosis, cyclic neutropenia
- Acute leukemia
- Thrombocytopenic purpura
- Infectious mononucleosis

Treatment

- Antibiotics, corticosteroids.
- Blood transfusion, bone marrow–stimulating agents.
- Bone-marrow transplantation.

Thrombocytopenic Purpura

Definition

- Thrombocytopenic purpura is a hematological disorder characterized by a markedly decreased number of circulating blood platelets.

Etiology

- Idiopathic cases have been described, but drugs, virus infections, malignancies, immunological disorders, human immunodeficiency virus (HIV) infection, and radiation are the most common causes.

Occurrence in children

- Rare. The idiopathic form is commonly seen during childhood.

Clinical features

- The clinical manifestations of the disease usually appear when the platelet level falls below 50 000–20 000/mm^3. In addition, the severity of the disorder is closely related to the extent of platelet reduction.

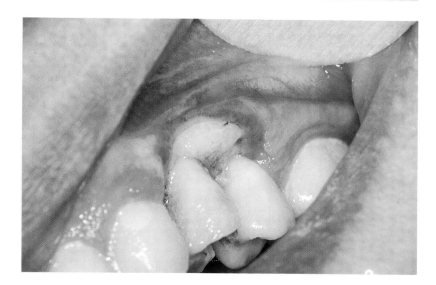

Fig. 19.**10** Agranulocytosis. Deep ulcer on the gingiva

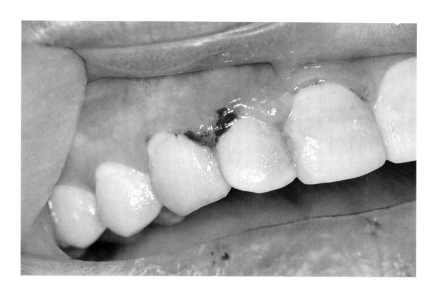

Fig. 19.**11** Aplastic anemia. Gingival bleeding

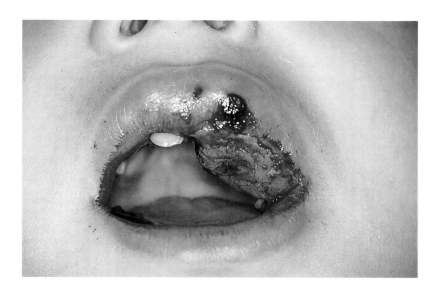

Fig. 19.**12** Aplastic anemia. Severe necrotic ulcer on the upper lip

- The oral manifestations are early and common. They are characterized by petechiae, ecchymoses, and hematomas of the oral mucosa (Fig. 19.**13**). Gingival hemorrhage, spontaneous or following minor trauma, is a constant early sign.
- Purpuric skin rash and bleeding usually occur.
- Bleeding episodes from the gastrointestinal and urinary tracts and epistaxis are frequent. Cerebral bleeding may rarely occur in children.

Laboratory tests

- Complete blood count.

Differential diagnosis

- Aplastic anemia
- Leukemia

Treatment

- Corticosteroids, infusions of plasma.

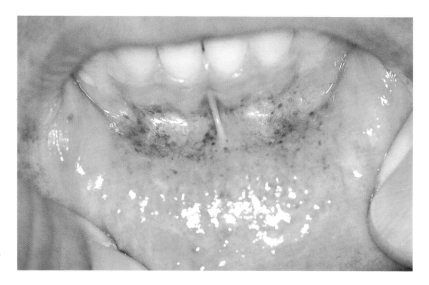

Fig. 19.**13**   Thrombocytopenic purpura. Petechiae on the oral mucosa

20 Metabolic Diseases

Hurler's Syndrome

Definition
- The mucopolysaccharidoses are a heterogeneous group of metabolic disorders usually inherited as autosomal recessive traits. About eight forms have been described.
- Hurler's syndrome is the most common and severe form of mucopolysaccharidosis, and often leads to death around 10–12 years of age.

Etiology
- The basic defect is the lack of the enzyme alpha-L-iduronidase, resulting in the accumulation and deposition of dermatan sulfate and heparan sulfate within the tissues, with excessive excretion in the urine.

Occurrence in children
- Rare; approximately one per 100 000 births.
- It develops during the first year of age.

Localization
- All body tissues.

Clinical features
- The oral manifestations include macrocheilia, macroglossia, open mouth with protruding tongue, hyperplastic gingivitis, numerous impacted teeth, large interdental spaces, tooth abrasion, tooth dislocation, disturbances in the jaw development, diminished temporomandibular joint mobility, multiple radiolucencies of the jaws detected radiographically (Fig. 20.**1**).
- Craniofacial malformations, characteristic facies (macrocephaly with frontal bulging, flattened nasal bridge with a saddle-shaped appearance, hypertelorism, protuberant tongue) (Fig. 20.**2**).
- Corneal clouding, scoliosis, dwarfism, chondrodystrophy, mental retardation, liver and spleen enlargement.
- Cardiac failure, hypertension, and respiratory tract infections are common complications.

Laboratory tests
- Histochemical evaluation of alpha-L-iduronidase in white blood cells, in bone-marrow cells, in the plasma, and in fibroblast tissue cultures.
- Radiographic examination.
- Determination of dermatan sulfate and heparan sulfate in the urine.

Differential diagnosis
- Other forms of mucopolysaccharidosis.

Treatment
- Supportive. There is no effective treatment.
- Common management for dental problems.

Glycogen Storage Disease Type Ib

Definition
- The glycogen storage diseases are a group of genetic disorders related to the glycogen metabolism.
- Type Ib is a disease variant with a severe prognosis, which is inherited as an autosomal recessive trait.

Etiology
- The cause of type Ib is a defect of the microsomal glucose-6-phosphate translocase. The disorder coexists with neutropenia and neutrophil dysfunction.

Occurrence in children
- Rare. It occurs early in childhood.

Localization
- Many organs; frequent oral involvement.

Clinical features
- The oral manifestations include gingivitis, periodontitis and recurrent ulcers. The oral ulcers appear as discrete, deep, punched-out lesions a few millimeters to several centimeters in size, usually covered by whitish pseudomembranes (Fig. 20.**3**). A high-arched palate may also be seen (Fig. 20.**4**). Recurrent oral infections are common complications.
- Characteristic facies (doll's face) (Fig. 20.**5**).
- Neutropenia and recurrent bacterial infections.

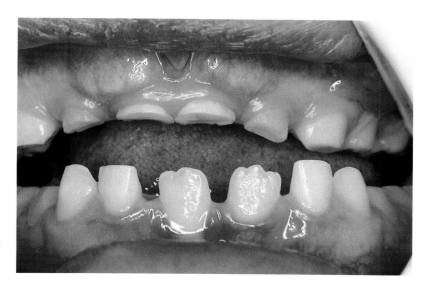

Fig. 20.**1** Hurler's syndrome. Large interdental spaces and teeth abrasion

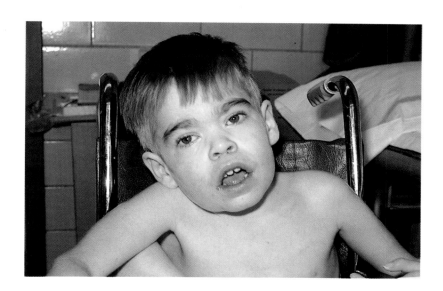

Fig. 20.**2** Hurler's syndrome. Characteristic facies

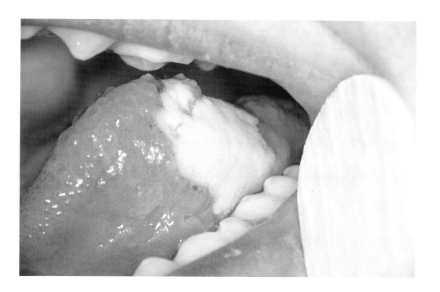

Fig. 20.**3** Glycogen storage disease type Ib. Large ulcer on the lateral surface of the tongue

- Liver and kidney enlargement.
- Bleeding diathesis, hypoglycemia, and hyperlipidemia.
- Delayed growth retardation, enlarged kidneys.

Laboratory tests
- Liver biopsy and histopathological examination.
- Biochemical evaluation (increased lactate, cholesterol, triglyceride, and uric acid).
- Hematological examination.

Differential diagnosis
- Congenital neutropenia
- Cyclic neutropenia, agranulocytosis
- Hypophosphatasia, acatalasia
- Diabetes mellitus
- Chediak–Higashi syndrome

Treatment
- Symptomatic. Proper diet, good oral hygiene, and antibiotics for oral complications.

Lipoid Proteinosis

Definition
- Lipoid proteinosis, also known as hyalinosis cutis et mucosae or Urbach–Wiethe syndrome, is a chronic genetic disorder characterized by the deposition of an amorphous, hyaline-like material (glycoproteins) in the skin and mucous membranes.

Etiology
- Genetic. It is inherited as an autosomal recessive trait.

Occurrence in children
- Rare. The disorder may appear early in childhood, and aggravates with aging.

Localization
- Oral mucosa (tongue, frenulum, palate, lips).
- Other mucosae (larynx, pharynx, esophagus, vulva, rectum).
- Skin (face, eyelid margin and other areas) and rarely other organs.

Clinical features
- The oral manifestations are early, common, and usually become more severe with aging. The oral lesions consist of pallor of the oral mucosa and induration of the labial mucosa and the posterior part of the tongue. Progressively, the lip, tongue, and buccal mucosa become nodular, thickened, and enlarged, with a yellowish-white color (Fig. 20.**6**). The lingual frenulum becomes indurated, thick, and short, resulting in reduced mobility of the tongue. Finally, the oral mucosa becomes firm and glossy, with increased fissures and scarring. Oral infections, ulcers, recurrent parotid swelling, dysphagia, hypodontia, and enamel hypoplasia may also occur.
- Hoarseness is the most characteristic symptom, present from infancy or early childhood, and is due to vocal-cord involvement.
- The skin changes appear as yellowish-white papules, nodules, and pustules. Yellow, waxy, atrophic scars and hyperkeratotic plaques in areas exposed to pressure or trauma usually appear progressively (Fig. 20.**7**).

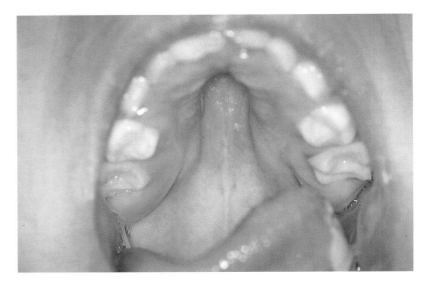

Fig. 20.**4**   Glycogen storage disease type Ib. High-arched palate

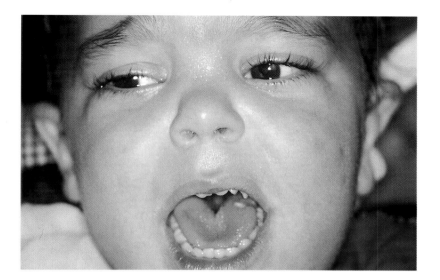

Fig. 20.**5** Glycogen storage disease type Ib. Characteristic facies (doll's face)

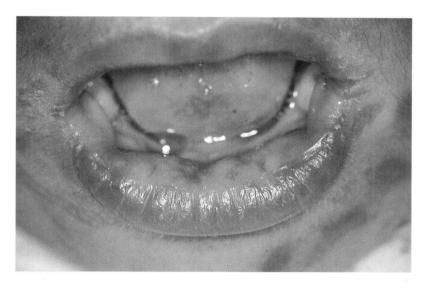

Fig. 20.**6** Lipoid proteinosis. Multilobulated and scarred lower lip

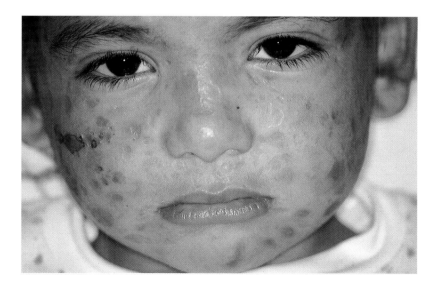

Fig. 20.**7** Lipoid proteinosis. Atrophic scars of the skin of the face

- Alopecia, hypohidrosis, hypertrichosis, and skin ulceration may occur (Fig. 20.**8**).
- Intracranial calcification is relatively common.

Laboratory tests

- Histopathologic examination of the skin and other mucosae reveals the deposition of a homogeneous, hyaline-like amorphous material (positive on the periodic acid–Schiff test) in the upper dermis, around the blood vessels, hair follicles, sweat glands, and erector pili muscles.

Differential diagnosis

- Hurler's syndrome
- Porphyria
- Amyloidosis

Treatment

- Symptomatic.

Cystic Fibrosis

Definition

- Cystic fibrosis is a hereditary, multisystemic, life-threatening disorder characterized by a dysfunction of the exocrine glands.

Etiology

- The pathological gene is located on chromosome 7, and produces a protein (CFTR) that causes a disturbance in chloride ion transport across the cell membranes. The condition is inherited as an autosomal recessive trait.

Occurrence in children

- Relatively common, approximately one in 2000 live births or more.

Localization

- All exocrine glands.
- Salivary gland involvement is relatively rare.

Clinical features

- Clinical manifestations from the pulmonary tract, gastrointestinal tract, and sweat glands are the main features.
- The oral manifestations are mild, and appear as lip enlargement or erythema, and gingival redness and mild dryness of the mouth (Figs. 20.**9,** 20.**10**).
- Pancreatic and liver insufficiency, deficiency of fat-soluble vitamins.
- Coughing is the most constant symptom of the pulmonary involvement. Pulmonary infections (*Staphylococcus aureus, Pseudomonas aeruginosa,* and *Hemophilus influenza*), extensive bronchiolitis, atelectasis, hemoptysis, pneumothorax, and cor pulmonale are common complications.
- Malabsorption, bulky, greasy stool, and failure to gain weight even with food intake are common findings. Abdominal pain and distension, intussusception, fecal impaction of the cecum, and rectal prolapse may occur.
- Sweating, with characteristic salty taste.
- Clubbing is a late sign (Fig. 20.**11**).

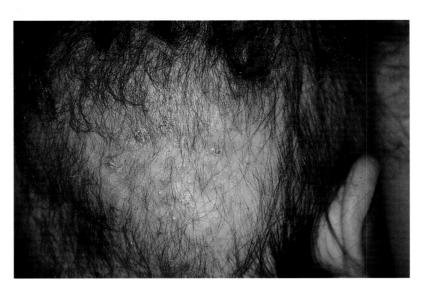

Fig. 20.**8** Lipoid proteinosis. Scarring and alopecia

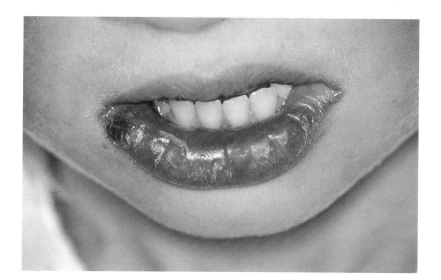

Fig. 20.**9** Cystic fibrosis. Enlargement of the lower lip and dryness

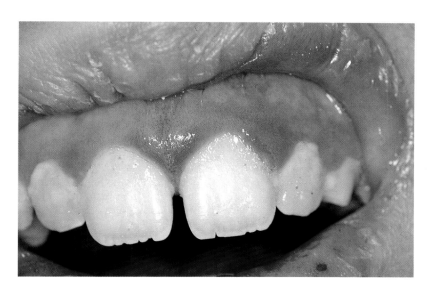

Fig. 20.**10** Cystic fibrosis. Gingival redness and dryness

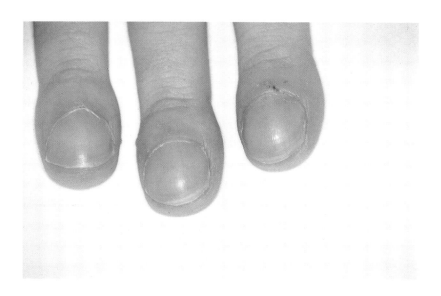

Fig. 20.**11** Cystic fibrosis. Clubbing

Laboratory tests

- Histopathological examination of the lip and minor salivary glands.
- Increased chloride, sodium and potassium levels in sweat.
- Absence of pancreatic enzymes in the intestinal fluid.
- Chest radiographic examination.

Differential diagnosis

- Cheilitis glandularis
- Cheilitis granulomatosa
- Lipoid proteinosis

Treatment

- High-calorie diet.
- Symptomatic.

Porphyria

Definition

- The porphyrias represent a group of disorders resulting from an abnormal porphyrin metabolism.

Etiology

- The disorders are caused by inborn enzymatic defects in the heme biosynthetic pathway. Each type of the disease is associated with a specific enzymatic defect that results in an excess of a specific porphyrin.
- Most types are inherited as autosomal dominant traits, and some as an autosomal recessive trait.

Classification

- On the basis of the principal site of the enzymatic defect, the porphyrias are classified into three major groups, each with several types: *erythropoietic, hepatic,* and *erythropoietic–hepatic*.

Occurrence in children

- Rare.
- The most common forms are the erythropoietic and the erythropoietic–hepatic.

Localization

- Skin, internal organs, nervous system.
- Rarely, the oral mucosa and teeth.

Clinical features

- In the oral cavity, a reddish-brown discoloration of the dentition is observed. Under ultraviolet light, the affected teeth show a characteristic reddish-pink fluorescence (congenital porphyria or Günther's disease).
- Erythema of the oral mucosa, atrophy, vesicles and ulcerations, especially on the lips and the vestibular gingiva, are rarely seen (in congenital erythropoietic porphyria and occasionally in porphyria cutanea tarda) (Figs. 20.**12,** 20.**13**).
- Skin lesions are common, and are characterized by photosensitivity, skin fragility, erythema, vesicles, bullae, ulcerations, milia atrophy and scar formation, hyperpigmentation, hypertrichosis (Figs. 20.**14**–20.**16**). Light-exposed areas of the skin are primarily affected.
- Neuropathy, psychosis, and signs and symptoms from various organs may occur.

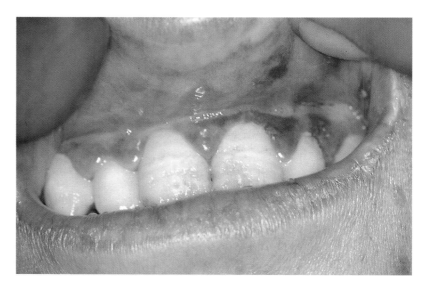

Fig. 20.**12** Porphyria cutanea tarda. Redness of the vestibular gingiva and atrophy of upper labial mucosa

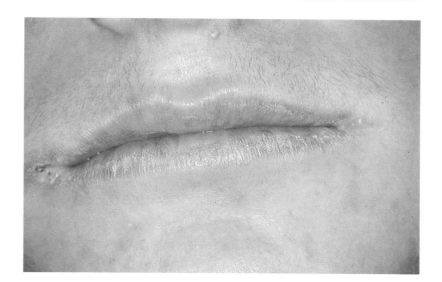

Fig. 20.**13**   Porphyria cutanea tarda. Angular cheilitis, telangiectasia, and scaling of the lips

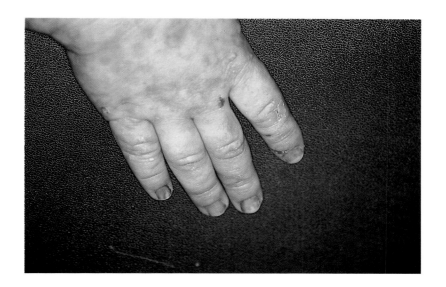

Fig. 20.**14**   Porphyria cutanea tarda. Scarring of the hand

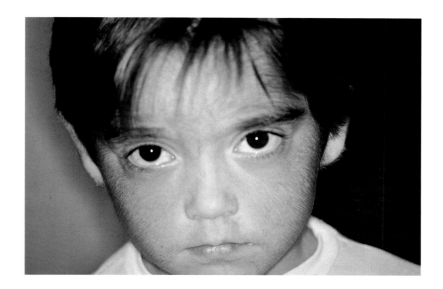

Fig. 20.**15**   Porphyria cutanea tarda. Facial hypertrichosis

Laboratory tests	• Biochemical tests (urine, fecal, erythrocytes). • Histopathological examination of skin biopsy. • Photobiological tests. • Direct immunofluorescence.
Differential diagnosis	• Epidermolysis bullosa • Chronic skin-blistering diseases • Lipoid proteinosis, pellagra
Treatment	• Protection from sun exposure. • Avoidance of alcohol drinks. • Antimalarial drugs, phlebotomy.

Acrodermatitis Enteropathica

Definition	• Acrodermatitis enteropathica is a rare hereditary nutritional disorder.
Etiology	• Zinc deficiency, due to defective absorption from the intestine. • It is inherited as an autosomal recessive trait.
Occurrence in children	• Exclusively. Usually appears a few weeks after birth.
Localization	• Skin (periorificial and acral), hair, and nails. • Oral mucosa and gastrointestinal tract.
Clinical features	• The oral manifestations usually include cheilitis, and less commonly, erythema, edema, and erosions of the oral mucosa. • The skin manifestations are characteristic, and begin with small, moist, erythematous lesions, classically located around the body orifices (mouth, eyes, nose, ears, congenital area) and symmetrically on the scalp, buttocks, extensor surface of the major joints and extremities. Vesiculobullous eruptions arise from an erythematous base, and in a few days become crusted and scaly, showing a psoriasiform pattern (Figs. 20.**17**, 20.**18**). Secondary infection with *Candida albicans* is common. • Hair loss, nail dystrophy, diarrhea, irritability, photophobia, and failure to thrive are common. • Growth retardation and, rarely, mental changes may also be seen.
Laboratory tests	• Serum zinc levels less than 50. • Low serum alkaline phosphatase levels.
Differential diagnosis	• Epidermolysis bullosa • Chronic skin-blistering diseases • Acquired immune deficiency syndrome (AIDS), premature infants with low zinc storage • Cystic fibrosis
Treatment	• Zinc administration. • Specific diet.

Diabetes Mellitus

Definition	• Diabetes mellitus represents a heterogeneous group of disorders in carbohydrate, protein, and lipid metabolism, resulting in macrovascular and specific microvascular complications.
Etiology	• The basic problem is either decreased production of insulin, or tissue resistance to the effects of insulin, or a combination of the two.
Classification	• Type 1 diabetes. • Type 2 diabetes. • Gestational diabetes. • Other types.
Occurrence in children	• Common.
Clinical features	• The oral manifestations associated with diabetes mellitus are variable and non-specific. They are usually seen in patients with poorly controlled diabetes.

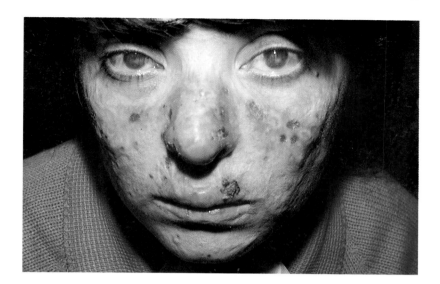

Fig. 20.**16**   Congenital erythropoietic porphyria. Ulcers and scarring of the face

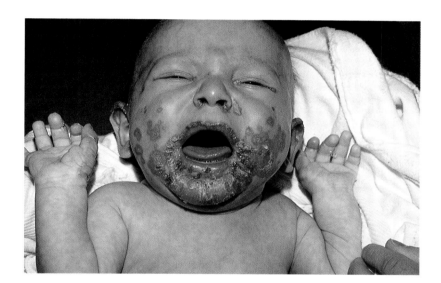

Fig. 20.**17**   Acrodermatitis enteropathica. Typical lips and perioral
and face lesions

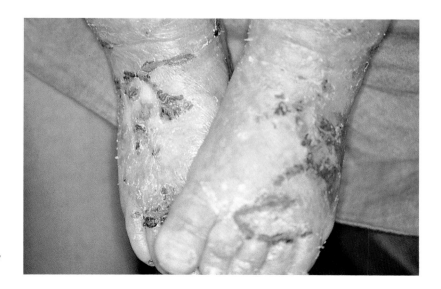

Fig. 20.**18**   Acrodermatitis
enteropathica. Erosions covered by
scaling

- Gingivitis, periodontitis, and increased incidence of caries are common (Figs. 20.**19,** 20.**20**).
- Xerostomia, salivary gland enlargement.
- Small erosions, retardation of wound healing.
- Oral candidiasis and other bacterial infections.
- Burning mouth syndrome and taste disorders.

Treatment
- Treatment of the oral lesions includes a high standard of oral hygiene and periodontal therapy.

Amyloidosis

Definition
- Amyloidosis is a rare metabolic disorder characterized by the extracellular deposition of amyloid, a fibrillary proteinaceous material, in various tissues and organs.

Etiology
- Unknown.

Classification
- *Primary, secondary, familial, senile,* and several subtypes.

Occurrence in children
- Very rare, mainly the secondary and familial forms.

Localization
- Many tissues and organs; oral involvement is extremely rare.

Clinical features
- The oral manifestations include petechiae, ecchymoses, nodules or tumors, and ulcers.
- Induration and enlargement of the tongue and of the major, and less frequently of the minor, salivary glands.
- Characteristic red color of the lesions.

Laboratory tests
- Histopathological examination and specific dyes (Congo red, thioflavine-T, and crystal violet).

Differential diagnosis
- Lipoid proteinosis
- Epidermolysis bullosa
- Macroglossia

Treatment
- Symptomatic.

Langerhans Cell Histiocytosis

Definition
- Langerhans cell histiocytosis, or histiocytosis X, represents a clinically heterogeneous disorder characterized by proliferation of Langerhans cells.

Etiology
- Remains obscure.

Classification
- The spectrum of Langerhans cell histiocytosis traditionally includes three clinical forms: Letterer–Siwe disease, Hand–Schüller–Christian disease, and eosinophilic granuloma.

Occurrence in children
- Common.

Localization
- Bones, skin, oral mucosa, visceral, bone marrow.

Clinical features
- *Letterer–Siwe disease* is the acute disseminated form of the disease, characterized by fever, chills, lymphadenopathy, hepatomegaly and splenomegaly, osteolytic bone lesions, generalized skin eruption (petechiae, scaly papules, nodules, vesicles, ulcers) and oral manifestations (Figs. 20.**21**). The oral lesions include ecchymoses, ulcerations, gingivitis, periodontitis, bone involvement, and loose teeth (Figs. 20.**22,** 20.**23**). The disease mainly occurs in infants, and has a severe prognosis.

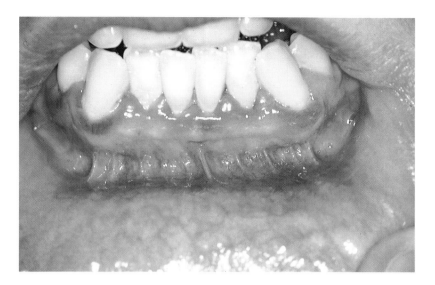

Fig. 20.**19**   Diabetes mellitus. Periodontitis

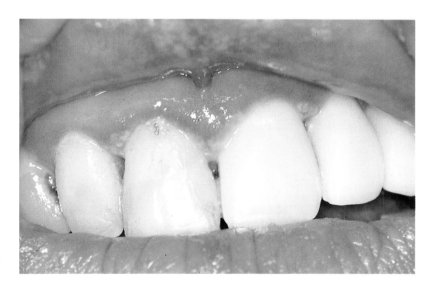

Fig. 20.**20**   Diabetes mellitus. Periodontitis and candidiasis

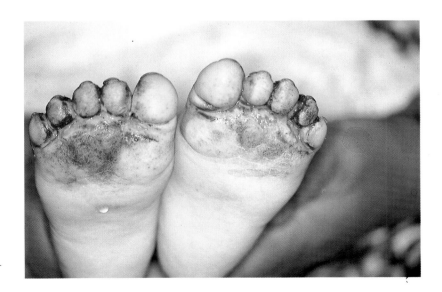

Fig. 20.**21**   Letterer–Siwe disease.
Necrotic ulcers of the feet

● *Hand–Schüller–Christian disease* is the chronic disseminated form of the disease, which is characterized by the classic triad: osteolytic bone lesions, diabetes insipidus, and exophthalmos (Fig. 20.**24**). Otitis media, onycholysis, skin rash, and oral manifestations may occur (Fig. 20.**25**). The oral lesions include ulcers, edema, gingival hyperplasia and necrosis, bone jaw lesions and loosening of the teeth, taste disturbances, halitosis, and retardation of wound healing (Fig. 20.**26**). The disease affects children between three and six years old, and generally has a good prognosis.

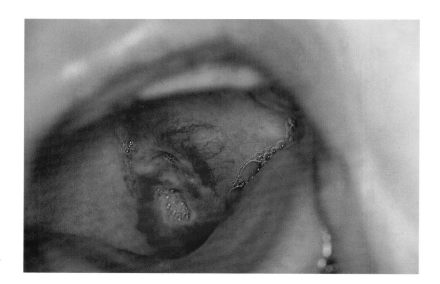

Fig. 20.**22** Letterer–Siwe disease. Deep ulcers on the soft palate

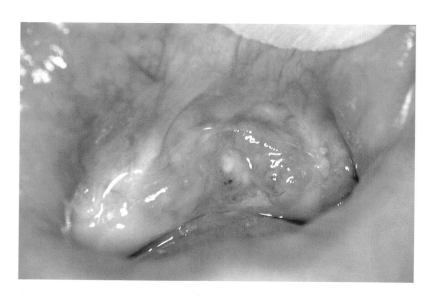

Fig. 20.**23** Letterer–Siwe disease. Irregular ulcers and disfigurement of the upper lip and alveolar mucosa

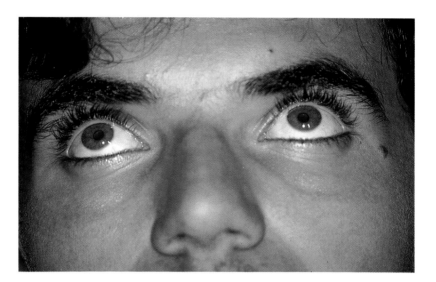

Fig. 20.**24**   Hand–Schüller–
Christian disease. Exophthalmos

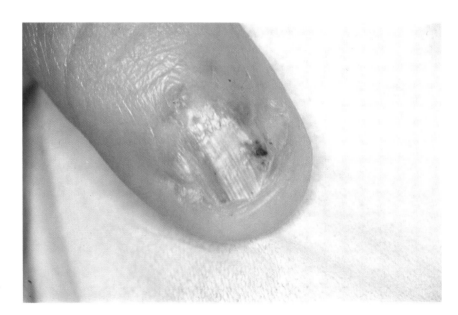

Fig. 20.**25**   Hand–Schüller–Christian disease. Onycholysis

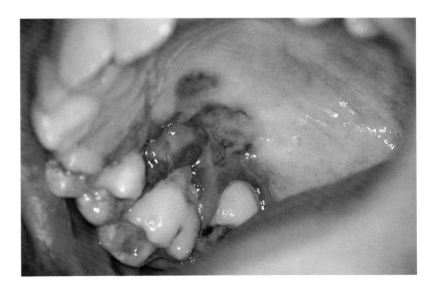

Fig. 20.**26**   Hand–Schüller–Christian disease. Multiple irregular ulcers and bone destruction on the
palate and gingiva

- *Eosinophilic granuloma* represents the localized benign form of the disease, usually characterized by asymptomatic solitary or multiple bone lesions. The jaws are frequently affected, resulting in bone destruction, loosening of the teeth, or even tooth loss. Ulcerations on the gingiva and palate may also be seen (Fig. 20.**27**). This form of the disease commonly develops in puberty or in young adults, and has a good prognosis.

Laboratory tests

- The histopathological examination is of diagnostic significance, and shows a proliferation of histiocytes, numerous eosinophils, and other cell types that contribute to the mechanism of inflammation (Fig. 20.**28**). In addition, monocytes, phagocytes, and multinucleated giant cells are seen, as well as areas of necrosis.
- Immunohistochemically, Langerhans cells stain positively for S-100 protein.
- The radiographic examination usually reveals sharply punched-out or ill-defined radiolucencies.

Differential diagnosis

- Eosinophilic ulcer
- Juvenile periodontitis
- Acatalasia
- Hypophosphatasia

Treatment

- Radiotherapy.
- Curettage, corticosteroids, and chemotherapeutic drugs.

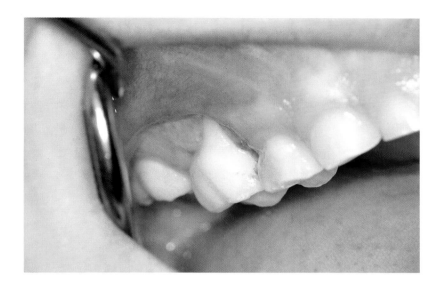

Fig. 20.**27**   Eosinophilic granuloma. Ulcer on the gingiva and bone destruction

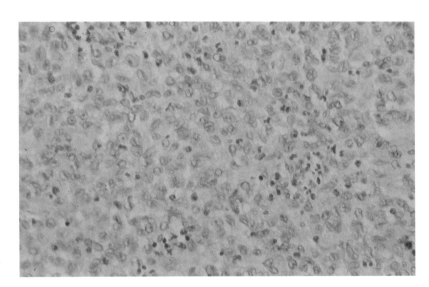

Fig. 20.**28**   Langerhans cell histiocytosis. Histiocytes and numerous eosinophils, in the typical histological pattern of the disease

21 Bacterial Infections

Scarlet Fever

Definition
- Scarlet fever, or scarlatina, is an acute infectious disease.

Etiology
- It is caused by group A β-hemolytic streptococci, which produce an erythrogenic toxin.

Occurrence in children
- Common in children under 10 years of age.

Localization
- Skin (trunk, neck, axillae, extremities, and face).
- Mouth (cheeks, tongue, lips, palate, and pharynx).

Clinical features
- After an incubation period of two to four days, the disease presents with fever (39–40 °C) and chills, headache, malaise, nausea, vomiting, pharyngitis, and submandibular lymphadenopathy.
- One to two days later, the skin rash appears. It is a diffuse, confluent macular erythema, with characteristic pallor of the perioral region.
- The oral mucosa is erythematous and edematous. Characteristically, the tongue is covered with a thick white coating, which later exfoliates. The uncovered fungiform papillae are enlarged, giving the tongue a characteristic strawberry appearance (Figs. 21.**1,** 21.**2**).
- The diagnosis is based on clinical criteria, and bacteriological confirmation is rarely required.

Differential diagnosis
- Measles
- Infectious mononucleosis
- Kawasaki's disease
- Drug reactions

Treatment
- Penicillin or erythromycin.

Actinomycosis

Definition
- Actinomycosis is a chronic granulomatous infectious disease.

Etiology
- The anaerobic Gram-positive bacterium *Actinomyces israelii*.

Occurrence in children
- Rare. Mainly the cervicofacial form.

Localization
- Mandibular angle and submandibular region; rarely the soft tissues of the mouth.

Clinical forms
- Cervicofacial
- Thoracic
- Abdominal

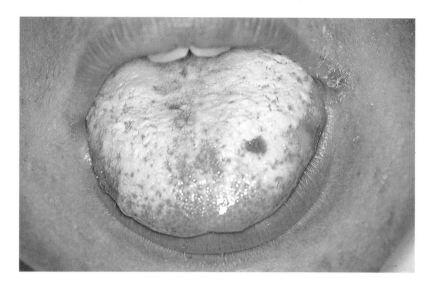

Fig. 21.**1**   Scarlet fever. Enlarged fungiform papillae of the tongue

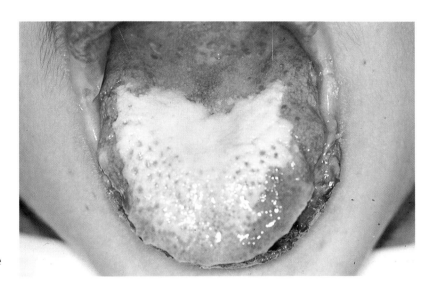

Fig. 21.**2**   Scarlet fever. Enlarged fungiform papillae, erythema, and white coating of the dorsum of the tongue

Clinical features

- The cervicofacial is the most common form.
- Painless, slow-growing hard swelling, erythema, trismus.
- Multiple abscesses and draining sinuses on the skin of the face and upper neck (Figs. 21.**3**, 21.**4**).
- Exudation of yellow purulent material, bearing the characteristic "sulfur granules," which consist of *Actinomyces* colonies.
- Rarely, the regional lymph nodes and the thyroid are involved.

Laboratory tests

- Culture of the exudate and isolation of the actinomyces.
- Biopsy and histopathological examination (Fig. 21.**5**).

Differential diagnosis

- Dental and periodontal abscess
- Tuberculosis
- Systemic mycoses

Treatment

- Penicillin, erythromycin or tetracyclines.
- Surgical debridement is necessary in most cases.

Tuberculosis

Definition

- Tuberculosis is a chronic granulomatous infectious disease.

Etiology

- *Mycobacterium tuberculosis*, and rarely *M. bovis*, *M. africanum*, and *M. microti*.
- The disease is usually transmitted by inhalation of infected droplets that have been expelled into the air by a person with active disease.

Occurrence in children

- Relatively frequent, and rising worldwide.

Localization

- Most commonly the lungs, but another organ in the body may be involved.
- The mouth is secondarily involved, usually from pulmonary tuberculosis.
- The tongue, palate, gingivae, lips, and tonsils are the oral sites most frequently affected.

Clinical features

- The typical lesion is a vegetating, usually painless and irregular ulcer.
- The ulcer has a thin, undermined border 1–5 cm in diameter.
- The surface of the ulcer is usually covered by a gray-yellowish exudate, and the surrounding tissues are mildly indurated with inflammation.
- Nodular, granular, and white lesions may be seen less often.
- Tuberculous osteomyelitis of the jaws and periapical tuberculous granuloma may also occur.
- Submandibular and cervical lymphadenopathy are frequent, occasionally with fistula (scrofula) formation (Figs. 21.**6**, 21.**7**).

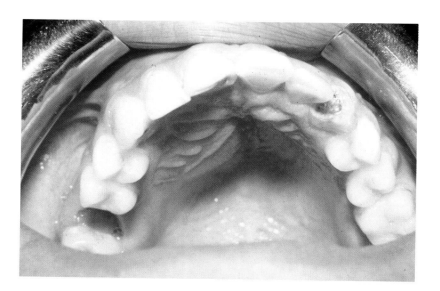

Fig. 21.**3**   Actinomycosis. Abscess and swelling of the palate

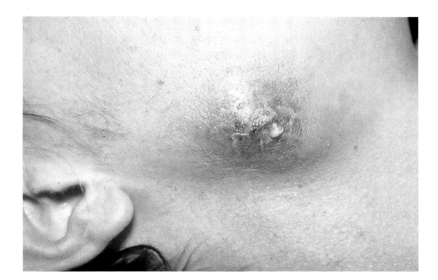

Fig. 21.**4** Actinomycosis. Inflammation and draining fistula on the skin at the angle of the mandible

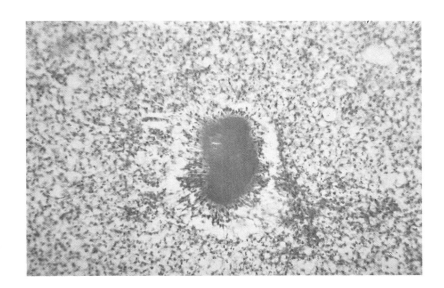

Fig. 21.**5** Actinomycosis. Colony of *Actinomyces*, surrounded by polymorphonuclear leukocytes

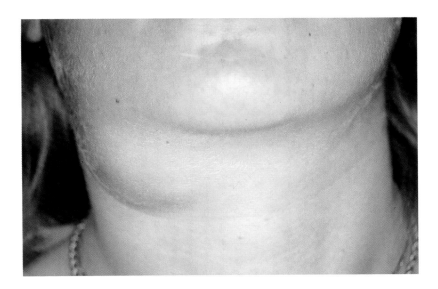

Fig. 21.**6** Tuberculosis. Submandibular and cervical lymph-node swelling

Laboratory tests

- Mantoux tuberculin skin test.
- Chest radiographs.
- Bacterial examination of sputum, urine, body fluids, and tissues.
- Histopathological examination of the oral lesions reveals granulomatous inflammation, usually with caseation.

Differential diagnosis

- Aphthous ulcers
- Traumatic ulcers
- Squamous-cell carcinoma
- Necrotizing sialadenometaplasia
- Systemic mycoses
- Actinomycosis
- Syphilis

Treatment

- Antituberculous multiple-drug regimens.

Syphilis

Definition

- Syphilis is a sexually transmitted disease.

Etiology

- *Treponema pallidum.*

Occurrence in children

- Rare.
- The disease may be transmitted congenitally from an infected mother to her offspring, transplacentally during gestation, or through contact with perigenital lesions during labor.
- Adolescents may be infected during early unprotected sexual contacts with high-risk partners.

Classification

- Syphilis is classified as *early* or *late*. Early syphilis is defined as having been present for one year or less after the initial infection, whereas late syphilis is present for more than one year.
- Syphilitic stigmata are dysplastic lesions of congenital etiology, in the absence of active disease. Stigmata occur frequently in the mouth.

Clinical features

- *Primary syphilis*
- This is characterized by the appearance of the *syphilitic chancre* at the site of inoculation of the spirochete, usually three weeks post-inoculation.
- The chancre is usually round and covered with whitish exudate. It has a slightly raised border, and is relatively hard on palpation (Fig. 21.**8**).
- Atypical primary chancres, taking the form of erosions, are frequent (Fig. 21.**9**).
- The most commonly involved oral site is the tongue, followed by the lips, palate, and the floor of the mouth. Ipsilateral painless regional lymphadenopathy is always present.
- This phase of the disease lasts for three to eight weeks.
- *Secondary syphilis*
- The lesions of secondary syphilis become apparent six to eight weeks after the appearance of the primary ulcer.
- *Syphilitic mucosal plaques* are the most frequent oral lesions. They take the form of slightly raised plaques with a whitish surface.

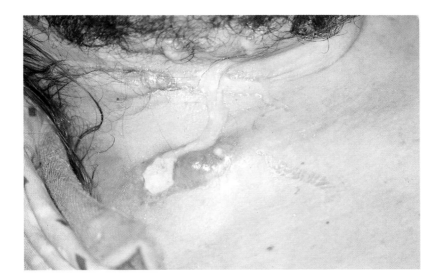

Fig. 21.**7** Tuberculosis. Cervical lymphadenopathy with numerous fistulas (scrofula)

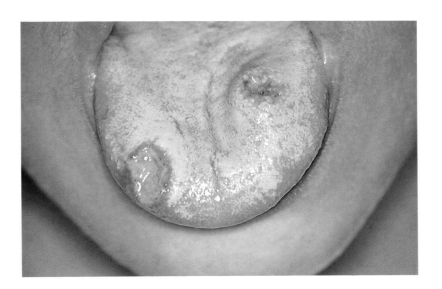

Fig. 21.**8** Primary syphilis. Two syphilitic chancres on the tongue

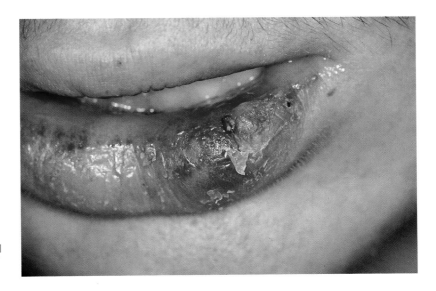

Fig. 21.**9** Primary syphilis. Atypical chancre on the vermilion border of the lower lip

- The lesions are most often painless and multiple, involving the palate, buccal mucosa, tongue, palate, gingiva, floor of the mouth, tonsils, etc. (Fig. 21.**10**).
- The glans penis is a frequent extraoral location (Fig. 21.**11**).
- *Condylomata lata* are hypertrophic papules, appearing in the perirectal region and rarely at the angles of the lips (Fig. 21.**12**).
- *Syphilitic papules* are the most frequent finding in secondary syphilis, and occur on the palms, soles, and trunk.
- *Generalized lymphadenopathy* is a characteristic sign of secondary syphilis.
- *Congenital syphilis*
- *Oral syphilitic stigmata* are dental abnormalities such as: notched, screwdriver-shaped incisors (Hutchinson's incisors), and tubercular molars (mulberry molars, Moon's molars) (Fig. 21.**13**).
- Enamel dots may also occur.
- Arched palate, short mandible, narrow palatal vault, atrophic glossitis, and perioral rhagades (fissures) may also occur.

Laboratory tests

- Dark-field microscopy in a smear material from active primary or secondary lesions of syphilis.
- Serological testing: rapid plasmin reagin (RPR), Venereal Disease Research Laboratory (VDRL) test, fluorescent treponemal antibody (FTA).

Differential diagnosis

- Dysplastic teeth of congenital or other etiology
- Traumatic ulcers
- Aphthous ulcers
- Herpetic ulcers
- Candidiasis
- Infectious mononucleosis

Treatment

- Penicillin.
- Erythromycin.
- Cephalosporins.

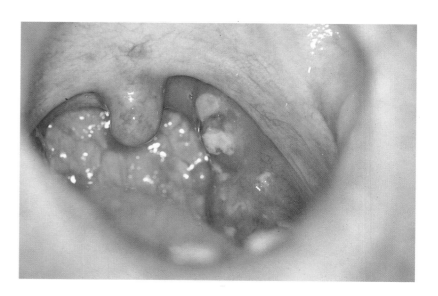

Fig. 21.**10** Secondary syphilis. Numerous mucosal plaques on the tonsil

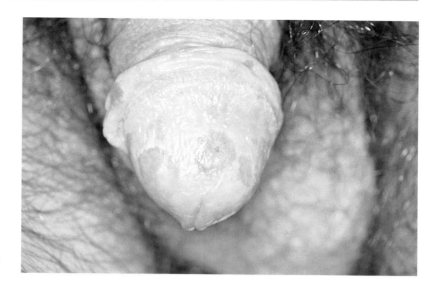

Fig. 21.**11** Secondary syphilis. Numerous mucosal plaques on the glans penis

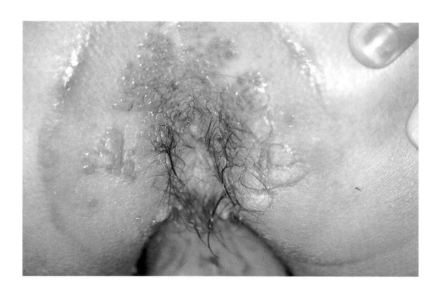

Fig. 21.**12** Secondary syphilis. Condylomata lata of the perirectal area

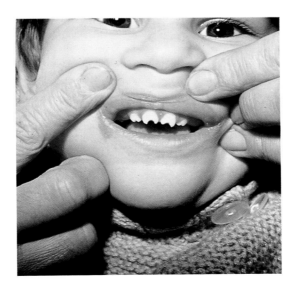

Fig. 21.**13** Congenital syphilis. Typical Hutchinson's incisors

22 Viral Infections

Measles

Definition
- Measles is an acute, eruptive, highly contagious disease of childhood.

Etiology
- It is caused by an RNA paramyxovirus.
- The virus is acquired via droplets that enter the respiratory tract.

Occurrence in children
- Common. Measles is an obligatory disease of childhood.

Localization
- Skin (face, neck, trunk, limbs).
- Mouth (buccal mucosa, lip mucosa, tongue gingiva).

Clinical features
- The incubation period is 8–12 days.
- The disease is heralded three to four days prior to the eruption by a prodrome consisting of moderate fever, chills, cough, myalgias, catarrh, photophobia, and conjunctivitis.
- Koplik's spots, whitish specks on a red base, appear on the buccal mucosa adjacent to the molar teeth one or two days prior to the eruption.
- Redness of the oral mucosa, petechiae, and small, round ulcerations may also appear (Fig. 22.**1**).
- The characteristic maculopapular dull red skin eruption first appears on the face, and then spreads to the neck, trunk and limbs over the next two days (Fig. 22.**2**).
- The diagnosis is based on clinical criteria.

Differential diagnosis
- Infectious mononucleosis
- Varicella
- Herpetiform ulcers
- Herpetic stomatitis

Treatment
- Symptomatic.
- Preventive vaccination is strongly recommended in pediatric guidelines.

Varicella

Definition
- Varicella or chickenpox is an eruptive, benign, highly contagious infection in children.

Etiology
- Varicella-zoster virus (VZV), a member of the herpes group of viruses.

Occurrence in children
- Almost exclusively.

Localization
- Skin (face, head, trunk)
- Mouth (palate, lip mucosa, buccal mucosa).

Clinical features
- The incubation period is 10–20 days.
- A prodrome of fever and headache heralds the onset of varicella.
- Small vesicles appear in the mouth, which rupture soon after their appearance, leaving small, round, shallow erosions surrounded by a red halo with a whitish bottom (Fig. 22.**3**).

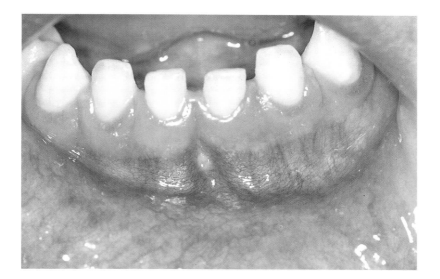

Fig. 22.**1**   Measles. Small, round ulcer on the labial frenulum

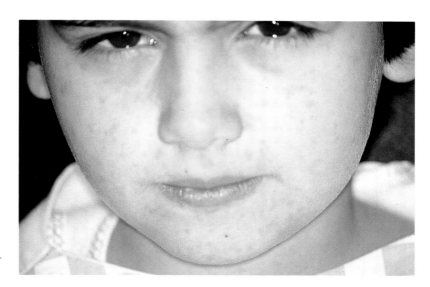

Fig. 22.**2**   Measles. Maculopapular eruption on the face

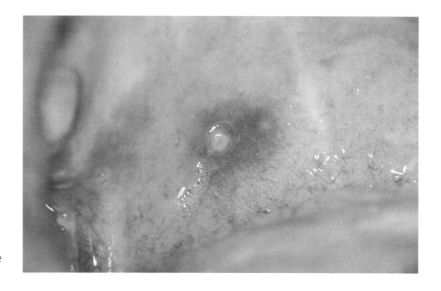

Fig. 22.**3**   Varicella. Small, round erosions surrounded by a red zone on the palate

- The characteristic variegated maculopapular, vesicular eruption spreads over the skin surfaces of the face, trunk, and head, with new elements appearing every two to three days during the course of the disease (Fig. 22.**4**).
- The vesicles and pustules rupture, and are covered with brownish crusts that later exfoliate.
- Rare complications of varicella are encephalitis (more common and severe in adults), pneumonitis, and Reye's syndrome.
- The diagnosis is based on clinical criteria.

Differential diagnosis
- Primary and secondary herpetic stomatitis
- Hand, foot, and mouth disease
- Measles

Treatment
- Symptomatic; acyclovir.

Infectious Mononucleosis

Definition
- Infectious mononucleosis is an acute, self-limited infectious disease.

Etiology
- Epstein–Barr virus (EBV). It is transmitted via the saliva or respiratory droplets, usually by kissing ("kissing disease").

Occurrence in children
- Common.

Localization
- Skin, lymph nodes, spleen, liver.
- Mouth (soft palate, uvula, tonsils, gingiva).

Clinical features
- The incubation period is 5–30 days, followed by low-grade fever that persists for one to two weeks; fatigue, malaise, mild headache, anorexia, and sore throat also occur.
- Generalized lymphadenopathy begins early, and is the most consistent sign.
- The oral manifestations are early and frequent, with the most constant sign being palatal petechiae (Fig. 22.**5**).
- Uvular edema, tonsillar exudate, gingivitis, pericoronitis, diffuse erythema, and rarely ulcerations may also occur.
- A maculopapular exanthem, usually on the trunk and arms, is present in 5–15% of cases (Figs. 22.**6**, 22.**7**).

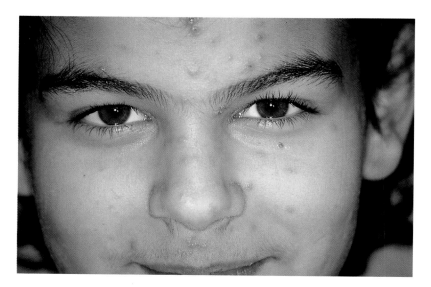

Fig. 22.**4** Varicella. Vesicular and maculopapular eruption on the face

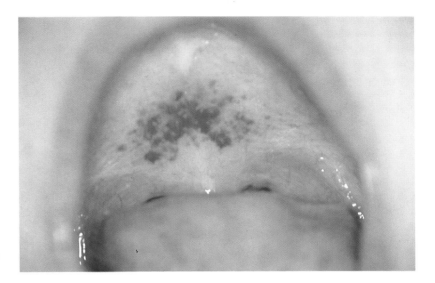

Fig. 22.**5**   Infectious mononucleosis. Petechiae on the palate

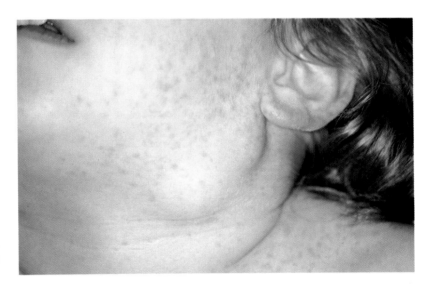

Fig. 22.**6**   Infectious mononucleosis. Maculopapular eruption on the skin and lymph-node enlargement

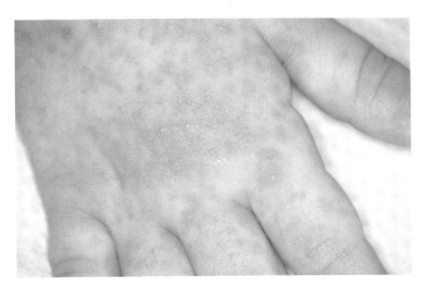

Fig. 22.**7**   Infectious mononucleosis. Diffuse maculopapular eruption on the hand

- Splenomegaly, hepatomegaly, and rarely central nervous system involvement may occur.
- The clinical diagnosis should be confirmed by specific laboratory tests.

Laboratory tests
- Mononucleosis spot test
- Paul–Bunnel test
- EBV IgM test

Differential diagnosis
- Herpetic gingivostomatitis
- Streptococcal oropharyngitis
- Vincent's infection
- Diphtheria
- Leukemia
- Drug reaction

Treatment
- There is no specific treatment. It is mainly supportive.

Hand, Foot, and Mouth Disease

Definition
- Hand, foot, and mouth disease is an acute epidemic enterovirus infection.

Etiology
- Usually coxsackievirus A16, and occasionally with A4, A5, A9, A10, or other types.

Occurrence in children
- Common.

Localization
- Mouth (buccal mucosa, labial mucosa, soft palate, uvula, tongue).
- Hand and foot (the lateral and dorsal surfaces of the fingers and toes, palms and soles).
- Rarely, the buttocks and other regions may be involved.

Clinical features
- An incubation period of three to six days, usually with mild prodromal symptoms (low-grade fever, malaise, headache) precedes the oral and skin manifestations.
- The oral lesions are almost always present, and are characterized by small vesicles that soon rupture, leaving painful, shallow ulcers surrounded by a red halo (Fig. 22.**8**).
- The number of the lesions varies from two to 20 or more, and they are usually 2–8 mm in diameter.
- The skin lesions present as multiple small vesicles surrounded by a narrow red halo (Figs. 22.**9**, 22.**10**).
- The disease lasts five to eight days.
- The diagnosis is based on clinical criteria.

Laboratory tests
- Viral cultures and serological investigations are recommended only in doubtful cases.

Differential diagnosis
- Aphthous ulcers
- Herpetic ulcers
- Herpangina
- Erythema multiforme

Treatment
- Symptomatic.

Mumps

Definition
- Mumps, or epidemic parotitis, is an acute viral infection that primarily involves the salivary glands.

Etiology
- Paramyxovirus.

Occurrence in children
- Common.

Localization
- Parotid gland.
- Less often, the submandibular and sublingual glands may also be involved.

Clinical features
- After an incubation period of 16–18 days, low-grade fever, chills, headache, malaise, and sore throat develop, and are accompanied by pain in the parotid area.

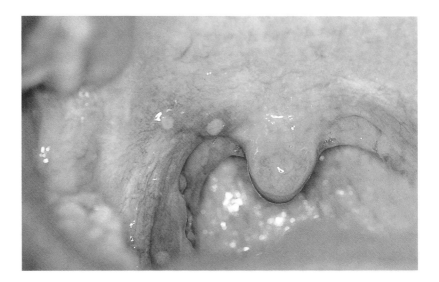

Fig. 22.**8**   Hand, foot, and mouth disease. Round shallow ulcers on the soft palate

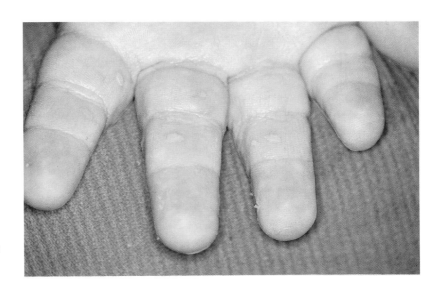

Fig. 22.**9**   Hand, foot, and mouth disease. Small vesicles on the fingers

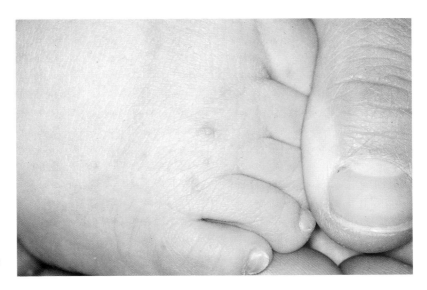

Fig. 22.**10**   Hand, foot, and mouth disease. Small vesicle of the dorsum of the foot

- Tender, rubbery, and edematous swelling of one or both of the parotids is the presenting sign, and lasts for about a week (Fig. 22.**11**).
- The opening of the parotid duct is frequently erythematous and edematous.
- Pain on chewing and on pressure beneath the angle of the mandible are common findings.
- The most common complications are orchitis and epididymitis, and rarely meningoencephalitis and pancreatitis.
- The diagnosis is usually based on clinical criteria.

Laboratory tests

- Viral cultures and serological examination may be helpful for the diagnosis.

Differential diagnosis

- Acute suppurative parotitis
- Angioedema
- Calculi in the salivary duct
- Buccal cellulitis
- Other viral infections
- Parotid gland emphysema
- Sjögren's syndrome

Treatment

- Vaccination against mumps is indicated for all children, with a high rate of protection.
- Symptomatic, including bed rest during the febrile period, and analgesics.

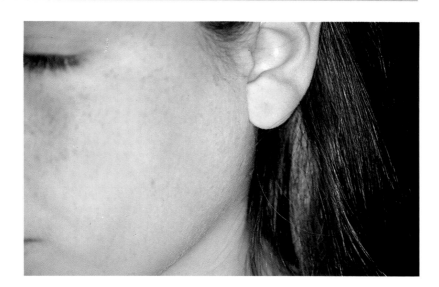

Fig. 22.**11**   Mumps. Parotid swelling

23 HIV Infection and AIDS

Herpes Simplex

Definition
- Herpes simplex is a relatively common viral infection in patients infected with human immunodeficiency virus (HIV).
- It may be primary or secondary.

Etiology
- Usually, herpes simplex virus type 1 (HSV-1), and rarely type 2 (HSV-2).

Occurrence in children
- Relatively common, either as primary or secondary form.

Localization
- Gingiva, lips, palate, tongue, perioral skin.

Clinical features
- The clinical features are similar to those in non–HIV-infected children (Fig. 23.**1**).
- However, recurrences are more frequent, and the duration of lesions is usually longer and more severe.
- The diagnosis is usually based on clinical criteria.

Differential diagnosis
- Aphthous ulcers
- Herpangina
- Hand, foot, and mouth disease
- Erythema multiforme
- Acute necrotizing ulcerative gingivitis
- Linear gingival erythema

Treatment
- Symptomatic. Also, systemic acyclovir.

Hairy Leukoplakia

Definition
- Hairy leukoplakia is one of the most common features of HIV infection.
- Rarely, it can appear in immunosuppressed patients after organ transplantation.

Etiology
- Epstein–Barr virus (EBV).

Occurrence in children
- Rare.

Localization
- Lateral border of the tongue, often bilateral.
- Less often, it may spread to the dorsum and the ventral surface of the tongue.

Clinical features
- White, asymptomatic, often elevated and unremovable patch.
- Typically, the surface of the lesions is corrugated, with a vertical orientation (Figs. 23.**2**, 23.**3**).
- Smooth and flat lesions may also occur.
- The lesions may be superinfected with *Candida albicans*.
- The lesion is not precancerous.

Laboratory tests
- Histopathological examination.
- Demonstration of EBV by in-situ hybridization or polymerase chain reaction (PCR).
- Electron microscopy.

Differential diagnosis
- Candidiasis
- Lichen planus
- Geographic tongue
- Leukoedema
- Chronic biting
- White sponge nevus
- White lesions due to restorative material
- Cinnamon contact stomatitis

Treatment
- Usually not needed.
- In severe cases, systemic acyclovir.

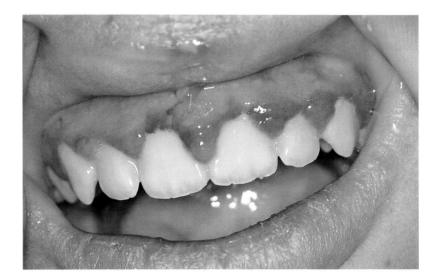

Fig. 23.**1**   HIV infection. Herpetic gingivitis

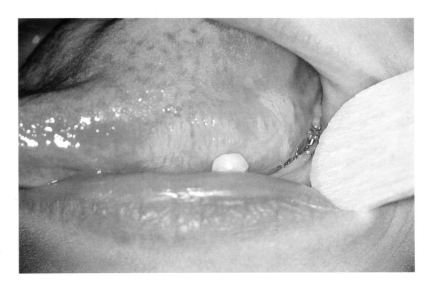

Fig. 23.**2**   HIV infection. Hairy leukoplakia on the lateral border of the tongue in a nine-year-old boy

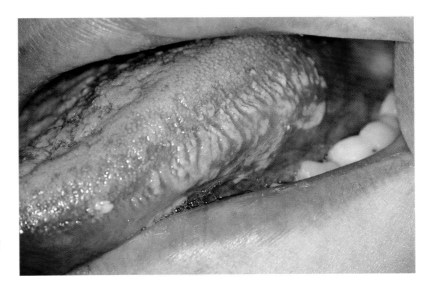

Fig. 23.**3**   HIV infection. Hairy leukoplakia on the lateral border of the tongue in a 17-year-old hemophiliac boy

Candidiasis

Definition
- Candidiasis is one of the most common opportunistic infections in HIV-infected patients.

Etiology
- Often *Candida albicans,* and less often other *Candida* species.

Occurrence in children
- Common. It is the most common early lesion in HIV-infected children.

Localization
- Buccal mucosa, soft palate, tongue, commissures, lips.

Clinical features
- Four forms of oral candidiasis have been recorded in HIV-infected patients: *pseudomembranous, erythematous, angular cheilitis,* and *hyperplastic.* Mucocutaneous candidiasis may also occur.
- The *pseudomembranous* form is the most common in HIV-infected children, and less often the erythematous. It presents as creamy-white or yellowish plaques or spots on a red or normal-colored mucosa (Figs. 23.**4,** 23.**5**). On scraping, the lesions are usually removed, leaving a red surface.
- The *erythematous* form presents as fiery red, ill-demarcated patches.
- The lesions may be localized or disseminated.
- Xerostomia and a burning sensation may occur.
- Diagnosis is usually based on clinical criteria.

Laboratory features
- Direct microscopic examination of smears.
- Culture.

Differential diagnosis
- Hairy leukoplakia
- Lichen planus
- Chronic biting
- Leukoedema

Treatment
- Topical (nystatin, amphotericin B, miconazole), or systemic (ketoconazole, fluconazole, itraconazole), antifungal agents.

Linear Gingival Erythema

Definition
- Linear gingival erythema is a unique gingival manifestation of HIV-infected patients.

Etiology
- Plaque microflora.
- *Candida* species play an important role.

Occurrence in children
- Rare.

Localization
- Along the margin of the gingiva, usually localized.

Clinical features
- It presents as a fiery red band along the margin of the gingiva, 2–4 mm in width (Fig. 23.**6**).
- Punctate erythema of the alveolar gingiva may also occur.
- Swollen interdental papillae may be present.
- Gingival bleeding, spontaneously or on brushing.
- Poor response to plaque control measures.
- The lesion is usually superinfected with *Candida albicans.*
- The diagnosis is based on clinical criteria.

Differential diagnosis
- Chronic gingivitis
- Herpetic gingivitis

Treatment
- Good oral hygiene.
- Mouth rinsing with providone iodine 10% or 0.1–0.2% chlorhexidine gluconate.
- Topical antifungal agents (nystatin, myconazole).

Kaposi's Sarcoma

Definition
- Kaposi's sarcoma is a multicentric neoplastic process, probably of endothelial origin.
- It is the most common tumor associated with acquired immune deficiency syndrome (AIDS).

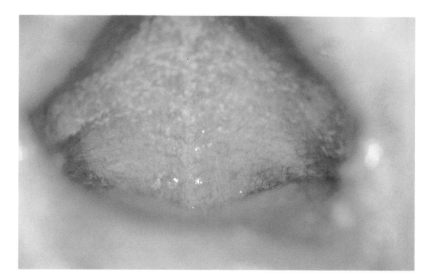

Fig. 23.**4**   HIV infection. Acute pseudomembranous candidiasis on the palate

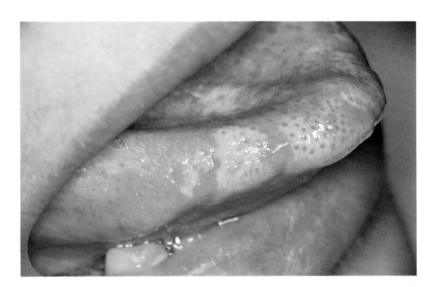

Fig. 23.**5**   HIV infection. Chronic pseudomembranous candidiasis on the tongue

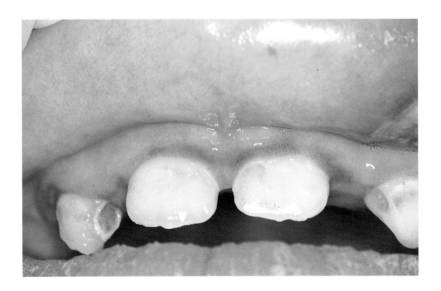

Fig. 23.**6**   HIV infection. Linear gingival erythema

Etiology
- Presumably herpesvirus type 8, immunodeficiency.

Classification
- Classic, African (endemic), immunosuppression-associated, and AIDS Kaposi's (epidemic).

Occurrence in children
- Very rare.

Localization
- Skin (head and neck, trunk, arms).
- Oral mucosa (common palate and gingiva). Less commonly, buccal mucosa, lips, tongue.
- Lymph nodes, viscera.

Clinical features
- AIDS-related Kaposi's sarcoma primarily involves the skin, oral and other mucosae, lymph nodes, and viscera.
- The size of the lesions varies from a few to several centimeters.
- The skin lesions are usually darker and larger (Fig. 23.**7**).
- Oral lesions may present as asymptomatic multiple or solitary reddish, brownish-red, or bluish macules or patches.
- In later stages, the lesions may become elevated, often lobulated, and ulcerated and tender (Fig. 23.**8**).
- The clinical diagnosis should be confirmed by a biopsy.

Laboratory tests
- The histopathological features consist of bands of spindle cells and plump endothelial cells and atypical vascular channels.
- Hemorrhage, hemosiderin deposition, lymphocytes and plasma-cell infiltratrion, and scattered mitoses of the spindle cells are common.

Differential diagnosis
- Pyogenic granuloma
- Peripheral giant-cell granuloma
- Bacillary angiomatosis
- Hemangioma
- Angiosarcoma

Treatment
- Alpha-interferon, chemotherapy, radiotherapy, and occasionally surgery.

Salivary Gland Enlargement

Definition
- Salivary gland enlargement, mainly parotid, is a relatively common manifestation in HIV-infected children.
- The prevalence varies from 10% to 20%.
- The parotid swelling may be unilateral or bilateral, and occurs late during the infection.
- The swelling may be persistent or transient, and usually reccurs.
- It is usually painless, and may rarely be associated with xerostomia.

Etiology
- The etiology is unknown. However, it has been suggested that cytomegalovirus infection may be responsible.

Treatment
- Treatment is symptomatic and empirical.

Other Lesions

- As the numbers of HIV-infected children have increased dramatically during the last few decades, the prevalence and spectrum of oral manifestations is increasing.
- The spectrum of oral lesions in HIV-infected children differs from that in adults. It is necessary to pay more attention to pediatric AIDS in order to record all the oral lesions and their significance for the diagnosis and prognosis of HIV infection.
- In addition to the common oral manifestations in HIV-infected children (candidiasis, herpes simplex, parotid enlargement, linear gingival erythema), several other lesions have also been recorded, including the following:
- Atypical ulcerations (Figs. 23.**9**, 23.**10**).
- Exfoliative cheilitis.
- Hairy tongue (Fig. 23.**11**).

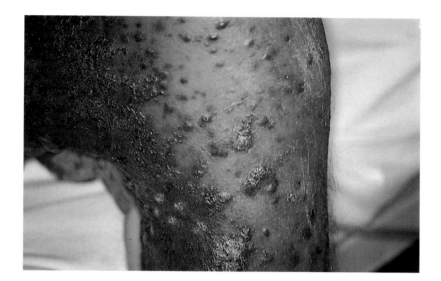

Fig. 23.**7**   AIDS. Kaposi's sarcoma on the leg in a 17-year-old hemophiliac boy

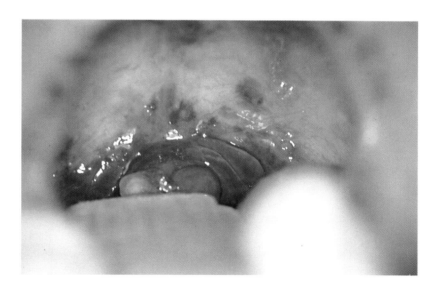

Fig. 23.**8**   AIDS. Kaposi's sarcoma on the soft palate and uvula (same patient as in Fig. 23.**7**)

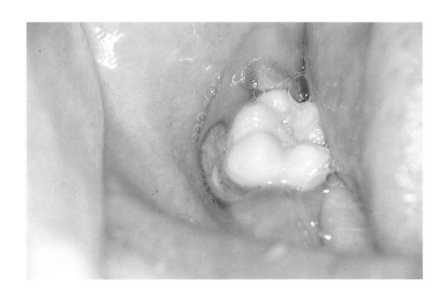

Fig. 23.**9**   HIV infection. Atypical ulcer on the gingiva

- Dysplastic lesions of the teeth (Fig. 23.**12**).
- Ulcerations due to rare bacterial infection in the oral cavity, e.g. *Pseudomonas aeruginosa* (Fig. 23.**13**).
- Clubbing (Fig. 23.**14**).

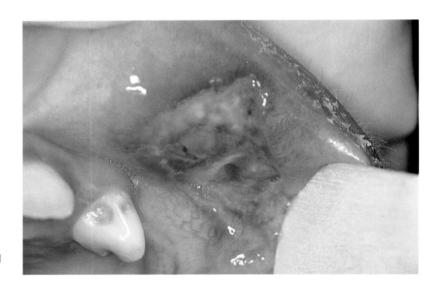

Fig. 23.**10**   HIV infection. Atypical large ulcer on the buccal mucosa

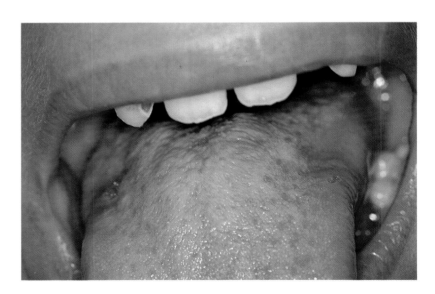

Fig. 23.**11**   HIV infection. Hairy tongue

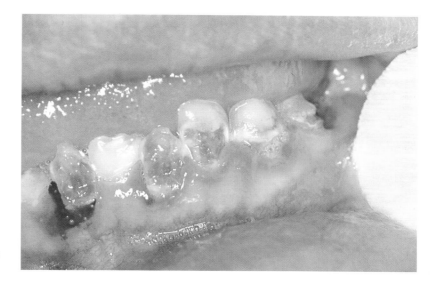

Fig. 23.**12** HIV infection. Multiple dental caries

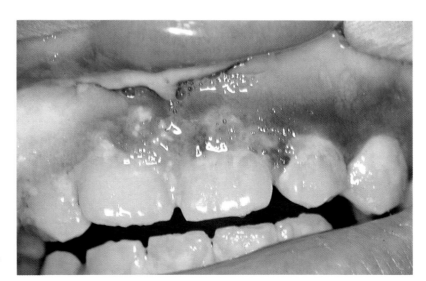

Fig. 23.**13** HIV infection. Large ulcer on the gingiva due to *Pseudomonas aeruginosa*

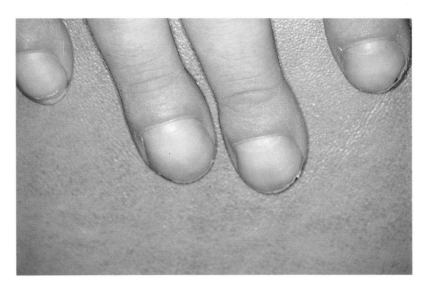

Fig. 23.**14** HIV infection. Clubbing

24 Systemic Mycoses

General aspects
- Systemic mycoses involve many organs and systems.
- Oral tissues have rarely been involved in systemic mycoses. However, over the past few years, oral manifestations have increased, particularly in immunocompromised patients.
- The oral cavity is a common site for infection by some mycoses (aspergillosis, cryptococcosis, histoplasmosis, mucormycosis), and it is the most common site in children with neoplasias.
- Some of the systemic mycoses are endemic in certain areas—e.g., histoplasmosis (Ohio and Mississippi valleys in the United States), blastomycosis (Mississippi, Missouri, and Ohio river valleys and in Southern Canada), coccidioidomycosis (arid parts of America), paracoccidioidomycosis (South America).
- Others—e.g., aspergillosis, cryptococcosis, histoplasmosis, and mucormycosis—more often affect immunosuppressed and immunocompromised patients.

Etiology
- Aspergillosis (*Aspergillus* species, particularly *A. fumigatus* and *A. flavus*).
- Histoplasmosis (*Histoplasma capsulatum*).
- Cryptococcosis (*Cryptococcus neoformans*).
- Mucormycosis (mainly *Mucor* and *Rhizopus*).
- Coccidioidomycosis (*Coccidioides immitis*).
- Paracoccidioidomycosis (*Paracoccidioides brasiliensis*).
- Blastomycosis (*Blastomyces dermatitidis*).

Occurrence in children
- Rare.

Localization
- Palate, buccal mucosa, tongue, gingiva, maxillary antrum.

Clinical features
- Oral mycotic lesions often appear as nodules and chronic vegetating ulcers, with a tendency to increase in size (Fig. 24.**1**).
- Yellow-black, necrotic ulcers are also common (aspergillosis, mucormycosis).
- Nasal and/or paranasal sinus signs and symptoms are common in some mycoses (mucormycosis, aspergillosis).
- Important for the diagnosis is a history of travel in endemic areas, or an immunocompromising state.
- The final diagnosis should be based on laboratory examination.

Laboratory tests
- Smear examination.
- Biopsy and histopathological examination.
- Culture of the affected tissues.

Differential diagnosis
- Oral tuberculosis
- Squamous-cell carcinoma
- Non-Hodgkin's lymphoma
- Eosinophilic ulcer
- Malignant granuloma
- Wegener's granulomatosis

Treatment
- Amphotericin is the drug of choice for most systemic mycoses.
- Itraconazole, ketoconazole, and fluconazole are also useful in some cases.
- Surgical debridement may be used in mucormycosis.

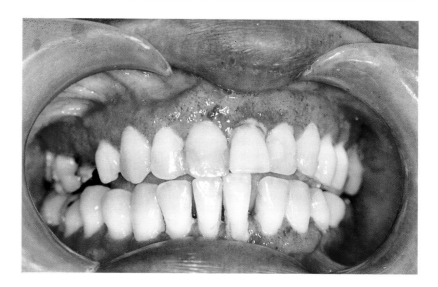

Fig. 24.**1**   Paracoccidioidomycosis.
Vegetating ulcers on the gingiva

25 Benign Tumors

Oral Squamous Papilloma

Definition
- Squamous papilloma is a relatively common benign proliferation of the oral stratified squamous epithelium.

Etiology
- Presumably human papillomavirus (HPV).

Occurrence in children
- Relatively common.

Localization
- Palate, uvula, tongue, lips, gingiva.

Clinical features
- Exophytic well-circumscribed, usually pedunculated, painless growth with characteristic numerous small finger-like projections, tending to produce a cauliflower surface formation (Figs. 25.**1**–25.**3**).
- The lesions are usually white, but they may be slightly red or normal in color.
- The size varies from a few millimeters to 0.5–1.0 cm in diameter. The lesions are usually solitary, although they may develop in multiple sites.
- The diagnosis is usually made clinically.

Histopathology
- It is characterized by keratinized stratified squamous epithelium, proliferating in a finger-like pattern with a delicate, fibrous connective-tissue core.
- Koilocytosis of the epithelial cells and variable degrees of chronic inflammatory change in the connective tissue may be found.

Differential diagnosis
- Verruca vulgaris
- Condyloma acuminatum
- Verruciform xanthoma
- Focal dermal hypoplasia syndrome

Treatment
- Surgical removal.

Traumatic Fibroma

Definition
- Traumatic fibroma, or irritation fibroma, is the most common "tumor" of the oral mucosa.
- In the great majority of cases, the lesion is a reactive focal fibrous hyperplasia of the connective tissue.
- The true neoplasm is thought to be very rare.

Etiology
- Chronic trauma.

Occurrence in children
- Relatively rare.

Localization
- Buccal mucosa, tongue, labial mucosa.

Clinical features
- The lesion typically presents as a painless, well-defined, firm, sessile or pedunculated tumor with a smooth surface of normal epithelium (Figs. 25.**4**, 25.**5**).
- The size ranges from 0.5 cm to 2 cm in diameter.
- The surface may occasionally be traumatically ulcerated.
- The clinical diagnosis should be confirmed by a biopsy.

Histopathology
- Dense and collagenized excess production of connective tissue.
- The covering epithelium is often thin and hyperkeratotic.
- Scattered, sparse inflammation may be seen.

Differential diagnosis
- Neurofibroma
- Schwannoma
- Granular-cell tumor
- Lipoma
- Peripheral ossifying fibroma
- Mucocele

Treatment
- Surgical removal

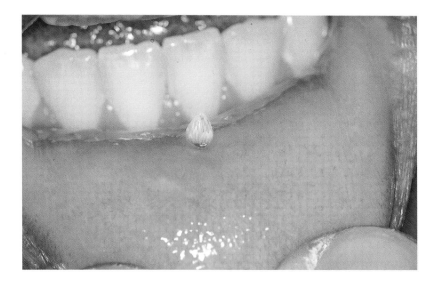

Fig. 25.**1**   Papilloma of the lower lip mucosa

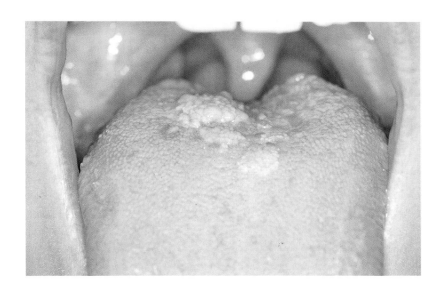

Fig. 25.**2**   Papillomas of the dorsum of the tongue

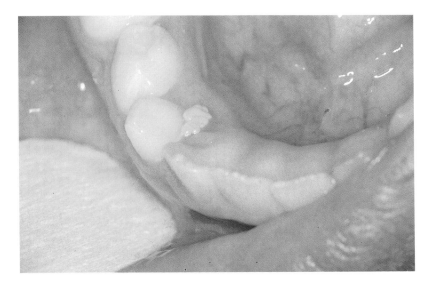

Fig. 25.**3**   Papilloma of the gingiva

Peripheral Ossifying Fibroma

Definition

- Peripheral ossifying fibroma is a relatively common reactive gingival growth.

Etiology

- Unknown; local irritation may play a role.
- It is probably derived from cells of the periodontal ligament or the periosteum.

Occurrence in children

- Relatively common.

Localization

- Exclusively on the gingiva, usually in the incisor–cuspid region of both jaws.

Clinical features

- It presents as a well-defined, firm, sessile, or pedunculated tumor, which often starts from the interdental papilla and is covered by normal epithelium (Fig. 25.**6**).
- The surface is frequently ulcerated, due to mechanical trauma.
- The size varies from 0.5 cm to 2.0 cm in diameter.
- The clinical diagnosis should be confirmed by a biopsy.

Histopathology

- Fibrous cellular proliferation associated with the formation of dystrophic calcifications, cementum-like components, bone, or osteoid.
- Multinucleated giant cells may occasionally be seen.
- Chronic inflammatory cells may be present at the periphery of the lesion.
- The covering epithelium is usually thin, or may be ulcerated.

Differential diagnosis

- Traumatic fibroma
- Pyogenic granuloma
- Peripheral giant-cell granuloma

Treatment

- Surgical removal.

Schwannoma

Definition

- Schwannoma, or neurilemoma, is a benign neural tumor.

Etiology

- Unknown.
- It derives from the Schwann cells of the nerve sheath.

Occurrence in children

- Very rare.

Localization

- Often the tongue, and rarely the palate, buccal mucosa, floor of the mouth, gingiva, and lips.

Clinical features

- The lesion presents as a slow-growing, well-circumscribed, encapsulated submucosal tumor, usually covered by normal epithelium (Fig. 25.**7**).
- It is usually asymptomatic, fairly firm on palpation, and may range from a few millimeters to 2 cm in size.
- The clinical diagnosis should be confirmed by a biopsy.

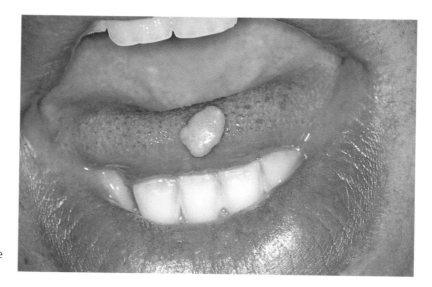

Fig. 25.**4** Traumatic fibroma of the tongue

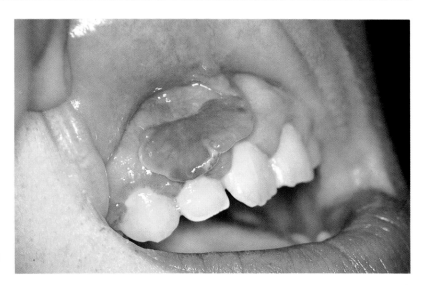

Fig. 25.**5**   Traumatic fibroma of the alveolar mucosa

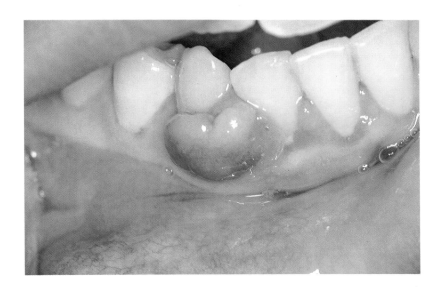

Fig. 25.**6**   Peripheral ossifying fibroma of the gingiva

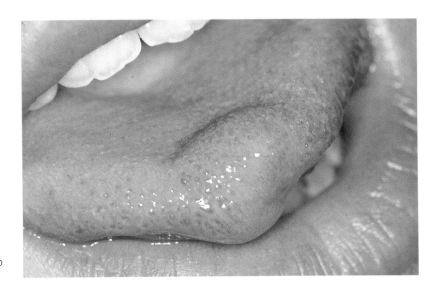

Fig. 25.**7**   Schwannoma on the tip of the tongue

Histopathology
- Encapsulated spindle cells that assume two different patterns, *Antoni A* and *Antoni B*.
- *Antoni A* consists of spindle cells organized in a palisaded pattern, frequently surrounding a cellular eosinophilic area (Verocay bodies).
- *Antoni B* consists of spindle cells randomly distributed in a loose fibrillar stroma (Fig. 25.**8**).

Differential diagnosis
- Fibroma
- Neurofibroma
- Granular-cell tumor
- Leiomyoma
- Traumatic neuroma

Treatment
- Surgical removal.

Neurofibroma

Definition
- Neurofibroma is a benign overgrowth of nerve tissue origin.

Etiology
- Unknown.
- Schwann cells and perineural fibroblasts are the cells of origin.

Occurrence in children
- Rare.

Localization
- The tongue and buccal mucosa are the areas most commonly affected.

Clinical features
- It may appear either as a solitary tumor or as multiple lesions, representing a manifestation of neurofibromatosis (von Recklinghausen's disease).
- Solitary neurofibroma presents as a slow-growing, painless, well-defined submucosal firm tumor, covered by normal epithelium (Fig. 25.**9**).
- The size varies from several millimeters to several centimeters.
- The clinical diagnosis should be confirmed by a biopsy.

Histopathology
- It consists of spindle-shaped cells with fusiform or wavy nuclei in a dedicate connective-tissue matrix, which may be myxoid.
- Mast cells are characteristically found scattered through the connective tissue.

Differential diagnosis
- Schwannoma
- Granular-cell tumor
- Fibroma
- Lipoma
- Neurofibromatosis

Treatment
- Surgical removal.

Granular-Cell Tumor

Definition
- Granular-cell tumor, or granular-cell myoblastoma, is an uncommon, benign lesion.

Etiology
- Unknown.
- It is currently believed to originate from Schwann cells; another possibility is that it is derived from undifferentiated mesenchymal cells.

Occurrence in children
- Rare.

Localization
- Tongue, buccal mucosa.

Clinical features
- It presents as an asymptomatic, well-defined, sessile nodule, which may be slightly elevated (Figs. 25.**10**, 25.**11**).
- The nodule is firm on palpation, with a whitish, reddish, or yellowish color.
- The size varies from 0.5 cm to 2.0 cm in diameter.
- The lesion is usually solitary, but multiple lesions may rarely be seen.
- The clinical diagnosis should be confirmed by a biopsy.

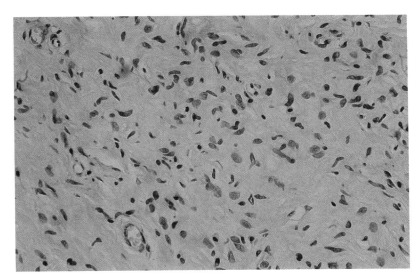

Fig. 25.**8**   Schwannoma. Spindle cells randomly distributed in a loose fibrillar stroma (Antoni B)

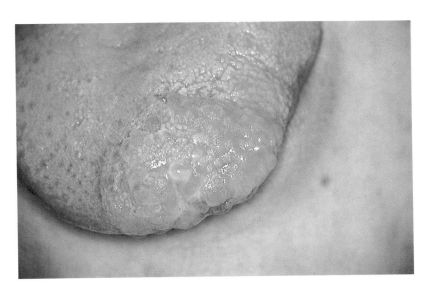

Fig. 25.**9**   Neurofibroma on the tip of the tongue

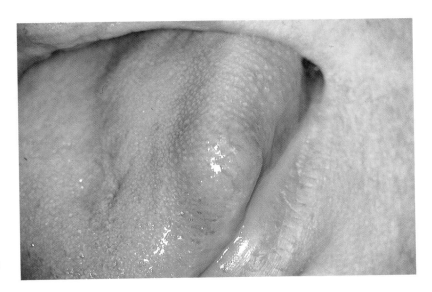

Fig. 25.**10**   Granular-cell tumor on the left border of the tongue

Histopathology

- It consists of large polygonal cells with pale eosinophilic granular cytoplasm and small nuclei. Pseudoepitheliomatous hyperplasia of the covering epithelium is a common finding (Fig. 25.**12**).
- Immunohistochemically, the tumor cells contain S-100 protein.

Differential diagnosis

- Schwannoma
- Neurofibroma
- Fibroma
- Rhabdomyoma
- Granular-cell tumor of the newborn

Treatment

- Surgical removal.

Granular-Cell Tumor of the Newborn

Definition

- Granular-cell tumor of the newborn, or congenital epulis, is a unique tumor that occurs only in newborns.

Etiology

- Unknown.
- The histogenesis is unclear, but it may be of pericyte origin or primitive mesenchymal cell origin.

Occurrence in children

- Rare.

Localization

- Exclusively on the alveolar ridges of newborns.

Clinical features

- It presents at birth as an asymptomatic, usually pedunculated, tumor of normal or reddish color, with a smooth surface (Fig. 25.**13**).
- It is usually solitary, but multiple lesions may occur (Fig. 25.**14**).
- The size ranges from 0.5 cm to 2.0 cm or more in diameter.
- The tumor is found about nine times more frequently in girls than in boys, and the maxillary ridge in the canine–incisor region is more commonly affected.
- The clinical diagnosis should be confirmed histopathologically.

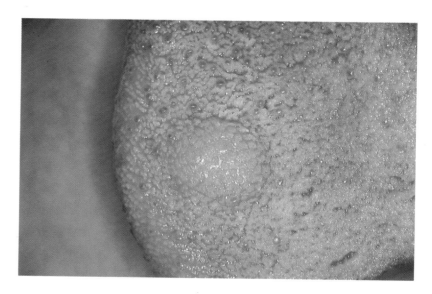

Fig. 25.**11** Granular-cell tumor on the dorsum of the tongue

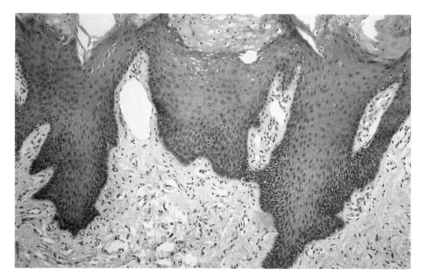

Fig. 25.**12**   Granular-cell tumor.
Pseudoepitheliomatous hyperplasia
of the epithelium and large polygonal cells, with eosinophilic granular cytoplasm in the corium

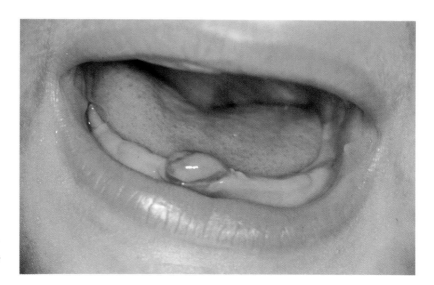

Fig. 25.**13**   Granular-cell tumor of
the newborn, on the alveolar ridge
of the mandible

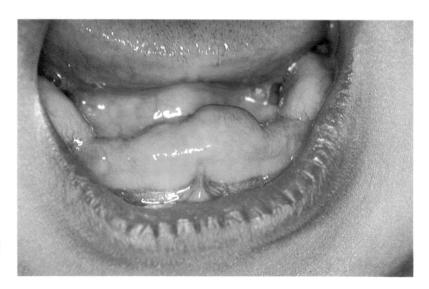

Fig. 25.**14**   Granular-cell tumors of
the newborn, on the alveolar ridge
of the mandible

Histopathology

- The lesion consists of sheets of large polygonal cells with pale, granular eosinophilic cytoplasm and round, small nuclei (Fig. 25.**15**).
- Characteristically, the overlying epithelium is thin, with atrophy of the rete ridges (Fig. 25.**16**).
- Immunohistochemical staining for S-100 protein is negative.

Differential diagnosis

- Melanotic neuroectodermal tumor of infancy
- Hamartomas
- Pyogenic granuloma
- Gingival cysts

Treatment

- Surgical removal.

Lymphangioma

Definition

- Lymphangioma is a benign disorder of the lymphatic vessels.

Etiology

- It is a developmental malformation rather than a true neoplasm.

Occurrence in children

- Common. About 50% of lymphangiomas are usually present at birth, and about 80–90% appear during the first three years of life.

Localization

- The dorsum of the tongue is the most common location; less often it may be found on the lips, buccal mucosa, soft palate, and floor of the mouth.
- Cervical lesions are also common.

Clinical features

- Lymphangiomas are classified into three forms: capillary lymphangioma, cavernous lymphangioma, and cystic hygroma, depending on the size of the lymphatics.
- Superficial lesions present as small, soft, elevated nodules that resemble a cluster of small "vesicles" with normal or yellow-grayish or red color due to secondary hemorrhage into the lymphatic spaces (Figs. 25.**17**–25.**19**).
- Deep lesions present as a soft, diffuse mass without color alteration.
- The size ranges from a few millimeters to extremely large lesions that cause organ deformities.
- Large, diffuse soft swelling may develop on the neck, extending to the submandibular, sublingual area and the parotid, producing facial swelling (cystic hygroma) (Fig. 25.**20**).

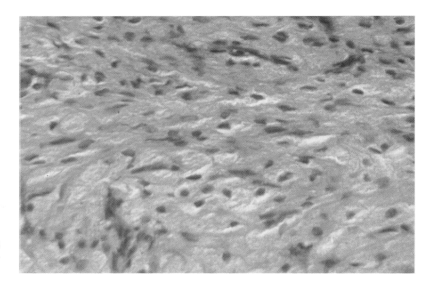

Fig. 25.**15** Granular-cell tumor of the newborn. Large polygonal cells with pale, granular eosinophilic cytoplasm and small, round nuclei

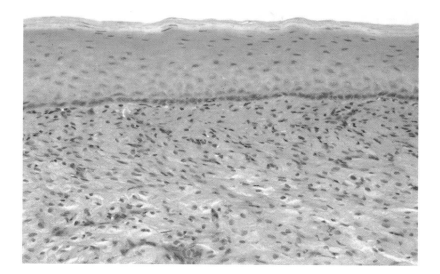

Fig. 25.**16** Granular-cell tumor of the newborn. Thin covering epithelium without rete ridges

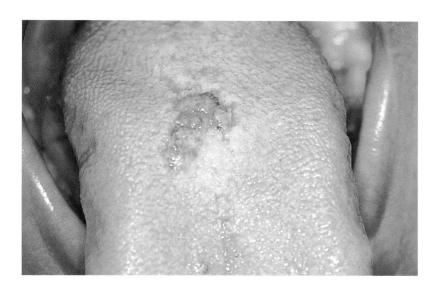

Fig. 25.**17** Lymphangioma. Localized lesion on the dorsum of the tongue

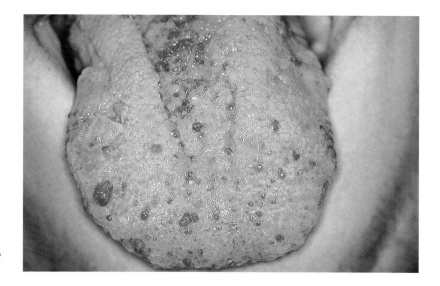

Fig. 25.**18** Lymphangioma. Scattered lesions on the dorsum of the tongue

- The lesions are usually asymptomatic. However, when they become larger, they may cause pain and discomfort during speech, chewing, and swallowing, or macroglossia.
- Recurrent infection of the lesion is common.
- The diagnosis is usually made clinically.

Histopathology

- The lesion consists of multiple dilated lymphatic vessels that are lined by thin endothelium located just beneath the epithelial surface (Fig. 25.**21**).
- The spaces are filled by lymphocytes, proteinaceous fluid, and occasionally red blood cells.

Differential diagnosis

- Hemangioma
- Median rhomboid glossitis
- Lingual thyroid
- Branchial cyst
- Mucocele
- Deep lymphangioma should be differentiated from other mesenchymal tumors.

Treatment

- Surgical removal. Recurrence is common.

Hemangioma

Definition

- Hemangiomas represent a benign proliferation of blood vessels.

Etiology

- It is a developmental malformation rather than a true neoplasm.

Occurrence in children

- Common. It is primarily a lesion of childhood, and is usually present at birth.

Localization

- Lips, tongue, buccal mucosa, alveolar mucosa, and gingiva.

Clinical features

- Two main forms of oral hemangioma are recognized: *capillary* and *cavernous.*
- *Capillary hemangioma* is the most common form, and it appears clinically as a flat, bright red area that may progressively become slightly elevated (Figs. 25.**22**, 25.**23**). After approximately two to three years, it may undergo slow, spontaneous resolution.

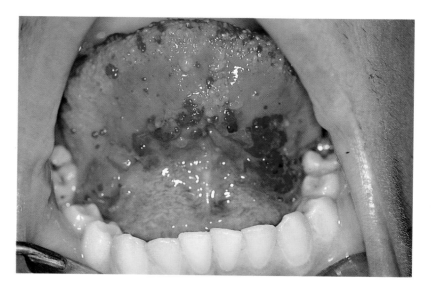

Fig. 25.**19** Lymphangioma on the ventral surface of the tongue

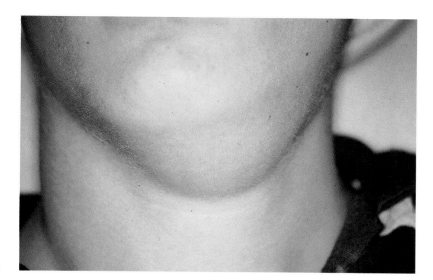

Fig. 25.**20**   Cystic hygroma. Sublingual and submandibular swelling

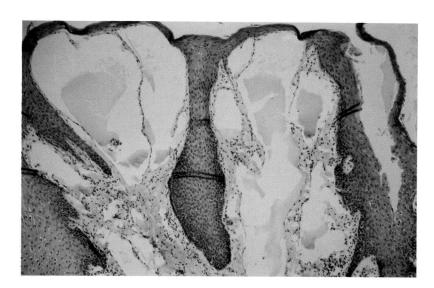

Fig. 25.**21**   Lymphangioma. Multiple dilated lymphatic vessels just beneath the epithelial surface

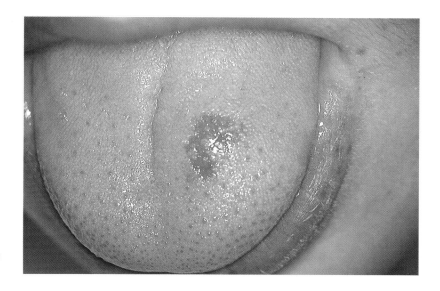

Fig. 25.**22**   Capillary hemangioma on the tongue

- *Cavernous hemangioma* is less common, and clinically appears as an elevated large lesion of deep red color (Figs. 25.**24**, 25.**25**). It usually involves deeper structures, and rarely undergoes spontaneous regression.
- The characteristic clinical sign in both forms is that the red color disappears on pressure, and returns when the pressure is released.
- The size ranges from a few millimeters to extensive lesions that may cause organ deformities (e.g. macroglossia, macrocheilia).
- Hemorrhage is the most common complication.
- Combined lesions with features of hemangioma and lymphangioma are not uncommon.
- Rarely, jaw lesions may occur.
- The diagnosis is usually made clinically.

Histopathology

- Capillary hemangioma consists of multiple capillary vascular spaces.
- Cavernous hemangioma consists of multiple large dilated sinuses filled with blood.
- Occasionally, a mixture of capillary and cavernous blood vessels may occur.

Differential diagnosis

- Pyogenic granuloma
- Peripheral giant-cell granuloma
- Leiomyoma
- Bacillary angiomatosis
- Kaposi's sarcoma
- Several syndromes with oral vascular lesions (e.g. Rendu–Osler–Weber, Maffucci's, Sturge–Weber, Klippel–Trenaunay–Weber).

Treatment

- Surgical removal.
- Laser therapy.
- Embolization, injection of sclerosing agents.

Pyogenic Granuloma

Definition

- Pyogenic granuloma is a common non-neoplastic tumor-like lesion.

Etiology

- It presumably represents an exaggerated tissue reaction to mild irritation or trauma.

Occurrence in children

- Relatively common.

Localization

- The gingiva is the most common site (70–75%). Less common sites are the tongue, lips, and buccal mucosa.

Clinical features

- It appears as a painless, nodular, light red mass that is pedunculated or sessile.
- The surface may be smooth or lobulated, and is often ulcerated, covered by a white-yellowish pseudomembrane (Figs. 25.**26**, 25.**27**).

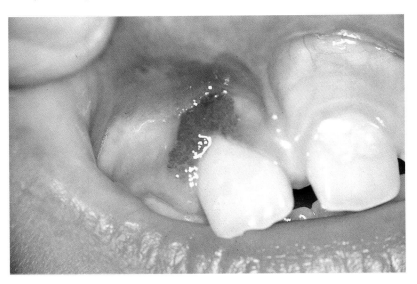

Fig. 25.**23** Capillary hemangioma on the gingiva

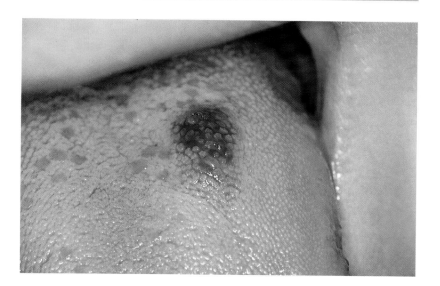

Fig. 25.**24**   Cavernous hemangioma on the tongue

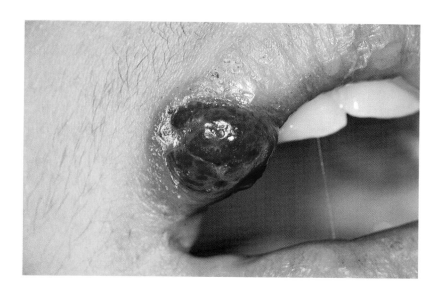

Fig. 25.**25**   Cavernous hemangioma on the upper lip

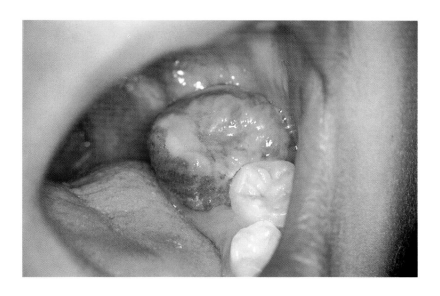

Fig. 25.**26**   Large pyogenic granuloma on the lower gingiva

- The lesion is soft on palpation, with a tendency to hemorrhage spontaneously or after slight irritation (Fig. 25.**28**).
- It grows rapidly, and its size usually ranges between 0.5 cm and 1.0 cm in diameter.
- The clinical diagnosis should be confirmed histologically.

Histopathology

- It consists of lobular masses of granulation tissue.
- Numerous endothelium-lined vessels are formed.
- Chronic inflammatory cell infiltration of neutrophils, lymphocytes and plasma cells are common.
- The surface is frequently ulcerated, and is covered by a fibrinous, purulent pseudomembrane.

Differential diagnosis

- Peripheral giant-cell granuloma
- Peripheral ossifying fibroma
- Bacillary angiomatosis
- Kaposi's sarcoma
- Hemangioma

Treatment

- Surgical removal.

Peripheral Giant-Cell Granuloma

Definition

- Peripheral giant-cell granuloma is a tumor-like overgrowth of the oral cavity.

Etiology

- It is a tissue reaction to local irritation or trauma rather than a true neoplasm.

Occurrence in children

- Common, particularly during mixed dentition.
- It appears with equal frequency in children of both sexes.

Localization

- Exclusively on the gingiva or edentulous alveolar ridge.

Clinical features

- It appears as a well-circumscribed, pedunculated or sessile, nodular mass, dark red in color (Figs. 25.**29**–25.**31**).
- The lesion is often ulcerated, and hemorrhage is common.
- On palpation, it is elastic, and the size usually ranges from 0.5 cm to 2.0 cm in diameter.
- The mandible is affected slightly more often than the maxilla.
- The clinical diagnosis should be confirmed histologically.

Histopathology

- It consists of abundant granulation tissue with numerous scattered multinucleated giant cells.
- Hemorrhage and hemosiderin deposition are common findings.
- The surface is frequently ulcerated.
- Chronic inflammatory cell infiltration is common.

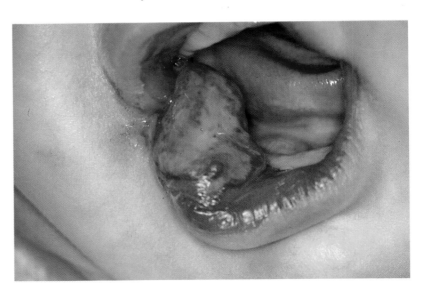

Fig. 25.**27** Large pyogenic granuloma on the labial and buccal mucosa

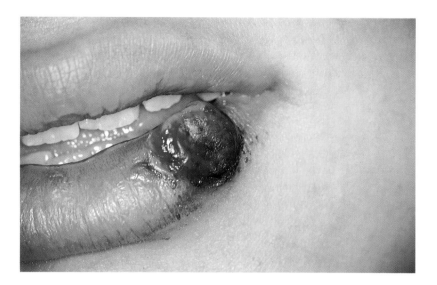

Fig. 25.**28**   Pyogenic granuloma on the lower lip

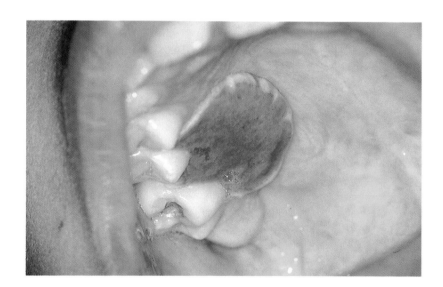

Fig. 25.**29**   Peripheral giant-cell granuloma on the palatal gingiva

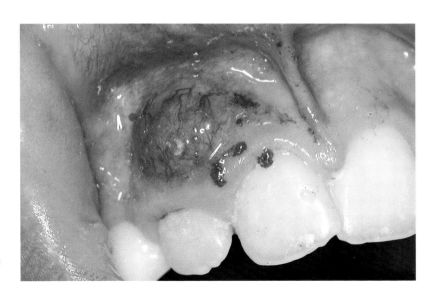

Fig. 25.**30**   Peripheral giant-cell granuloma on the buccal aspect of the gingiva and alveolar mucosa of the maxilla

Differential diagnosis	<ul><li>Pyogenic granuloma</li><li>Peripheral ossifying fibroma</li><li>Bacillary angiomatosis</li><li>Kaposi's sarcoma</li><li>Hemangioma</li><li>"Brown tumor" of hyperparathyroidism</li></ul>
Treatment	<ul><li>Surgical removal.</li></ul>

Riga–Fede Granuloma

Definition	<ul><li>Riga–Fede granuloma is a unique granulomatous ulceration of infants.</li></ul>
Etiology	<ul><li>Chronic trauma from the primary incisors, usually during breast feeding and the instinctive process of sucking.</li></ul>
Occurrence in children	<ul><li>Relatively rare, exclusively in infants.</li></ul>
Localization	<ul><li>The tip and the inferior surface of the tongue or the lingual frenulum.</li></ul>
Clinical features	<ul><li>It appears as an exophytic, ulcerated, granulomatous mass covered by a yellowish pseudomembrane (Fig. 25.**32**).</li><li>The lesion is painful, producing difficulties during chewing.</li><li>The size varies from 1 cm to 2 cm in diameter.</li><li>The age at the time of diagnosis ranges from one week to 12 months.</li><li>The diagnosis is usually based on the history and the clinical features.</li></ul>
Histopathology	<ul><li>The lesion consists of granulation tissue with numerous histiocytes and eosinophils (Fig. 25.**33**).</li><li>The ulcerated surface is covered by a fibrinopurulent membrane containing fibrin intermixed with neutrophils and degenerated cells.</li></ul>
Differential diagnosis	<ul><li>Eosinophilic ulcer</li><li>Pyogenic granuloma</li><li>Traumatic ulcer</li></ul>
Treatment	<ul><li>Construction of a protective shield.</li><li>Discontinuation of breast-feeding.</li><li>Surgical excision in case of failure of the above measures.</li></ul>

Melanotic Neuroectodermal Tumor of Infancy

Definition	<ul><li>Melanotic neuroectodermal tumor of infancy is a rare benign pigmented tumor of infants.</li></ul>
Etiology	<ul><li>Unknown.</li><li>It is of neural crest origin.</li></ul>
Occurrence in children	<ul><li>Rare, exclusively in infants, usually during the first six months of life.</li></ul>
Localization	<ul><li>Anterior region of the maxilla (80%), particularly in tooth-bearing areas. Other sites include the mandible, skull, shoulder, skin, brain, and epididymis.</li></ul>

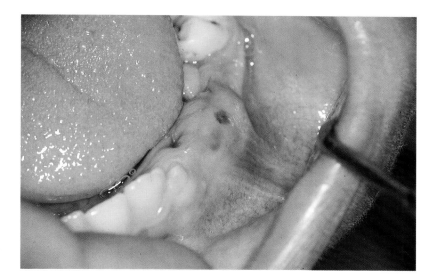

Fig. 25.**31** Peripheral giant-cell granuloma on the alveolar ridge of the mandible

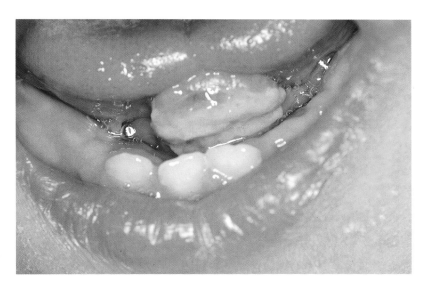

Fig. 25.**32** Riga–Fede granuloma on the lingual frenulum and inferior surface of the tongue

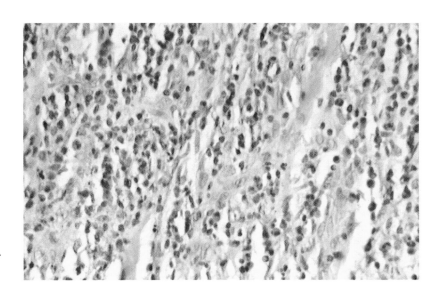

Fig. 25.**33** Riga–Fede granuloma. Granulation tissue with numerous eosinophils and histiocytes

Clinical features

- It appears as a rapidly growing, painless tumor that is usually red-brown to black (Fig. 25.**34**).
- The tumor often destroys the bone, and may cause displacement of the primary teeth.
- The rapid development and the bone resorption usually mimic a malignant tumor.
- The clinical diagnosis should be confirmed with laboratory tests.

Laboratory tests

- Histopathologically, the tumor consists of two cell populations embedded in fibrous connective tissue. The first cell type consists of nests or alveolar structures of cuboidal epithelioid cells, with vesicular nuclei and granules of melanin pigment. The second cell type consists of small round cells, with hyperchromatic nuclei and little cytoplasm (Fig. 25.**35**).
- Radiographic examination reveals bone destruction.
- Increased urinary levels of vanillylmandelic acid (VMA).

Differential diagnosis

- Granular-cell tumor of the newborn
- Neuroblastoma
- Odontogenic tumors
- Sarcomas
- Eruption cyst

Treatment

- Surgical removal.

Oral Melanotic Macules

Definition

- Oral melanotic macules are relatively rare oral mucosal lesions, analogous to skin freckles, due to focal increase of melanin production.

Etiology

- Unknown.
- Genetic and hormonal factors may be involved. Mechanical irritation and some drugs may also be responsible.
- Unlike skin freckles, the oral melanotic macules are not related to sun exposure.

Occurrence in children

- Rare.

Localization

- The vermilion border of the lower lip is the site most commonly involved. The buccal mucosa, palate, and gingiva are less commonly affected.

Clinical features

- The lesion appears usually as a solitary, asymptomatic, flat brown to black macule (Figs. 25.**36**, 25.**37**).
- It is round or oval in shape, and the size usually ranges from 0.5 cm to 2.0 cm in diameter.
- Oral melanotic macules cannot be distinguished clinically from other melanotic disorders.
- Biopsy is required for a definitive diagnosis.

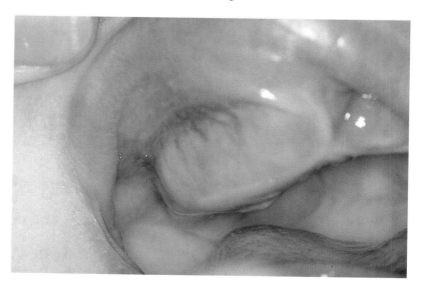

Fig. 25.**34** Melanotic neuroectodermal tumor of infancy on the anterior maxilla

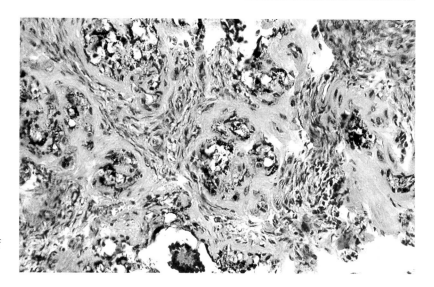

Fig. 25.**35** Melanotic neuroectodermal tumor of infancy. Nests of
small hyperchromatic round cells
and melanin pigment

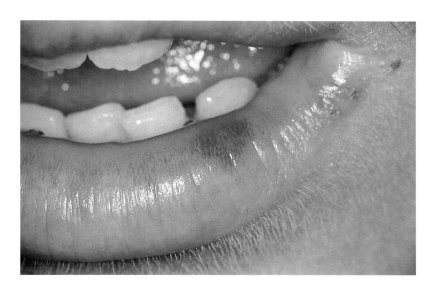

Fig. 25.**36** Freckle of the lower lip

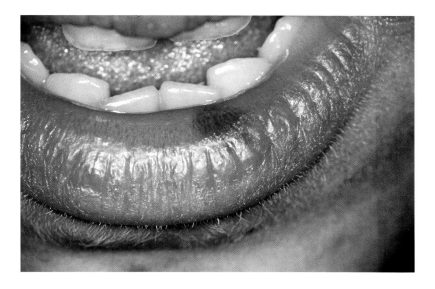

Fig. 25.**37** Freckle of the lower lip

Histopathology	• The lesion shows increased amounts of melanin in the basal cell layer and in the lamina propria (Fig. 25.**38**).
	• The number of melanocytes is normal.
Differential diagnosis	• Lentigo
	• Amalgam tattoo
	• Peutz–Jeghers syndrome
	• Melanocytic nevi
	• Melanoma
Treatment	• Usually, treatment is not needed except for aesthetic reasons.
	• Surgical removal and biopsy if there are diagnostic doubts.

Melanocytic Nevi

Definition	• Melanocytic nevi are developmental benign malformations originating from cells of the neural crest.
	• They may be acquired or congenital.
Etiology	• Developmental.
Occurrence in children	• Relatively uncommon.
	• Some nevi begin to develop during childhood, but most of them present later.
Localization	• Common on the skin.
	• Uncommon intraorally. The hard palate and the gingiva are the sites of predilection, followed by the lips and buccal mucosa.
Classification	• Based on histopathological criteria (location of nevus cells and the presence or absence of junctional activity) four types of oral nevi are recognized: *intramucosal, junctional, compound,* and *blue.*
Clinical features	• They present as asymptomatic flat or slightly raised spots or plaques of brown or brown-black color (Figs. 25.**39**, 25.**40**).
	• Rarely, non-pigmented lesions may be seen.
	• The size usually varies between 0.5 cm and 1.0 cm in diameter.
	• Intramucosal nevus is the most common type, followed by the compound and blue nevi. Junctional nevi are very rare.
	• Because of the clinical similarity of the nevi, the final diagnosis should always based on histopathological features.
	• The junctional nevus has a potential for malignant transformation.
Histopathology	• *Intramucosal:* consists of clusters (nests) of nevus cells within connective tissue, separated from the epithelium by a zone of collagen.
	• *Junctional:* consists of nests of nevus cells along the basal-cell layer of the epithelium. As the nevus cells proliferate, groups of them drop off into the underlying connective tissue, showing junctional activity.
	• *Compound:* consists of nests of nevus cells located both in the epithelium and in the underlying connective tissue (Fig. 25.**41**).
	• *Blue:* consists of multiple, elongated, slender, melanin-containing melanocytes arranged in a pattern parallel to the epithelium.
Differential diagnosis	• Melanotic macules
	• Lentigo
	• Melanoma
	• Amalgam tattoo
	• Peutz–Jeghers syndrome
Treatment	• Excisional biopsy.

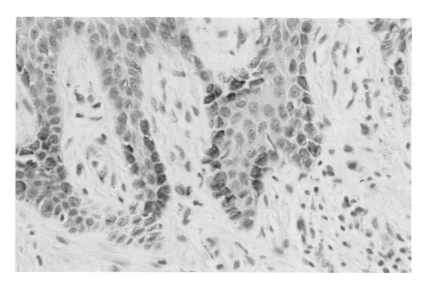

Fig. 25.**38**   Freckle. Increased melanin production in the basal-cell layer

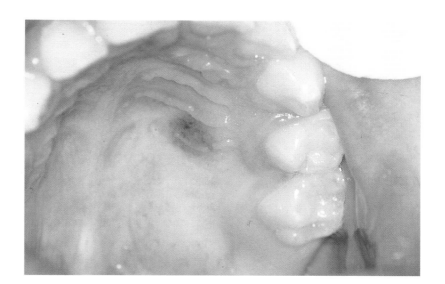

Fig. 25.**39**   Compound nevus on the palate

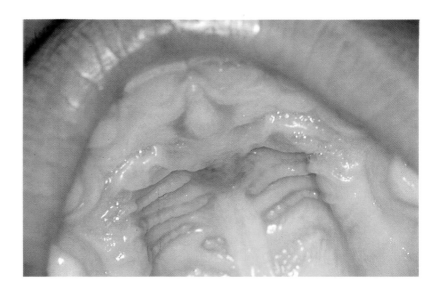

Fig. 25.**40**   Blue nevus on the palate

Spitz Nevus

Definition	• Spitz nevus, or spindle-cell and epithelioid-cell nevus is an uncommon benign melanocytic nevus with a unique histopathological pattern.
Etiology	• Developmental.
Occurrence in children	• Rare. • It appears exclusively during childhood.
Localization	• Skin. The most common site is the face, and less commonly the shoulder and legs. • It does not develop intraorally.
Clinical features	• It appears as a firm, usually smooth, dome-shaped, red or reddish-brown nodule (Fig. 25.**42**). The color is caused by the rich vascularity. • Characteristically, the lesion appears suddenly, grows rapidly, and can reach 1–2 cm in diameter. • Bleeding and crusting may rarely occur after minor irritation.
Histopathology	• The lesion histologically resembles a compound nevus. • It consists of spindle and epithelioid nevus cells, with giant and multinucleated cells among them (Fig. 25.**43**). • Mitotic figures may be seen, but abnormal mitoses are absent. • The epidermis may exhibit acanthosis and spongiosis.
Differential diagnosis	• Melanocytic nevi • Melanoma • Hemangioma • Pyogenic granuloma • Juvenile xanthogranuloma • Basal-cell carcinoma
Treatment	• Surgical removal.

Pleomorphic Adenoma

Definition	• Pleomorphic adenoma is the most common neoplasm of the major and minor salivary glands. • It represents 62–75% of tumors of the major salivary glands, and 42–70% of minor salivary gland tumors.
Etiology	• Unknown. • It originates from ductal and myoepithelial cells.
Occurrence in children	• Very rare. It usually appears after the age of 20.
Localization	• Major salivary glands: parotid gland, submandibular gland. • Minor salivary glands: soft palate, upper lip, and buccal mucosa.
Clinical features	• It appears as a painless, slow-growing, firm swelling. • The minor salivary gland tumor presents as a dome-shaped swelling covered by normal epithelium (Fig. 25.**44**). • It is rarely ulcerated by trauma, and is elastic on palpation. • The diameter at the time of diagnosis is 2–3 cm or more. • Intraoral tumors may cause swelling and difficulties in chewing and speaking.
Histopathology	• The lesion consists of a mixture of ductal epithelium cells and myoepithelial cells within a mesenchyme stroma. • The epithelial component often forms tubules, islands, or solid sheets of cells. • The myoepithelial cells usually appear as spindle cells, and less often look like plasma cells. • The stromal changes consist of intermixed mucoid, myxoid, chondroid, and hyaline material. • Rarely, osteoid and adipose tissues may also be seen.
Differential diagnosis	• Other salivary gland tumors • Necrotizing sialadenometaplasia

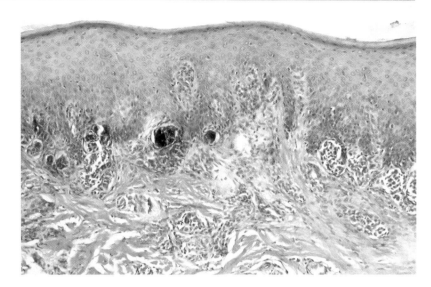

Fig. 25.**41** Compound nevus. Nests of nevus cells located both in the basal cell layer of the epithelium and in the underlying connective tissue

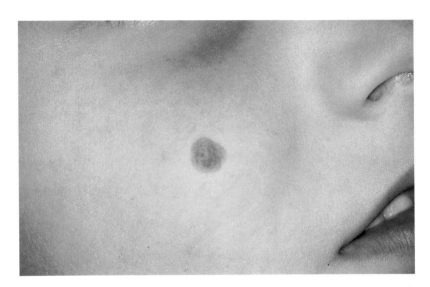

Fig. 25.**42** Spitz nevus on the skin of the face

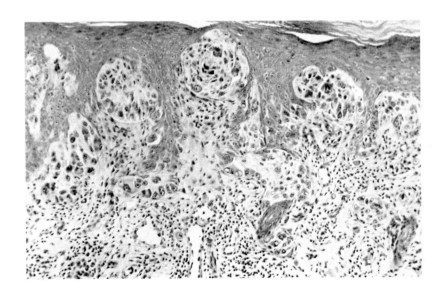

Fig. 25.**43** Spitz nevus. Nests of spindle cells and epithelioid nevus cells

- Lipoma
- Soft-tissue abscesses

Treatment

- Surgical removal.

Necrotizing Sialadenometaplasia

Definition

- Necrotizing sialadenometaplasia is a non-neoplastic, inflammatory, benign, and usually self-limiting disorder of the salivary glands.

Etiology

- The cause is unknown, although the concept of ischemic necrosis after local infarction seems possible.

Occurrence in children

- Rare.

Localization

- Posterior part of the hard palate (70–80%), usually unilateral, and rarely in other regions.

Clinical features

- It appears suddenly as a nodular swelling, which within two to three weeks leads to a painful, crater-like ulcer with an irregular border (Fig. 25.**45**).
- The diameter ranges from 1 cm to 6 cm.
- Both clinically and histologically, the lesion mimics a malignant neoplasm.
- The clinical diagnosis should be confirmed by a biopsy.

Histopathology

- It is characterized by acinar necrosis, followed by squamous metaplasia of the ductal epithelium (Fig. 25.**46**).
- The lobular structure of the salivary glands is usually preserved.
- Pseudoepitheliomatous hyperplasia of the overlying epithelium and periductal inflammatory infiltrate may occur.

Differential diagnosis

- Mucoepidermoid carcinoma
- Squamous-cell carcinoma
- Traumatic ulcer
- Malignant granuloma
- Salivary gland tumors

Treatment

- The lesion usually heals spontaneously within 4–10 weeks.
- Low-dose systemic corticosteroids (15–20 mg prednisolone) for about one week helps to heal the lesion quickly.

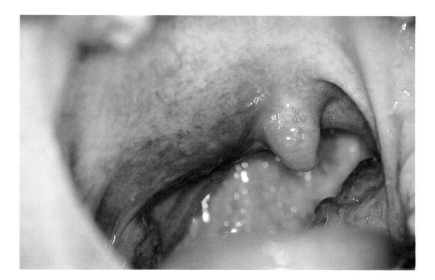

Fig. 25.**44**   Pleomorphic adenoma on the soft palate

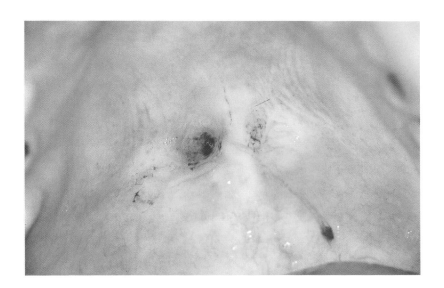

Fig. 25.**45**   Necrotizing sialade-nometaplasia on the palate

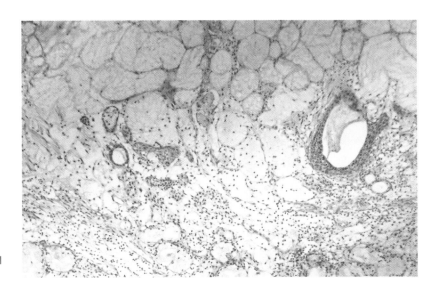

Fig. 25.**46**   Necrotizing sialade-nometaplasia. Acinar necrosis and squamous metaplasia of the ductal epithelium

26 Fibro-Osseous and Giant-Cell Lesions

Monostotic Fibrous Dysplasia

Definition
- Fibrous dysplasia is a benign developmental disorder, characterized by the replacement of normal bone by fibrous connective tissue containing trabeculae of non-lamellar immature bone.
- Two forms of the disorder are recognized, *monostotic* and *polyostotic*.

Etiology
- Unknown. In some cases, heredity may be responsible.

Occurrence in children
- Rare. The incidence is about one per million population per year.
- Most cases occur in children and adolescents.

Localization
- The maxilla and the mandible are affected with equal frequencies.

Clinical features
- The condition appears as a painless, slow-growing bone swelling (Figs. 26.**1,** 26.**2**).
- Rarely, aggressive, rapid-growing lesions may occur.
- The swelling may be firm, elastic, or hard on palpation, and may cause facial or intraoral bone deformity (Fig. 26.**3**).
- The overlying mucosa is normal, and displacement of the teeth may rarely be seen.
- Chronic osteomyelitis may occur rarely.
- The polyostotic form is characterized by involvement of many bones, café-au-lait skin spots, or hyperpigmentation, and occasionally by endocrine disorders of the pituitary, the parathyroids, and the thyroid gland (Fig. 26.**4**).
- Very rarely, osteosarcoma may arise in the monostotic type of fibrous dysplasia.

Laboratory tests
- Histopathologically, abundant cellular fibrous connective tissue is present, usually in a whorled pattern. Woven bone formation in varying amounts may occur in the fibrous stroma. Characteristically, the bone trabeculae display an irregular outline, likened to Chinese characters. The abnormal bone usually fuses to normal bone at the periphery. Osteoclasts and cementum-like structures may occasionally be seen.

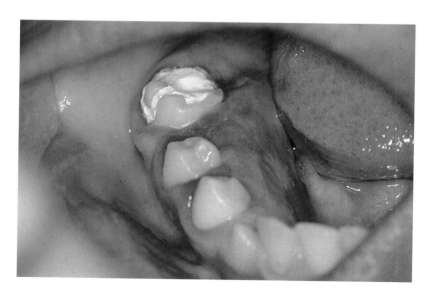

Fig. 26.**1** Monostotic fibrous dysplasia. Bone swelling of the right lingual aspect of the mandible

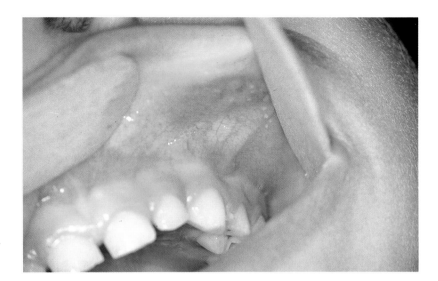

Fig. 26.**2**   Monostotic fibrous dysplasia. Swelling of the left buccal
aspect of the maxilla

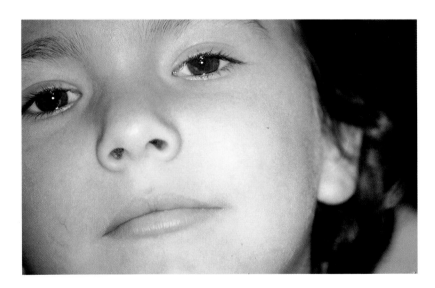

Fig. 26.**3**   Monostotic fibrous dysplasia. Facial swelling on the left
side

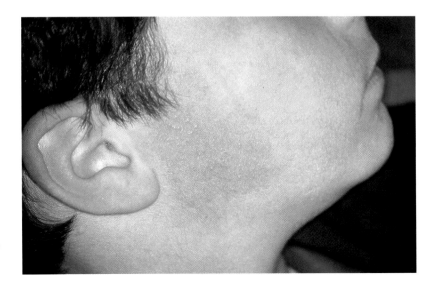

Fig. 26.**4**   Monostotic fibrous dysplasia. Hyperpigmented patch of
the skin

- Radiographically, the classic pattern is multilocular opaque lesions with a ground-glass appearance (Fig. 26.**5**). The lesions are poorly defined, and the cortical bone may become thin due to expansion of the bone.

Differential diagnosis

- Cherubism
- Ossifying fibroma
- Odontogenic tumors
- Chronic osteomyelitis
- Ewing's sarcoma
- Osteosarcoma

Treatment

- Small asymptomatic and inactive lesions may not require treatment.
- Surgical correction is necessary in lesions that produce cosmetic and functional problems.

Cherubism

Definition

- Cherubism is a benign fibro-osseous disorder of the jaws.

Etiology

- Hereditary. It is transmitted as an autosomal dominant trait.
- Sporadic cases may occur without a family history.

Occurrence in children

- Rare. It appears exclusively in children, usually below 10 years of age.

Localization

- The mandible and, less commonly, the maxilla are affected.

Clinical features

- The condition appears as a painless symmetrical bilateral expansion of the jaw bones and cheeks, producing a round facies (Figs. 26.**6**, 26.**7**).
- In severe cases with extensive maxillary involvement, retraction of the lower eyelids and exposure of the sclera below the irises may occur, creating the cherubic appearance.
- The teeth are displaced, and sometimes fail to erupt.
- Occasionally, unilateral lesions may occur.

Laboratory tests

- Histopathologically, the lesion consists of vascular fibrous stroma with variable numbers of multinucleated giant cells. Hemorrhagic areas are commonly found.
- Radiographically, the lesions present as multilocular radiolucencies with osseous expansion (Fig. 26.**8**). The jaw lesions may be associated with unerupted and displaced teeth.

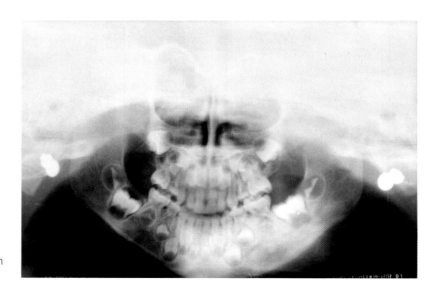

Fig. 26.**5**   Monostotic fibrous dysplasia. Multilocular opaque lesions with a ground-glass appearance on the mandible

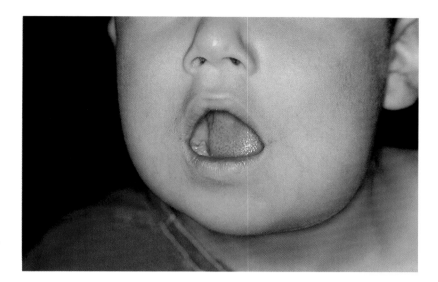

Fig. 26.**6** Cherubism. Bilateral expansion of the jaw bones and cheeks

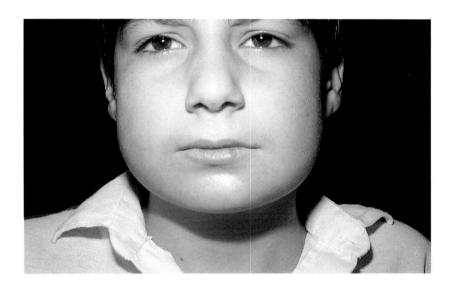

Fig. 26.**7** Cherubism. Typical round facies

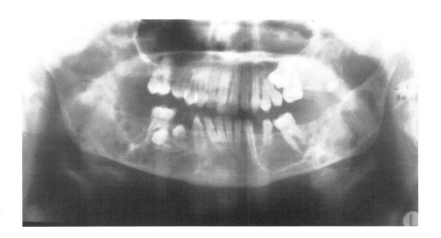

Fig. 26.**8** Cherubism. Multilocular radiolucencies with osseous expansion

Differential diagnosis	• Fibrous dysplasia • Odontogenic cysts and tumors • Gorlin's syndrome • Central giant-cell granuloma • Osteosarcoma
Treatment	• Some lesions tend to regress after puberty. • Surgical reconstruction and curettage is recommended after stabilization of the size of the lesions.

Central Giant-Cell Granuloma

Definition	• Central giant-cell granuloma is a non-neoplastic lesion of the jaws.
Etiology	• Unknown.
Occurrence in children	• Rare. The incidence is about one or two per million population per year. • It mainly develops in children, adolescents, and young adults.
Localization	• Common in the mandible, and less common in the maxilla. • The lesions occur more often in the anterior portions of the jaws. • Lesions beyond the jaw bones are very rare.
Clinical features	• It appears as a painless slight swelling or expansion of the affected jaw, occasionally with increased mobility of the teeth. • Rarely, cortical bone perforation with extension into the oral soft tissues, pain, and paresthesia may occur. • The diagnosis should be based on laboratory tests.
Laboratory tests	• Histopathologically, the stroma of the lesions consists of fibroblasts and shows abundant capillary proliferation. Characteristically, multinucleated giant cells are present in varying numbers throughout the connective-tissue stroma. Extravasated erythrocytes, hemosiderin-laden macrophages, and sometimes foci of new bone formation may be observed. • Radiographically, the lesions appear as multilocular or unilocular radiolucencies of the jaws (Fig. 26.**9**). The cortical bone may expand or rarely perforate. The size of the radiolucencies may vary from 0.5 cm to 10 cm. The radiographic features are not diagnostic.
Differential diagnosis	• Peripheral giant-cell granuloma • "Brown tumor" of hyperparathyroidism • Cherubism • Odontogenic tumors • Odontogenic cysts • Giant-cell tumor of the bone
Treatment	• Surgical removal and extensive curettage.

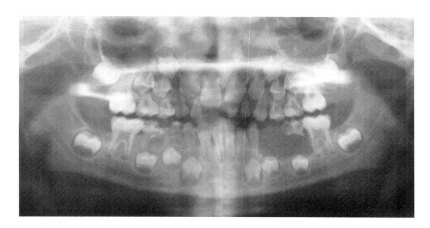

Fig. 26.**9** Central giant-cell granuloma. Unilocular radiolucency on the left side of the mandible

27 Malignant Neoplasms

Squamous-Cell Carcinoma

Definition
- Squamous-cell carcinoma is the most common malignant neoplasm of the oral cavity in adults.
- It accounts for 90–92% of oral cancers.

Etiology
- The exact etiology remains unknown. Multifactorial intrinsic and extrinsic factors play a role.
- Oncogenes and tumor-suppressor genes may be involved.

Occurrence in children
- Very rare in patients below 19 years.

Localization
- Tongue, lower lip, buccal mucosa, palate, gingiva.

Clinical features
- In the early stages, it may appear as an asymptomatic erosion or superficial ulcer, a red or white patch, or both.
- In the advanced stages, it may appear as a deep, painful ulcer with an irregular or papillary surface, elevated borders, and a hard base, or as an exophytic ulcerated mass (Figs. 27.**1**, 27.**2**).
- Clinically, oral squamous-cell carcinoma may mimic a variety of oral lesions or diseases.
- The clinical diagnosis must always be confirmed by a biopsy.
- The prognosis depends on the size and location of the lesion, histological grading, lymph-node involvement, and distant metastases.

Histopathology
- It is characterized by invasive islands and cords or solid masses of malignant epithelial cells penetrating into the corium and the underlying tissues.
- Varying degree of cellular and nuclear pleomorphism are present.
- Depending on the degree of malignant cell differentiation, three grades are recognized; well-differentiated, moderately differentiated, and poorly differentiated.

Differential diagnosis
- Traumatic ulcer
- Aphthous ulcer
- Tuberculous ulcer
- Eosinophilic ulcer.
- Necrotizing sialadenometaplasia
- Systemic mycoses

Treatment
- Surgical excision is the treatment of choice.
- Radiotherapy may also be given, usually in association with surgery.

Mucoepidermoid Carcinoma

Definition
- Mucoepidermoid carcinoma is one of the most common malignant neoplasms of the salivary glands originating from the ductal epithelium.

Etiology
- Unknown.

Occurrence in children
- Relatively rare. However, it is the most common malignant salivary gland neoplasm of childhood.

Localization
- Parotid gland.
- Minor salivary glands of palate, retromolar area, lower lip, buccal mucosa, tongue.

Clinical features
- The intraoral tumor usually appears as a painless, rubbery swelling, which may be ulcerated (Fig. 27.**3**).
- The color is red or blue, and the lesion may be fluctuant, with an exudation of mucous material on pressure, mimicking a mucocele.
- The prognosis of the tumor is somewhat better in children than in older patients.
- The clinical diagnosis should be confirmed by a biopsy.

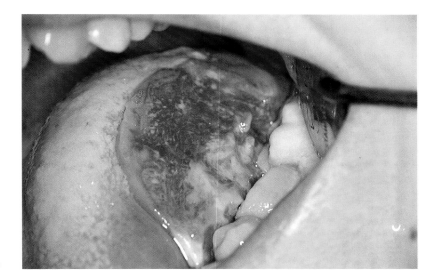

Fig. 27.**1**   Squamous-cell carcinoma on the border of the tongue

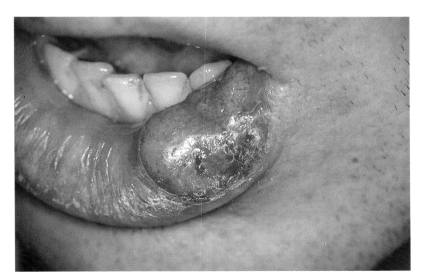

Fig. 27.**2**   Spindle-cell carcinoma (a variety of squamous-cell carcinoma) on the lower lip

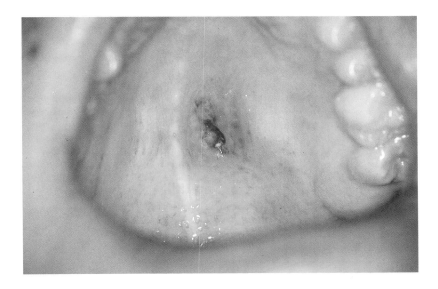

Fig. 27.**3**   Mucoepidermoid carcinoma on the palate

Histopathology	• Histopathologically, the lesion is composed of atypical epidermoid, mucus-producing and intermediate cells. • Cystic spaces lined by mucin-containing cells, and solid cellular masses of cells are common findings. • Depending on the cellular population, the tumor is divided into three forms; low-grade, intermediate, and high-grade.
Differential diagnosis	• Mucocele • Necrotizing sialadenometaplasia • Pleomorphic adenoma • Other salivary gland tumors
Treatment	• Surgical removal. • Radiotherapy may also be given.

Leukemias

Definition	• The leukemias are a heterogeneous group of malignant neoplastic disorders of the blood-forming tissues, characterized by defects of leukocyte maturation and proliferation.
Etiology	• The etiology in most cases remains obscure, although both genetic and environmental factors may be involved.
Classification	• Depending on the cell type primarily affected, leukemias are classified into *non-lymphocytic* and *lymphocytic*, and depending on the natural history of the disease, into *acute* and *chronic*. • Several subtypes of leukemias are defined, depending on the cell morphology.
Occurrence in children	• Leukemias are the most common form of malignant neoplasia in childhood. • They account for approximately one-third of new cancer cases diagnosed per year. • The acute lymphocytic leukemias affect children primarily, and account for about 75% of the cases, with a peak incidence around four years of age. Acute non-lymphocytic leukemia accounts for about 15–20% of cases of leukemia in children. The chronic forms of the disease are very rare in children.
Clinical features	• Over 75% of children with acute lymphocytic leukemia have had signs and symptoms of the disease for less than two to three months at the time of diagnosis. • Early symptoms are anorexia, irritability, fatigability, pallor, bleeding, and fever (Fig. 27.**4**). • Common oral manifestations are petechiae and bleeding, particularly from the gingiva. Mild gingival enlargement and non-specific oral ulcerations may also occur (Figs. 27.**5**–27.**8**).

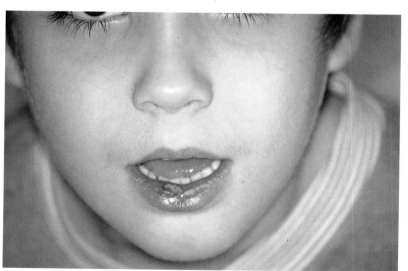

Fig. 27.**4** Acute lymphocytic leukemia. Pallor of the face

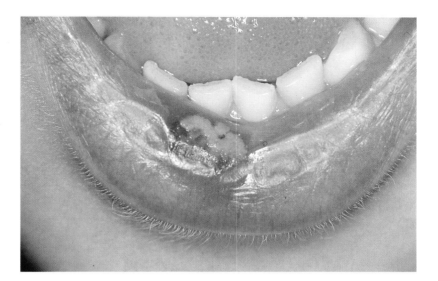

Fig. 27.**5**   Acute lymphocytic
leukemia. Ulcer of the lower lip

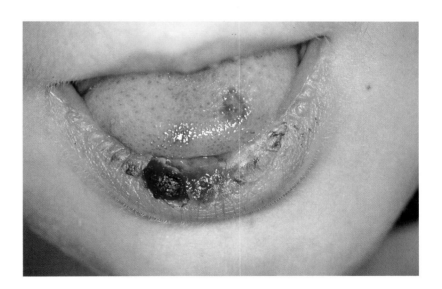

Fig. 27.**6**   Acute lymphocytic
leukemia. Ulcers of the lower lip
and tongue

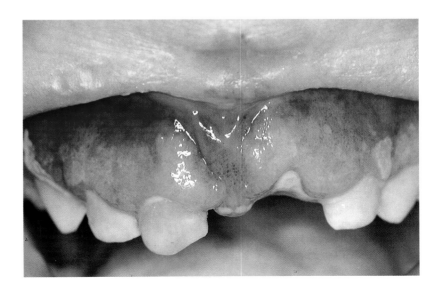

Fig. 27.**7**   Acute lymphocytic
leukemia. Moderate gingival enlargement

- During chemotherapy, oral ulcerations and bacterial, viral, and *Candida* infections are frequent (Figs. 27.**9**–27.**11**).
- Lymphadenopathy, splenomegaly, and hepatomegaly may be present in about 70–80% of patients. Less common are arthralgia and bone pain.
- The clinical diagnosis should always be confirmed by laboratory tests.

Laboratory tests

- Peripheral blood smear examination
- Bone marrow examination and genetic typing
- Extramedullary tissue examination

Differential diagnosis

- Infectious mononucleosis
- Cyclic neutropenia
- Agranulocytosis
- Myelic aplasia

Treatment

- Chemotherapy.
- Supportive care (administration of blood products and infections management).
- Radiotherapy for specific indications (e.g., testicular localization, central nervous system protective radiation, etc.).

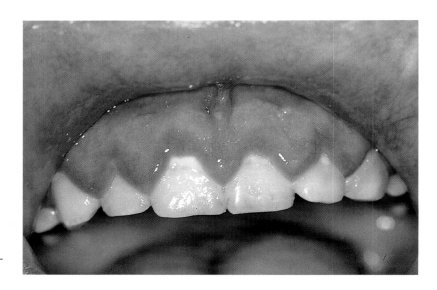

Fig. 27.**8** Acute non-lymphocytic leukemia. Gingivitis and mild gingival enlargement

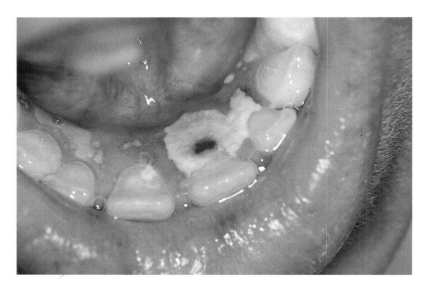

Fig. 27.**9** Acute non-lymphocytic leukemia. Candidiasis on the gingiva, during chemotherapy

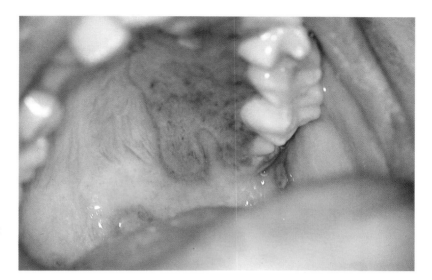

Fig. 27.**10**   Acute non-lymphocytic leukemia and non-Hodgkin's lymphoma. Large ulcer on the palate and gingiva, during chemotherapy

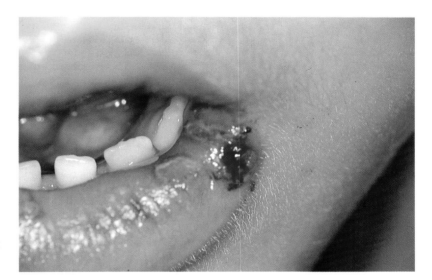

Fig. 27.**11**   Acute non-lymphocytic leukemia. Ulcers and bleeding of the lower lip

Hodgkin's Disease

Definition
- Hodgkin's disease is a malignant lymphoproliferative disorder caused by neoplastic transformations of lymphoid cells.

Etiology
- The exact etiology remains obscure. However, genetic factors, environmental factors, and viruses may be associated with the development of the disease.

Occurrence in children
- Relatively common, usually after the age of five years, with a peak at 15–18 years.
- In childhood, about 70–80% of the patients are boys.

Localization
- The cervical lymph nodes are the most frequently affected site.
- The axillary, supraclavicular, inguinal, and mediastinal lymph nodes may also be affected.
- Extranodular locations may rarely occur.

Clinical features
- Depending on the extent of the disease, four stages (I–IV) are recognized. Patients are further categorized as B and A, depending on the presence or absence, respectively, of systemic symptoms.
- The most frequent presenting feature is enlargement of the cervical lymph nodes (single or multiple) (Fig. 27.**12**). The involved lymph nodes are firm, mobile, and usually non-tender.
- Most patients with Hodgkin's disease have few or no symptoms at the time of diagnosis. The most common symptoms include low-grade unexplained fever, which can be associated with recurrent night sweats, weight loss of more than 10%, fatigue, anorexia, malaise, weakness, and pruritus.
- Extranodal oral mucosal involvement is very rare.
- The prognosis and treatment in Hodgkin's disease are dependent on the stage of the disease.
- The diagnosis should be confirmed by a biopsy.

Laboratory tests
- The cornerstone to the histopathological diagnosis is the presence of the Reed–Sternberg cell (a large cell with a bilobar or multilobulated nucleus with prominent inclusion-like nucleoli) and variants (Hodgkin cells, lacunar cells, etc.) (Fig. 27.**13**). However, the diagnosis depends on additional cellular and architectural findings in the tissues.
- Four histological subtypes of Hodgkin's disease are recognized: *lymphocyte-predominant, nodular sclerosis, mixed cellularity,* and *lymphocyte depletion.*
- Immunohistochemical examination is important for accurate diagnosis.
- Histopathological examination of the bone marrow.
- Radiography and computed tomography (CT).

Differential diagnosis
- Non-Hodgkin's lymphoma
- Leukemias
- Infectious mononucleosis
- Bacterial or viral pharyngitis
- Toxoplasmosis

Treatment
- Radiotherapy, chemotherapy, or both.
- Bone-marrow transplantation is used in a selected group of patients.

Non-Hodgkin's Lymphoma

Definition
- Non-Hodgkin's lymphoma is a heterogeneous group of neoplastic disorders that originate from lymphocytic cell lines (usually B-cell origin, and rarely T-cell origin).

Etiology
- Transforming genes or oncogenes and some viruses may play a role in the pathogenesis in some types of lymphomas.
- Congenital and acquired immunodeficiencies predispose to the development of the disease.

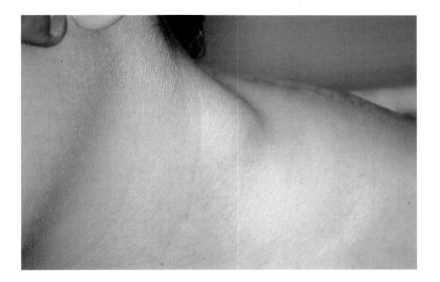

Fig. 27.**12** Hodgkin's disease. Swelling of cervical lymph nodes

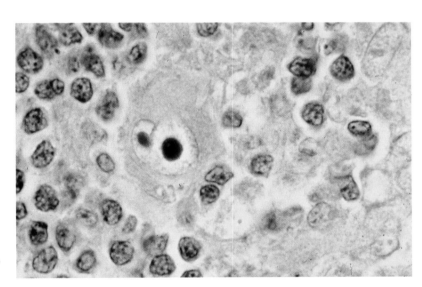

Fig. 27.**13** Hodgkin's disease. Typical Reed–Sternberg cell

Occurrence in children	• Relatively common. • Boys are three times more frequently affected than girls. • The non-Hodgkin's lymphomas are the third most common cause of cancer mortality in children under 15 years of age.
Localization	• Waldeyer's ring, head and neck, mediastinal and abdominal lymph nodes. • Extranodal involvement may also rarely occur in the oral cavity (base of the tongue, palate, posterior gingiva, buccal mucosa, jaws).
Clinical features	• A firm spherical lymph node larger than 1 cm that is not associated with an infection and persists for more than four to six weeks should be suspicious for non-Hodgkin's lymphoma, and must be biopsied. • The clinical features depend on the site of primary involvement and the extent of local and distant disease. • In the head and neck area, the lesion presents as a painless, unexplained mass that has been slowly increasing for months. As the disease progresses, the enlarged nodes become more numerous and fixed to surrounding tissues (Fig. 27.**14**). • Oral extranodal involvement is rare, and presents as painless reddish or purplish diffuse swellings with a soft consistency on palpation. The lesion may be ulcerated. • Weight loss, fever, and night sweats are less common in patients with non-Hodgkin's lymphoma than in patients with Hodgkin's disease. • The disease is classified into three groups: *low-grade, intermediate,* and *high-grade.* • The clinical diagnosis should always be confirmed by biopsy.
Laboratory tests	• Histopathological examination shows a proliferation of lymphocytic cells, which may exhibit varying degrees of differentiation, depending on the type of the disease (Figs. 27.**15**, 27.**16**). The histopathological diagnosis of non-Hodgkin's lymphoma can be reliably made on examination of lymph-node morphology. • Immunohistochemical examinations. • Histopathological examination of the bone marrow. • Radiography, CT.
Differential diagnosis	• Hodgkin's disease • Infectious mononucleosis • Human immunodeficiency virus (HIV) infection • Leukemias • Infectious lymph-node enlargement • Systemic mycoses • Eosinophilic ulcer
Treatment	• Chemotherapy, radiotherapy, or both.

Burkitt's Lymphoma

Definition	• Burkitt's lymphoma is a highly malignant B-cell lymphoma arising within germinal cells of the lymph nodes.
Etiology	• Epstein–Barr virus is strongly related to the development of the disease. In addition, cytogenetic chromosomal translocations, which may also be related to the lymphoma development, have been recorded.
Occurrence in children	• Very common, usually between three and eight years of age, in Africa. • Rare in Western countries, usually between 10 and 12 years of age.
Localization	• Frequently the jaws (60–70%). The maxilla is twice as often affected as the mandible. Oral soft tissues may rarely be affected. • The abdominal region, bone marrow, and central nervous system may affected.
Clinical features	• Two forms of the disease are recognized: the African, endemic form (common) and the American, non-endemic form (rare).

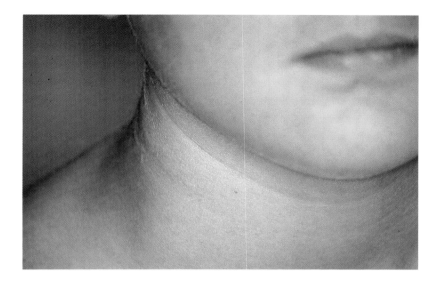

Fig. 27.**14**   Non-Hodgkin's lymphoma. Swelling of cervical lymph nodes

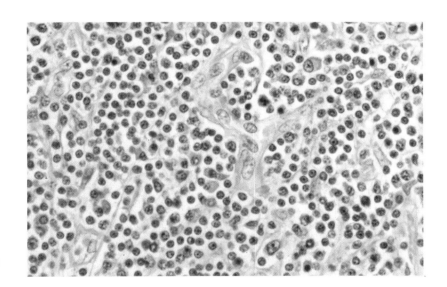

Fig. 27.**15**   Non-Hodgkin's lymphoma. Uniform population of dark, round, poorly differentiated cells of the lymphocytic series

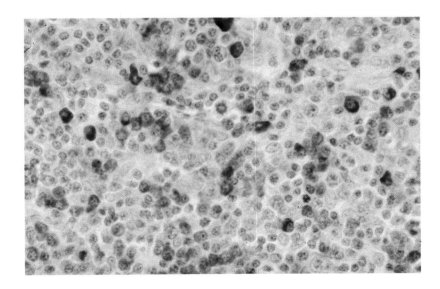

Fig. 27.**16**   Non-Hodgkin's lymphoma. Immunohistochemical demonstration of ϰ light chains

- Clinically, the tumor presents as a rapidly proliferative swelling of the jaws that may produce marked destruction of the facial bone and facial nerve paresis (Figs. 27.**17**–27.**19**).
- Jaw pain, tenderness, loose teeth, and paresthesia may occur.
- Rarely, an exophytic ulcerated mass may be seen in the oral soft tissues (Fig. 27.**20**).
- The progress of the tumor is usually rapid.
- The prognosis depends on the stage of the disease, and long-term survival ranges from 20% to 70%.

Laboratory tests

- Histopathologically, the lesion consists of broad sheets of monomorphous B-cell lymphocytes with small, round to oval, basophilic nuclei and numerous mitoses. There are multiple macrophages with abundant cytoplasm, which are less intensely stained compared to the surrounding cells, forming the typical "starry sky" pattern (Fig. 27.**21**).
- Immunohistochemical examination.
- Panoramic radiographic examination.
- CT.

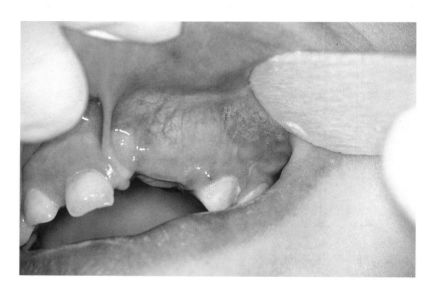

Fig. 27.**17** Burkitt's lymphoma. Swelling of the maxilla

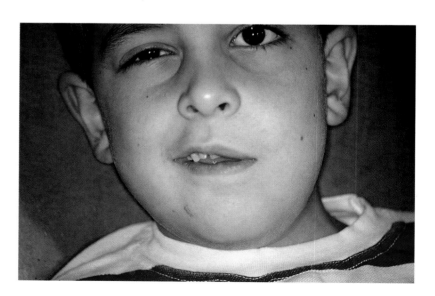

Fig. 27.**18** Burkitt's lymphoma. Facial swelling and facial nerve paresis

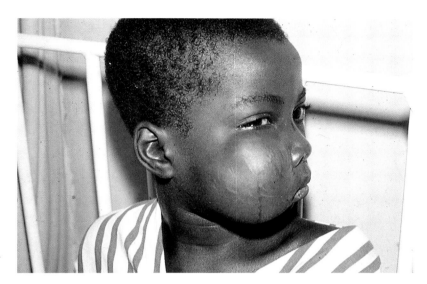

Fig. 27.**19**   Burkitt's lymphoma. Facial deformity

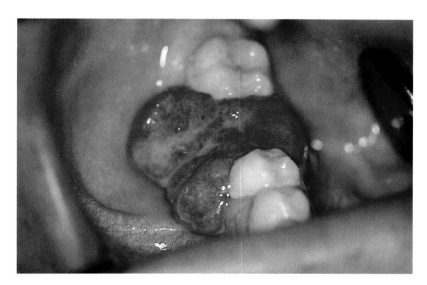

Fig. 27.**20**   Burkitt's lymphoma. Exophytic, ulcerated mass on the gingiva of the mandible

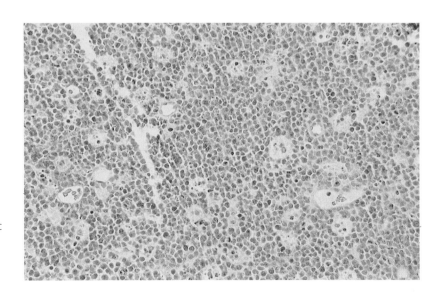

Fig. 27.**21**   Burkitt's lymphoma. Monomorphous B-cell lymphocytic population with small, round basophilic nuclei and numerous mitoses, and the typical "starry-sky" pattern

Differential diagnosis	● Other types of non-Hodgkin's lymphoma
	● Ewing's sarcoma
	● Odontogenic tumors
	● Central giant-cell granuloma
	● Fibrous dysplasia
	● Neuroblastoma
	● Embryonal rhabdomyosarcoma
Treatment	● Chemotherapy and radiotherapy.
	● Surgical resection.

Soft-Tissue Plasmacytoma

Definition	● Soft-tissue plasmacytoma, or extramedullary plasmacytoma, is a monoclonal neoplasm that consists of plasma cells indistinguishable from those seen in multiple myeloma.
Etiology	● Unknown.
Occurrence in children	● Very rare.
Localization	● It occurs most commonly in the nasopharynx, nasal cavity, paranasal sinuses, and tonsils.
	● The oral soft tissues (palate, floor of mouth, tongue, gingiva) are rarely involved.
Clinical features	● The oral tumor appears as a non-tender, solitary, well-circumscribed, soft swelling with a smooth, normal surface (Fig. 27.**22**). Rarely, the lesion may be ulcerated.
	● The size at the time of diagnosis varies from 1 cm to several centimeters in diameter.
	● The clinical features are non-specific, and the diagnosis should always be confirmed by a biopsy.
	● The prognosis is usually good. However, a number of patients may ultimately develop multiple myeloma.
Histopathology	● Histopathologically, the lesion is characterized by a dense, monotonous infiltrate of plasma cells that may show a broad morphological spectrum, ranging from mature-looking plasma cells to undifferentiated cells (Fig. 27.**23**).
	● Intracytoplasmic deposits of immunoglobulin in the form of globules positive on the periodic acid–Schiff test (Russell bodies) and nuclear inclusions (Dutcher bodies) can be seen.
	● The plasma cells show monotypic cytoplasmic immunoglobulin, and lack surface immunoglobulin.
Differential diagnosis	● Non-Hodgkin's lymphoma
	● Pleomorphic adenoma
	● Other salivary gland tumors
	● Abscesses
	● Oral soft-tissue cysts
Treatment	● Radiotherapy, alone or in combination with surgical excision, is the treatment of choice.

Rhabdomyosarcoma

Definition	● Rhabdomyosarcoma is a malignant soft-tissue neoplasm that is thought to arise from the same embryonic mesenchyme as striated skeletal muscle.
Etiology	● Unknown.
Occurrence in children	● It is the most common soft-tissue sarcoma in children.
	● There is an early peak of tumor occurrence before five years of age, and a later one around 15–20 years of age.
	● Boys are more commonly affected than girls.
Localization	● Usually, the head and neck area (40–50%), prostate, bladder, genitourinary tract, extremities.

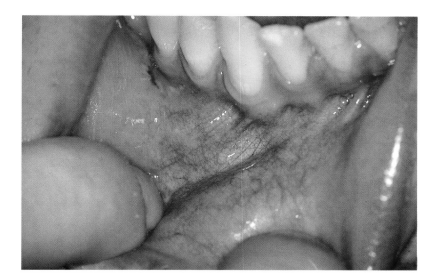

Fig. 27.**22**   Soft-tissue plasmacy-toma. Swelling of the alveolar–labial groove

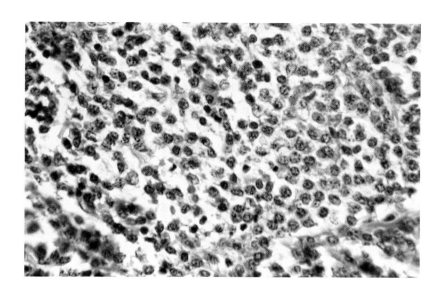

Fig. 27.**23**   Soft-tissue plasma-cytoma. Sheets of monotonous plasma cells, with varying degrees of differentiation

Clinical features

- The tumor usually appears as a rapidly growing infiltrative swelling mass, which may be painful.
- Head tumors may produce facial deformation (Fig. 27.**24**).
- Trismus, cranial nerve paralysis may also occur.
- Early diagnosis of the tumor requires an alert physician, and the clinical suspicion should always be confirmed by a biopsy.
- The prognosis of the tumor has improved significantly over the last two decades.

Laboratory tests

- Histopathologically, four subtypes are recognized: *embryonal* (accounts for about 66% of cases), *alveolar, pleomorphic,* and *undifferentiated* (Fig. 27.**25**).
- CT and radiography are also useful for diagnosis.

Differential diagnosis

- Neuroblastoma
- Lymphomas
- Other sarcomas
- Lymphangioma

Treatment

- Surgical excision, usually followed by chemotherapy and radiotherapy.

Ewing's Sarcoma

Definition

- Ewing's sarcoma is a unique round-cell malignant tumor of the bone, probably with a neuroectodermal origin.

Etiology

- Unknown.

Occurrence in children

- The tumor represents about 5–8% of primary bone malignancies.
- Relatively common. Approximately 70–80% of cases develop in patients below 18 years of age.
- Boys are more frequently affected than girls.

Localization

- Femur, pelvis, head, and trunk.
- Jaw involvement is rare, occurring in about 1–2% of cases. The ramus and the angle of the mandible one the most commonly affected areas.

Clinical features

- The most prominent presenting symptoms are bone swelling and pain, which may be accompanied by tenderness and fever.
- As the bone lesion enlarges, it progressively penetrates the cortex, forming a soft-tissue mass (Fig. 27.**26**), which usually becomes ulcerated.
- Loose teeth, paresthesias, and facial deformity are common findings.
- The jaw lesions may be primary or metastatic.
- The clinical diagnosis should be confirmed by a biopsy.

Laboratory tests

- Histopathologically, the tumor consists of uniformly packed, small round cells with scanty cytoplasm and little surrounding stroma (Fig. 27.**27**). The round to oval nuclei contain finely dispersed chromatin and inconspicuous nucleoli. The cell cytoplasm characteristically contains glycogen.

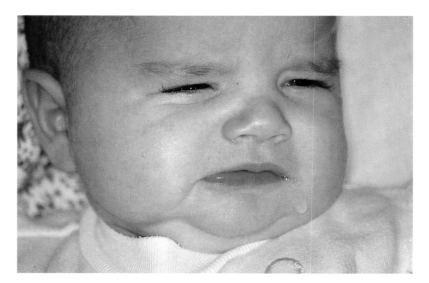

Fig. 27.**24** Rhabdomyosarcoma. Swelling of the right side of the face

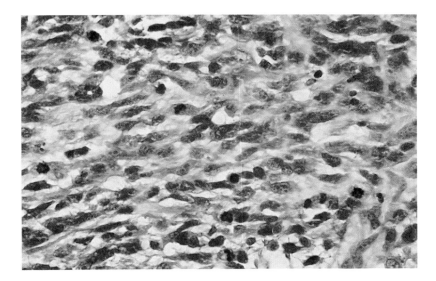

Fig. 27.**25** Rhabdomyosarcoma.
Atypical spindle cells, with nuclear
polymorphism and mitoses

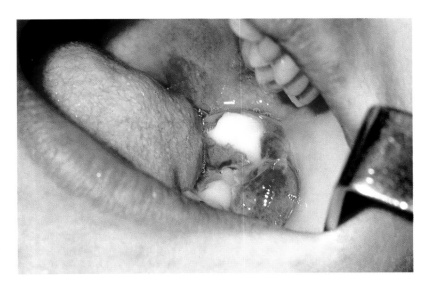

Fig. 27.**26** Ewing's sarcoma. Bone
swelling and an ulcerated mass on
the gingiva of the mandible

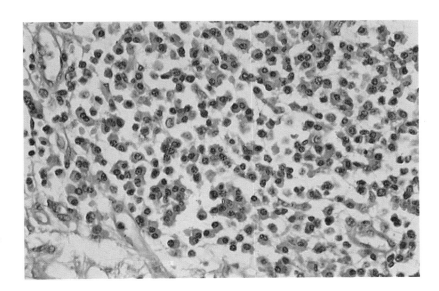

Fig. 27.**27** Ewing's sarcoma. Uniformly packed small, round cells
with scanty cytoplasm and little
stroma

- Radiographically, the jaw lesions are non-specific, and are characterized by irregular destructive radiolucency with ill-defined borders. A variable periosteal "onion-skin" reaction may be seen.
- CT.

Differential diagnosis

- Osteosarcoma
- Chondrosarcoma
- Neuroblastoma
- Odontogenic tumors
- Eosinophilic granuloma
- Osteomyelitis

Treatment

- Surgical excision in association with radiotherapy and chemotherapy.

Osteosarcoma

Definition

- Osteosarcoma is the most common primary malignant bone tumor, and the neoplastic cells produce osteoid.

Etiology

- Unknown.

Occurrence in children

- Relatively rare.
- Bone tumors have an annual incidence in children of about five cases per million.
- Jaws osteosarcoma in children is very rare.
- The onset is most frequent between 12 and 18 years.

Localization

- Distal femur, proximal humerus, proximal tibia.
- Approximately 3–5% of osteosarcomas occur in the jaws. The body and angle of the mandible, the ascending ramus, and the alveolar ridge of the maxilla are the most frequently affected areas.

Clinical features

- The most common initial finding is pain and swelling at the site of the tumor (Fig. 27.**28**).
- Loosening and displacement of teeth, and paresthesia may occur.
- Nasal obstruction may occur in maxillary osteosarcomas.
- An exophytic soft-tissue mass may also be noted.
- Osteosarcomas of the jaws frequently recur, often (20–40%) metastasizing to the lungs and brain and rarely to regional lymph nodes.

Laboratory tests

- Histopathologically, the tumor consists of malignant mesenchymal cells producing osteoid (the *osteoblastic* form). In addition, the malignant cells may produce chondroid material (the *chondroblastic* form) and fibrous material (the *fibroblastic* form).
- Radiographically, the findings can be variable, depending on the degree of calcification and progression of the lesions. Early lesions are characterized by localized periodontal ligament space widening and destruction of one or several teeth. Irregular, ill-defined radiolucent lesions, usually intermixed with areas of radiopacity, are common findings. The typical sun-ray radiopaque appearance caused by periosteal reaction may be observed in about 23–30% of jaw osteosarcomas.
- Serum alkaline phosphatase activity may be increased.

Differential diagnosis

- Chondrosarcoma
- Chronic osteomyelitis
- Ewing's sarcoma
- Giant-cell tumor of the bone
- Odontogenic tumors

Treatment

- Surgical excision.
- Radiotherapy and chemotherapy may also be used to treat recurrences.

Metastatic Neoplasms

Definition

- Metastatic neoplasms may be observed either in the jaws or in the oral soft tissues.

Etiology

- Same as the primary malignancy.

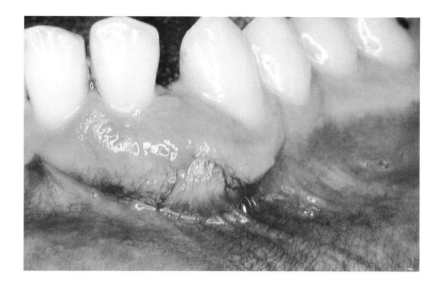

Fig. 27.**28** Osteosarcoma. Swelling of the mandible in the lateral incisor–canine area

Occurrence in children	• Very rare. • The primary neoplasm may be osteosarcoma, neuroblastoma, carcinoma of the gastrointestinal tract and thyroid, embryonic carcinoma, melanoma, undifferentiated carcinoma.
Localization	• Mandible, maxilla, gingiva, palate, tongue, buccal mucosa, lips.
Clinical features	• Oral metastatic tumors may remain asymptomatic for a long time. • Bone pain and swelling, teeth loosening, gingival swelling, and paresthesia are the most common findings in metastatic tumors to the jaws (Fig. 27.**29**). • Exophytic masses, usually ulcerated, as well as pain and hemorrhage are common in soft-tissue metastatic tumors. • The clinical features are usually non-diagnostic, and should be confirmed by laboratory tests.
Laboratory tests	• Biopsy and histopathological examination usually produce findings resembling those of the primary neoplasm (Figs. 27.**30**, 27.**31**). However, metastatic neoplasms are sometimes poorly differentiated, and it can be difficult to determine the precise origin. • Immunohistochemical studies. • Radiography. • CT.
Differential diagnosis	• Primary oral malignant tumors • Lymphomas • Peripheral giant-cell granuloma • Pyogenic granuloma • Melanotic neuroectodermal tumor of infancy • Granular-cell tumor of infancy
Treatment	• Treatment of the primary neoplasm, chemotherapy. • Surgical excision or radiotherapy of the metastatic focus.

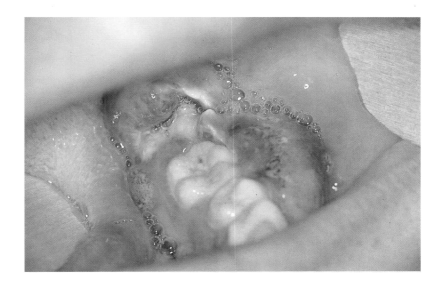

Fig. 27.**29** Metastatic carcinoma on the gingiva of the mandible, originating from the rectum

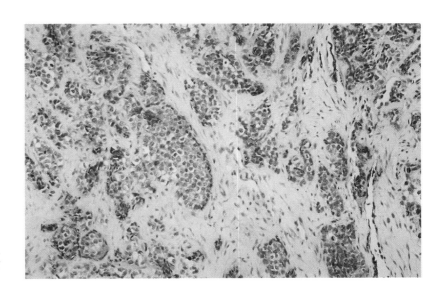

Fig. 27.**30** Metastatic carcinoma. Histological pattern at the primary site on the rectum

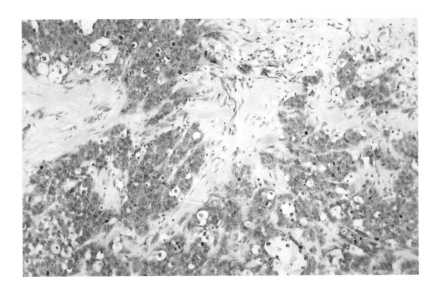

Fig. 27.**31** Metastatic carcinoma. Histological pattern in the gingiva, showing characteristics similar to those in the rectum (Fig. 27.**30**)

References

Part I   Local Diseases

Chapter 1
Dental Defects

Bhat M, Nelson KB. Developmental enamel defects in primary teeth in children with cerebral palsy, mental retardation, or hearing defects: a review. Adv Dent Res 1989; 3: 132–42.

Bixler D. Heritable defects affecting dentin. In: Stewart ER, Prescott HG, eds. Oral facial genetics. St. Louis: Mosby, 1976: 227–61.

Dixon GH, Stewart RE. Genetic aspects of anomalous tooth development. In: Stewart ER, Prescott HG, eds. Oral facial genetics. St. Louis: Mosby, 1976: 124–50.

Giunta JL. Dental changes in hypervitaminosis D. Oral Surg Oral Med Oral Pathol 1998; 85: 410–3.

Jorgenson RJ. Teeth. In: Stevenson RE, Hall JG, Goodman RM, eds. Human malformations and related anomalies. Oxford: Oxford University Press, 1993: 383–96.

Kalk WWI, Batenburg RHK, Vissink A. Dentin dysplasia type I. Oral Surg Oral Med Oral Pathol 1998; 86: 175–8.

Kamma J, Lygidakis NA, Nakou M. Subgingival microflora and treatment in prepubertal periodontitis associated with chronic idiopathic neutropenia: case report. J Clin Periodontol 1998; 25: 759–65.

Katsaris N, Lygidakis NA. Ankylosis of primary molars: literature review and case presentation. Pedodontia 1993, 8: 65–74.

Lau CE, Stavkin CH, Snead LM. Analysis of human enamel genes: insights into genetic disorders of enamel. Cleft Palate J 1990; 27: 121–30.

Lygidakis NA. Oral and teeth abnormalities in genetic disease [dissertation]. Oxford: University of Oxford, 1983.

Lygidakis NA. Collagen abnormalities in genetic dentine defects [dissertation]. London: Institute of Dental Surgery, University of London, 1984.

Lygidakis NA. Genetic anomalies of hard dental tissues, 1: genetic anomalies of enamel. Pedodontia 1995; 9: 61–9.

Lygidakis NA. Genetic anomalies of hard dental tissues, 2: genetic anomalies of dentine and cementum. Pedodontia 1995; 9: 123–33.

Lygidakis NA, Lindenbaum RH. Pitted enamel hypoplasia in tuberous sclerosis patients and first-degree relatives. Clin Genet 1987; 32: 216–21.

Lygidakis NA, Smith R, Oulis CI. Scanning electron microscopy of teeth in osteogenesis imperfecta type I. Oral Surg Oral Med Oral Pathol 1996; 81: 567–72.

Nikiforuk G, Fraser D. The etiology of enamel hypoplasia: A unifying concept. Pediatrics 1981; 98: 888.

Pindborg JJ. Disturbances in tooth formation etiology. In: Pindborg JJ, ed. Pathology of the dental hard tissues. Copenhagen: Munksgaard, 1970: 138–210.

Pindborg JJ. Aetiology of developmental enamel defects not related to fluorosis. Int Dent J 1991; 32: 115.

Poole AE, Redford-Badwal DA. Structural abnormalities of the craniofacial complex and congenital malformations. Pediatr Clin North Am 1991; 38: 1089.

Rowley R, Hill JF, Winter BG. An investigation of the association between anterior open-bite and amelogenesis imperfecta. Am J Orthod 1982; 81: 229–35.

Seow WK. Enamel hypoplasia in the primary dentition: a review. ASDC J Dent Child 1991; 58: 441–51.

Seow WK. Dental development in amelogenesis imperfecta: a controlled study. Pediatr Dent 1995; 17: 26–30.

Sundell S, Koch G. Hereditary amelogenesis imperfecta: epidemiology and clinical classification in a Swedish child population. Swed Dent J 1985; 9: 157–69.

Takagi Y, Fujita H, Katano H, et al. Immunochemical and biochemical characteristics of enamel proteins in hypocalcified amelogenesis imperfecta. Oral Surg Oral Med Oral Pathol 1998; 85: 424–30.

Thakkar NS, Sloan P. Dental manifestations of systemic disease. In: Jones JH, Mason DK, eds. Oral manifestations of systemic disease. 2nd ed. London: Baillière Tindall, 1990: 480–511.

Witkop CJ, Sauk JJ. Heritable defects of enamel. In: Stewart ER, Prescott HG, eds. Oral facial genetics. St. Louis: Mosby, 1976: 151–226.

Witkop CJ Jr. Amelogenesis imperfecta, dentinogenesis imperfecta and dentin dysplasia revisited: problems in classification. J Oral Pathol 1989; 7: 547–53.

Chapter 2
Developmental Anomalies

Daley TD. Intraoral sebaceous hyperplasia: diagnostic criteria. Oral Surg Oral Med Oral Pathol 1993; 75: 343–7.

Daley TD. Pathology of intraoral sebaceous glands. J Oral Pathol Med 1993; 22: 241–5.

Dedo MDD. Hemifacial atrophy: A review of an unusual craniofacial deformity, with a report of a case. Arch Otolaryngol 1978; 104: 538–43.

Eggen S, Natvig B. Concurrence of torus mandibularis and torus palatinus. Scand J Dent Res 1994; 102: 60–3.

Gorlin RJ, Cohen MM, Levin LS. Syndromes of the head and neck. 3rd ed. Oxford: Oxford University Press, 1990.

Grewe JM, McCombie F. Prevalence of cleft uvula in British Columbia. Angle Orthod 1971; 41: 336–9.

Kaufman FL. Managing the left lip and palate patient. Pediatr Clin North Am 1991; 38: 1127–47.

Mathewson RJ, Siegel MJ, McCanna DL. Ankyloglossia: a review of the literature and a case report. J Dent Child 1966; 33: 238–43.

Meskin LH, Gorlin RJ, Isaacson RJ. Abnormal morphology of the soft palate, 1: the prevalence of cleft uvula. Cleft Palate 1964; 1: 342–6.

Morgan AF, Stewart FW, Stein IJ. Double lip: report of a case. Oral Surg Oral Med Oral Pathol 1960; 13: 236–9.

Navas J, Rodriguez-Pichardo A, Camacho F. Ascher syndrome: a case study. Pediatr Dermatol 1991; 8: 122–3.

Notestine GE. The importance of the identification on ankyloglossia (short lingual frenulum) as a cause of breastfeeding problems. J Hum Lactation 1990; 6: 113–5.

Pensler JM, Murphy GF, Mulliken JB. Clinical and ultrastructural studies of Romberg's hemifacial atrophy. Plast Reconstr Surg 1990; 85: 669–74.

Precious DS, Delaire J. Clinical observations of cleft lip and palate. Oral Surg Oral Med Oral Pathol 1993; 75: 141–51.

Ridala AE, Ranta R. Lower lip sinuses, 1: epidemiology, microforms, and transverse sulci. Br J Plast Surg 1981; 34: 25–30.

Sedano HO. Congenital oral anomalies in Argentinian children. Comm Dent Oral Epidemiol 1975; 3: 61–3.

Sewerin I. The sebaceous glands in the vermilion border of the lips and in the oral mucosa of man. Acta Odontol Scand 1975; 33 (Suppl): 68.

Taylor WB, Mich AA, Lane DK. Congenital fistulas of the lower lip: associations with cleft lip–palate and anomalies of extremities. Arch Dermatol 1966; 94: 421–4.

Vanderas AP. Incidence of cleft lip, cleft palate and cleft lip and palate among races: a review. Cleft Palate J 1987; 24: 216–25.

Wallace AF. Tongue-tie. Lancet 1963; ii: 377–8.

Whyman RA, Doyle TCA, Harding WJ, Ferguson MM. An unusual case of hemifacial atrophy. Oral Surg Oral Med Oral Pathol 1992; 73: 564–9.

**Chapter 3
Mechanical and Electrical Injuries**

Barrett AP, Buckley DJ. Covert self-mutilation of oral tissues and skin by mechanical and chemical means. Oral Surg Oral Med Oral Pathol 1988; 65: 685–8.

Braham RL. Oral soft tissue lesions in children and adolescents. Practitioner 1984; 228: 319–25.

Buchner A, Hansen LS. Amalgam pigmentation (amalgam tattoo) of the oral mucosa. Oral Surg Oral Med Oral Pathol 1980; 49: 139–44.

Buker MD, Chiaviello C. Household electrical injuries in children: epidemiology and identification of avoidable hazards. Am J Dis Child 1989; 143: 59–62.

Comer RW, Fitchie JG, Caughman WF, Zwemer JD. Oral trauma: emergency care of lacerations, fractures, and burns. Postgrad Med 1989; 85: 34–7.

Linebaugh ML, Koka S. Oral electrical burns: etiology, histopathology, and prosthodontic treatment. J Prosthodont 1993; 2: 136–41.

Orban B. Discolorations of the oral mucous membrane by metallic foreign bodies. J Periodontol 1956; 17: 55–65.

Palin WE, Sadove AM, Jones JE, et al. Oral electrical burns in a pediatric population. J Oral Med 1987; 42: 17–27.

Regezi JA, Zarbo RJ, Daniels TE, Greenspan JS. Oral traumatic granuloma: characterization of the cellular infiltrate. Oral Surg Oral Med Oral Pathol 1993; 75: 723–7.

Scully CM, Welbury EE. Color atlas of oral diseases in children and adolescents. St. Louis: Mosby, 1993.

Stewart D, Kernohan D. Self-inflicted gingival injuries. Dent Pract 1972; 22: 418–26.

Svirsky JA, Sawyer DR. Dermatitis artefacta of the paraoral region. Oral Surg Oral Med Oral Pathol 1987; 64: 259–63.

Van Wyk CW, Staz J, Farman AG. The chewing lesion of the cheeks and lips: its features and prevalence among a selected group of adolescents. J Dent 1977; 5: 193–9.

**Chapter 4
Chemical Burns and Allergies**

Albright BW, Taylor CG. Hereditary angioneurotic edema: report of a case. J Oral Surg 1979; 37: 888.

Alford B, Harris H. Chemical burns of the mouth, pharynx and esophagus. Ann Otol 1959; 68: 122–7.

Chue PW. Acute angioneurotic edema of the lip and tongue due to emotional stress. Oral Surg Oral Med Oral Pathol 1976; 41: 734–8.

Claman HN. Mouth ulcers associated with prolonged chewing of gum containing aspirin. JAMA 1967; 202: 651–2.

Glick GL, Chafee RB, Salkin LM. Oral mucosal lesions associated with acetyl salicylic acid: two case reports. NY State Dent J 1975; 40: 475–8.

Greaves M, Lawlor F. Angioedema: manifestations and management. J Am Acad Dermatol 1991; 25: 155–65.

Kawashima Z, Flagg RH, Cox DE. Aspirin-induced oral lesion: report of a case. J Am Dent Assoc 1975; 91: 130.

Laskaris G. Color atlas of oral diseases. 2nd ed. Stuttgart: Thieme, 1994.

Maron FS. Mucosal burn resulting from chewable aspirin: report of case. J Am Dent Assoc 1989; 119: 279–89.

Mattingly G, Rodu B, Alling R. Quincke's disease: nonhereditary angioneurotic edema of the uvula. Oral Surg Oral Med Oral Pathol 1993; 75: 292–5.

Najjar TA. Harmful affects of „aspirin compounds." Oral Surg Oral Med Oral Pathol 1977; 44: 64–70.

Neumann-Jensen B. Angioneurotic edema of the tongue. Dan Dent J 1978; 82: 233–5.

Chapter 5
Foreign-Body Deposits

Blanton PL, Hurt WC, Largeut MD. Oral factitious injuries. J Periodontol 1977; 48: 33–7.

Cohen MM. Stomatologic alterations in childhood, 2. ASDC J Dent Child 1977; 44: 327–35.

Cristobal MC, Aguitar A, Urbina F, et al. Self-inflicted tongue ulcer: an unusual form of factitious disorder. J Am Acad Dermatol 1987; 17: 339–41.

Elzay RP. Traumatic ulcerative granuloma with stromal eosinophilia (Riga–Fede's disease and traumatic eosinophilic granuloma). Oral Surg Oral Med Oral Pathol 1983; 55: 497.

Luker J, Scully C. Paediatric oral medicine, 5: the oral mucosa (i). Dent Update 1988; 15: 292–8.

Mani NJ. Gingival tattoo: a hitherto undescribed mucosal pigmentation. Quintessence Int 1985; 16: 157–9.

Peters E, Gardner DG. A method of distinguishing between amalgam and graphite in tissue. Oral Surg Oral Med Oral Pathol 1986; 62: 73–6.

Severin I. A clinical and epidemiologic study of morsicatio buccarum–labiorum. Scand J Dent Res 1971; 79: 73.

Stewart DJ, Kernohan DC. Self-inflicted gingival injuries: gingivitis artefacta, factitial gingivitis. Dent Pract 1972; 22: 418–26.

Chapter 6
Periodontal Diseases

Aldred MJ, Bartold PM. Genetic disorders of the gingivae and periodontium. Periodontology 2000 1998; 18: 7–20.

Armitage GC, Van Dyke TE. Periodontal diseases of children and adolescents. J Periodontol 1996; 67: 57–62.

Bozzo L, Almeida O, Scully C, Aldred MJ. Hereditary gingival fibromatosis. Oral Surg Oral Med Oral Pathol 1994; 78: 452–4.

Burmeister AJ, Best AM, Palcanis GK, et al. Localized juvenile periodontitis and generalized severe periodontitis: clinical findings. J Clin Periodontol 1984; 11: 181–9.

Chung CP, Nisengard RJ, Slots J, Genco RJ. Bacterial IgG and IgM antibody titers in acute necrotizing ulcerative gingivitis. J Periodontol 1983; 54: 557–62.

Christersson LA, Zambon JJ. Suppression of *Actinobacillus actinomycetemcomitans* in localized juvenile periodontitis with systemic tetracycline. J Clin Periodontol 1993; 20: 345–401.

Cianciola LJ, Park BH, Bruck E, et al. Prevalence of periodontal disease in insulin-dependent diabetes mellitus (juvenile diabetes). J Am Dent Assoc 1982; 104: 653–60.

Corlin RJ, Cohen MM, Levin LS. Syndromes of the head and neck. 3rd ed. Oxford: Oxford University Press, 1990: 847–58.

Dongari A, McDonnell HT, Langlais RP. Drug-induced gingival overgrowth. Oral Surg Oral Med Oral Pathol 1993; 76: 543–8.

Genco RJ, Christersson LA, Zambon JJ. Juvenile periodontitis. Int Dent J 1986; 36: 168–73.

Goepferd SJ. Advanced alveolar bone loss in the primary dentition: a case report. J Periodontol 1981; 52: 753.

Jacombson L. Mouth breathing and gingivitis. J Periodontol 1973; 8: 269–75.

Laskaris G, Dimitriou N, Angelopoulos A. Immunofluorescent studies in desquamative gingivitis. J Oral Pathol 1981; 10: 398–402.

Laskaris G, Triantafyllou A, Economopoulou P. Gingival manifestations of childhood cicatricial pemphigoid. Oral Surg Oral Med Oral Pathol 1988; 66: 349–52.

Laskaris G, Potouridou E, Laskaris M, Stratigos J. Gingival lesions of HIV infection in 178 Greek patients. Oral Surg Oral Med Oral Pathol 1992; 74: 168–71.

Latcham NL, Powell RN, Jago JD, Seymour GJ, Aitken JF. A radiographic study of chronic periodontitis in 15-year-old Queensland children. J Clin Periodontol 1983; 10: 37–45.

Luker J, Scully C. Paediatric oral medicine, 4: the gingiva. Dental Update 1988; 15: 198–201.

Melnick SL, Roseman JM, Engel D, Cogen RB. Epidemiology of acute necrotizing ulcerative gingivitis. Epidemiol Rev 1988; 10: 191–211.

Nisengard R. Periodontal implications: mucocutaneous disorders. Ann Periodontol 1996; 1: 401–38.

Palmer RM, Eveson JW. Plasma-cell gingivitis. Oral Surg Oral Med Oral Pathol 1981; 51: 187–9.

Papapanou P. Epidemiology and natural history of periodontal disease. In: Lang N, Karring T, eds. Proceedings of the First European Workshop on Periodontology. Chicago: Quintessence, 1994: 23–41.

Plasschaert AJM, Folmer T, van den Heuvel JLM, et al. An epidemiologic survey of periodontal disease. Comm Dent Oral Epidemiol 1978; 6: 65–70.

Schenkein HA, Van Dyke TE. Early-onset periodontitis: systemic aspects of etiology and pathogenesis. Periodontology 2000 1994; 6: 7–25.

Scully C, Laskaris G. Mucocutaneous disorders. Periodontology 2000 1998; 18: 81–94.

Sklavounou A, Laskaris G. Frequency of desquamative gingivitis in skin diseases. Oral Surg Oral Med Oral Pathol 1983; 56: 141–4.

Sklavounou-Andrikopoulou A, Mortakis N, Katsadaki S. Plasma cell lesions: a rare oral inflammatory disease entity. Hell Dent J 1993; 3: 53–7.

Takagi M, Yamamoto H, Mega H, et al. Heterogeneity in the gingival fibromatosis. Cancer 1991; 68: 2202–12.

Tonetti M, Mombelli A. Early onset periodontitis. In: Lindhe J, Karring T, Lang N, eds. Clinical periodontology and implant dentistry. Copenhagen: Munksgaard, 1997: 226–57.

Vassilopoulou A, Laskaris G. Papillon–Lefèvre syndrome: report of two brothers. J Dent Child 1989; Sept/Oct: 388–91.

Williams RC. Periodontal disease. N Engl J Med 1990; 322: 373–82.

Wilson TC Jr, Kornman KS. Fundamentals of periodontics. Chicago: Quintessence, 1996.

Wolfe MD, Carlos JP. Periodontal disease in adolescents: epidemiologic findings in Navajo Indians. Comm Dent Oral Epidemiol 1987; 15: 33–40.

Chapter 7
Diseases of the Lips

Axell T, Skoglund A. Chronic lip fissures. Int J Oral Surg 1981; 10: 354–8.

Brooke RI. Exfoliative cheilitis. Oral Surg Oral Med Oral Pathol 1978; 4: 52–5.

Fisher AA. Allergic contact dermatitis from musical instruments. Cutis 1993; 51: 75–6.

Hayakawa R, Matsunaga K, Suzuki M, et al. Lipstick dermatitis due to C_{18} aliphatic compounds. Contact Dermat 1987; 16: 215–9.

Ohman SC, Dahlen G, Moller A, Ohman A. Angular cheilitis: a clinical and microbial study. J Oral Pathol 1986; 10: 354–8.

Reade PC, Sim R. Exfoliative cheilitis: a factitious disorder? Int J Oral Maxillofac Surg 1986; 15: 313–7.

Rosenquist B. Medial lip fissure: etiology and suggested treatment. Oral Surg Oral Med Oral Pathol 1991; 72: 10–4.

Sainsbury CPQ, Dodge JA, Walker DM, Aldred MJ. Orofacial granulomatosis in childhood. Br Dent J 1987; 163: 154–7.

Swerlick RA, Cooper PH. Cheilitis glandularis: a re-evaluation. J Am Acad Dermatol 1984; 10: 466–72.

Tyldesley WR. Exfoliative cheilitis. Br J Oral Surg 1973, 10: 357–9.

Williams PM. Management of cheilitis granulomatosa. Oral Surg Oral Med Oral Pathol 1991; 72: 436–9.

Worsaae N, Christensen KC, Schiodt M, Reibel J. Melkersson–Rosenthal syndrome and cheilitis granulomatosa: a clinical pathological study of thirty-three patients, with special reference to their oral lesions. Oral Surg Oral Med Oral Pathol 1982; 54: 404–13.

Zimmer WM, Rogers RS, Reeve CM, Sheridan PH. Orofacial manifestations of Melkersson–Rosenthal syndrome. Oral Surg Oral Med Oral Pathol 1992; 74: 610–9.

Chapter 8
Diseases of the Tongue

Baughman RA. Median rhomboid glossitis: a developmental anomaly? Oral Surg Oral Med Oral Pathol 1971; 31: 56–65.

Farman AG. Tongue fissures: a classification and comparative prevalence study among 825 European Caucasian and 605 Xhosa Negro schoolchildren. J Biol Buccal 1976; 4: 349–64.

Ghose LJ, Baghdady VS. Prevalence of geographic and plicated tongue in 6090 Iraqi schoolchildren. Comm Dent Oral Epidemiol 1982; 10: 214–6.

Hume WJ. Geographic stomatitis: a critical review. J Dent 1975; 3: 25–43.

Knapp MJ. Oral tonsils: location, distribution and histology. Oral Surg Oral Med Oral Pathol 1970; 29: 155–61.

Kullaa-Mikkonen A. Familial study of fissured tongue. Scand J Dent Res 1988; 96: 366–75.

Kuramoto Y, Tadaki T, Hatchome N, Tagami H. Geographic tongue in two siblings. Dermatologica 1987; 174: 298–302.

Laskaris G. Color atlas of oral diseases. 2nd ed. Stuttgart: Thieme, 1994.

Marks R, Radden BG. Geographic tongue: a clinicopathological review. Aust J Dermatol 1981; 22: 75–9.

Morris LF, Phillips CM, Binnie WH, et al. Oral lesions in patients with psoriasis: a controlled study. Cutis 1992; 49: 339–44.

Pollack RS. Median rhomboid glossitis: case report in an infant. Ann Surg 1954; 139: 250–2.

Rahaminoff P, Muksam HV. Some observations on 1246 cases of geographic tongue. Am J Dis Child 1957, 93: 514–25.

Sedano H, Freyre IC, De La Garza MLG, et al. Clinical orodental abnormalities in Mexican children. Oral Surg Oral Med Oral Pathol 1989, 68: 300–11.

Simpson HE. Lymphoid hyperplasia in foliate papillitis. J Oral Surg 1964, 22: 209–14.

Sklavounou A, Laskaris G. Oral psoriasis: report of a case and review of the literature. Dermatologica 1990; 180: 157–60.

Van der Waal I, Beemster G, van der Kwast WAM. Median rhomboid glossitis caused by *Candida*? Oral Surg Oral Med Oral Pathol 1979; 47: 31–5.

Chapter 9
Non-Odontogenic Cysts

Allard RHB. Thyroglossal cyst. Head Neck Surg 1982; 5: 134–9.

Black EE, Leathers RD, Younglood D. Dermoid cyst of the floor of the mouth. Oral Surg Oral Med Oral Pathol 1993; 75: 556–8.

Brown FH, Houston GD, Lubow RM, Sagan MA. Cyst of the incisive (palatine) papilla: report of a case. J Periodontol 1987; 58: 274–5.

Buchner A, Hansen LS. Lymphoepithelial cysts of the oral cavity: a clinicopathologic study of 38 cases. Oral Surg Oral Med Oral Pathol 1980; 50: 441–9.

Chaudhry AP, Yamane GM, Sharlock SE, et al. A clinicopathological study of intraoral lymphoepithelial cysts. J Oral Med 1984; 39: 79–84.

Crysdale WS, Mendelsohn JD, Conley S. Ranulas mucoceles of the oral cavity: experience in 26 children. Laryngoscope 1988; 98: 296–8.

Jensen JL. Superficial mucocele of the oral mucosa. Am J Dermatol 1990; 12: 88–92.

King RC, Smith BR, Burk JL. Dermoid cyst in the floor of the mouth: review of the literature and case reports. Oral Surg Oral Med Oral Pathol 1994; 78: 567–76.

Lowry RE, Tempero RM, Davis LF. Epidermoid cyst of the floor of the mouth. J Oral Surg 1979; 37: 271–3.

Lustmann J, Copelyn M. Oral cysticercosis: review of the literature and report of 2 cases. Int J Oral Surg 1981; 10: 371–5.

McClathecy KD, Appelblatt NH, Zarbo RJ, Merrel DM. Plunging ranula. Oral Surg Oral Med Oral Pathol 1984; 57: 408–12.

Ohishi M, Ishii T, Shinohara M, Horinouchi Y. Dermoid cyst of the floor of the mouth: lateral teratoid cyst with sinus tract in an infant. Oral Surg Oral Med Oral Pathol 1985; 60: 191–4.

Osborne TE, Haller JA, Levin LS, et al. Submandibular cystic hygroma resembling a plunging ranula in a neonate. Oral Surg Oral Med Oral Pathol 1971; 71: 16–20.

Oygur T, Dursun A, Uluoglu O, Dursum G. Oral congenital dermoid cyst in the floor of the mouth of a newborn. Oral Surg Oral Med Oral Pathol 1992; 74: 627–30.

Quick CA, Lowell SH. Ranula and the sublingual salivary glands. Arch Otolaryngol 1977; 103: 397–400.

Quinn JH, Robinson WC. Multiple congenital cysts of the floor of the mouth in a newborn infant. Oral Surg Oral Med Oral Pathol 1965; 20: 1–5.

Rees RT. Congenital ranula. Br J Dent 1979; 146: 345–6.

Romero de Leon E, Aguirre A. Oral cysticercosis. Oral Surg Oral Med Oral Pathol 1995; 79: 572–7.

Shear M. Cysts of the oral regions. Bristol: Wright, 1983.

Swanson KS, Kaugars GE, Cunsolley JC. Nasopalatine duct cyst: an analysis of 334 cases. J Oral Maxillofac Surg 1991; 49: 268–71.

Warnakulasuriya KA, Herath KB. Investigating a lingual thyroid. Int J Oral Maxillofac Surg 1992; 21: 227–9.

Yeschua R, Bab IA, Wexler MR, et al. Dermoid cyst of the floor of the mouth in an infant. J Maxillofac Surg 1977; 5: 211–3.

Chapter 10
Odontogenic Cysts

Altini M, Shear M. The lateral periodontal cyst: an update. J Oral Pathol Med 1992; 21: 245–50.

Andersen RA. Eruption cyst: a retrograde study. J Dent Child 1990; 57: 124–7.

Cataldo E, Berkman MD. Cysts of the oral mucosa in newborns. Am J Dis Child 1968; 116: 44–8.

Clark CA. A survey of eruption cysts in the newborn. Oral Surg Oral Med Oral Pathol 1962; 15: 917–22.

Dahl EC. Diagnosing inflammatory and non-inflammatory periapical disease. J Indiana Dent Assoc 1991; 70: 22–6.

Eliasson S, Isacsson G, Kondell PA. Lateral periodontal cysts: clinical, radiographic and histopathological findings. Int J Oral Maxillofac Surg 1989; 18: 191–3.

Fromm A. Epstein's pearls, Bohn's nodules and inclusion cysts of the oral cavity. J Dent Child 1967; 34: 275–87.

Gilhar A, Winterstein G, Godfried E. Gingival cysts of the newborn. Int J Dermatol 1988; 27: 261–2.

Heydt D, Thompson SH, Shakenovsky BN. Transition of apical periodontal cysts to intramedullary osteomyelitis: a clinicopathological analysis. J Endod 1985; 11: 67–70.

Jorgensen RJ, Shapira SD, Salinas CF, Levin LS. Intraoral findings and anomalies in neonates. Pediatrics 1982; 69: 577–82.

Seward MH. Eruption cyst: an analysis of its clinical features. J Oral Maxillofac Surg 1973; 31: 31–5.

Stockdale CR, Chandler NP. The nature of the periapical lesion: a review of 1108 cases. J Dent 1988; 16: 123–9.

Chapter 11
Recurrent Aphthous Ulcers

Addy M, Hunter ML, Kingdom A. A study of the prevalence of recurrent minor aphthous ulceration in a group of children aged 15–16 years. J Paediatr Dent 1990; 6: 29–33.

Esparza Gomez GC, Lopez-Arguello Illana C, Garcia Nunez JA, Moreno Lopez LA. Recurrent aphthous stomatitis: review and update. Medicina Oral 1998; 3: 18–35.

Field EA, Brookes V, Tyldesley WR. Recurrent aphthous ulceration in children: a review. Int J Paediatric Dent 1992; 2: 1–10.

Laskaris G. Recurrent aphthous stomatitis. In: Katsabas A, Lotti T, eds. European Handbook of Dermatological Treatments. Heidelberg: Springer, 1999: 51–55.

Lehner T. Immunologic aspects of recurrent oral ulcers. Oral Surg Oral Med Oral Pathol 1972; 33: 80–5.

Lehner T. Progress report: oral ulceration and Behçet's syndrome. Gut 1977; 18: 491–6.

Lucer J, Scully C. Paediatric oral medicine, 5: the oral mucosa (i). Dent Update 1988; 15: 292–8.

Pedersen A. Recurrent aphthous ulceration: virological and immunological aspects. APMIS 1993; 101 (Suppl 37): 5–37.

Rees TP, Binnie WH. Recurrent aphthous stomatitis. Dermatol Clin 1996; 14: 243–56.

Scully C, Porter SR. Recurrent aphthous stomatitis: current concepts of etiology, pathogenesis and management. J Oral Pathol Med 1989; 18: 21–7.

Ship JA. Recurrent aphthous stomatitis: an update. Oral Surg Oral Med Oral Pathol 1996; 81: 141–7.

Stratigos A, Laskaris G, Stratigos J. Behçet's disease. Semin Neurol 1992; 12: 346–57.

Woo SB, Sonis ST. Recurrent aphthous ulcers: a review of diagnosis and treatment. J Am Dent Assoc 1996; 127: 1202–13.

Chapter 12
Bacterial Infections

Chung CP, Nisengard RJ, Slots J, Genco RJ. Bacterial IgG and IgM antibody titers in acute necrotizing ulcerative gingivitis. J Periodontol 1983; 54: 557–62.

Fleisher G, Ludwing S, Campos J. Cellulitis: bacterial etiology, clinical features and laboratory findings. J Pediatr 1980; 97: 591–6.

Fox PC. Bacterial infections of salivary glands. Curr Opin Dent 1991; 1: 411–4.

Gill Y, Scully C. Orofacial odontogenic infections: review of microbiology and current treatment. Oral Surg Oral Med Oral Pathol 1990; 70: 155–8.

Hartnett AC, Shiloah J. The treatment of acute necrotizing ulcerative gingivitis. Quintessence Int 1991; 22: 95–100.

Holbrook WP. Bacterial infections of oral soft tissues. Curr Opin Dent 1991; 1: 404–10.

Johnson A. Inflammatory conditions of the major salivary glands. Ear Nose Throat 1989; 68: 94–102.

Johnson BD, Engel D. Acute necrotizing ulcerative gingivitis: a review of diagnosis, etiology and treatment. J Periodontol 1986; 57: 141–50.

Laskaris G. Oral manifestations of infectious diseases. Dent Clin North Am 1996; 40: 395–423.

Luker J, Scully C. Paediatric oral medicine, 2: bony lesions and deformities of the face. Dent Update 1988; 15: 15–25.

Saunders PR, Macpherson DW. Acute suppurative parotitis: a forgotten cause of upper airway obstruction. Oral Surg Oral Med Oral Pathol 1991; 72: 412–6.

Sklavounos A, Legakis N, Ioannidou H, Patrikiou A. Anaerobic bacteria in dentoalveolar abscesses. Int J Oral Surg 1986; 15: 288–91.

Stratigos J, Laskaris G. Skin and oral manifestations of AIDS. Athens: Zita, 1996.

Taiwo JO. Oral hygiene status and necrotizing ulcerative gingivitis in Nigerian children. J Periodontol 1993; 64: 1071–4.

Taylor CO, Carter JB. Buccal cellulitis in an infant due to ampicillin-resistant *Hemophilus influenzae*. J Oral Maxillofac Surg 1986; 44: 234–8.

Wannfors K, Hammarstrom L. Infectious foci in chronic osteomyelitis of the jaws. Int J Oral Surg 1985; 14: 493–503.

Wilson TC Jr, Kornman KS. Fundamental of periodontics. Chicago: Quintessence, 1996.

Yanagisawa S. Pathologic study of periapical lesions, 1: Periapical granuloma: clinical, histopathologic and immunohistopathologic studies. J Oral Pathol 1980; 9: 288–300.

Zhao-Ju Z, Song-Ling W, Jia-Rui Z, et al. Chronic obstructive parotitis: report on ninety-two cases. Oral Surg Oral Med Oral Pathol 1992; 73: 434–40.

Zou Z, Wang S, Zhu J, et al. Recurrent parotitis in children: a report of 102 cases. Clin Med J 1990; 103: 567–82.

Chapter 13
Viral Infections

Archard HO, Heck JW, Stanley HR. Focal epithelial hyperplasia: an unusual mucosal lesion found in Indian children. Oral Surg Oral Med Oral Pathol 1965; 20: 201–12.

Child Day Care Infectious Disease Study Group. Public health considerations of infectious diseases in child day care centers. J Pediatr 1984; 105: 683–701.

Eversole LR. Viral infections of the head and neck among HIV-seropositive patients. Oral Surg Oral Med Oral Pathol 1992; 73: 155–63.

Eversole LR, Laipis PJ, Merrell P, Choi E. Demonstration of human papillomavirus DNA in oral condyloma acuminatum. J Oral Pathol 1987; 16: 266–72.

Green TL, Eversole LE, Leider AS. Oral and labial verruca vulgaris: clinical, histologic and immunohistochemical evaluation. Oral Surg Oral Med Oral Pathol 1986; 62: 410–6.

Greenberg MS. Herpesvirus infections. Dent Clin North Am 1996; 40: 359–68.

Hahn A, Hundeiker M, Loning T. Ausgedehnte HPV-6-DNA-positive condylomata acuminata auf der Zunge. Aktuel Dermatol 1990; 16: 34–6.

Harris AM, Van Wyk CW. Heck's disease (focal epithelial hyperplasia): a longitudinal study. Community Dent Oral Epidemiol 1993; 21: 82–5.

Henke RD, Guerin R, Mile-Laugoch K, et al. In situ detection of human papillomavirus types 13 and 32 in focal epithelial hyperplasia of the oral mucosa. J Oral Pathol Med 1989; 18: 419–21.

Juretic M. Natural history of herpetic infection. Helv Pediatr Acta 1966; 21: 256–68.

Laskaris G. Color atlas of oral diseases. 2nd ed. Stuttgart: Thieme, 1994.

Laskaris G. Oral manifestations of infectious diseases. Dent Clin North Am 1996; 40: 395–423.

Laskaris G, Papanicolaou S, Angelopoulos A. Focal epithelial hyperplasia: the first reported case from Greece. Dermatologica 1981; 162: 254–9.

Mindel A. Herpes simplex virus. Berlin: Springer, 1989.

Nakayama T, Urano T, Osano M, et al. Outbreak of herpangina associated with coxsackievirus B3 infection. Pediatr Infect Dis J 1989; 8: 495–8.

Papadayachee A. Human papillomavirus (HPV) types 2 and 57 in oral verrucae demonstrated by in situ hybridization. J Oral Pathol Med 1994; 23: 413–7.

Schubert MM. Oral manifestations of viral infections in immunocompromised patients. Curr Opin Dent 1991; 1: 384–97.

Steigman AJ, Lipton MA, Braspemmcky H. Acute lymphonodular pharyngitis: a newly described condition due to coxsackie A virus. J Pediatr 1962; 61: 331–6.

Syrjanen SM. Human papillomavirus infections in the oral cavity. In: Syraonen KJ, Gissman L, Koss LG, eds. Papillomaviruses and human disease. Heidelberg: Springer, 1987.

Zunt SL, Tomich C. Oral condyloma acuminatum. J Dermatol Surg Oncol 1989; 15: 591–4.

Chapter 14
Fungal Infections

Challacombe SJ, Muir J, Howell SA, et al. Genetic variability of *Candida albicans* in HIV infection. Microbial Ecol Health Dis 1995; 8: 63–70.

Holmstrup P, Axell T. Classification and clinical manifestations of oral yeast infections. Acta Odontol Scand 1990; 48: 57–60.

Samaranayake LP. Superficial oral fungal infections. Curr Opin Dent 1991; 1: 415–22.

Samaranayake LP. Oral mycosis in HIV infection. Oral Surg Oral Med Oral Pathol 1992; 73: 171–80.

Samaranayake LP, MacFarlane TW, eds. Oral candidosis. London: Wright, 1990.

Schnell JD. Epidemiology and the prevention of peripheral mycoses. Chemotherapy 1982; 28 (Suppl 1): 66–72.

Scully C, Monteil R, Sposto MR. Infections and tropical diseases affecting the human mouth. Periodontology 2000 1998; 18: 47–70.

Sweet SP. Selection and pathogenicity of *Candida albicans* in HIV infection. Oral Dis 1997; 3 (Suppl 1): S88–95.

White TC, Pfaller MA, Rinaldi MG, et al. Stable azole drug resistance associated with a substrain of *Candida albicans* from an HIV-infected patient. Oral Dis 1997; 3 (Suppl 1): S102–9.

Part II   Systemic Diseases

Chapter 15
Genetic Disorders

Aloi FG, Molinero A. White sponge nevus with epidermolytic changes. Dermatologica 1988; 177: 323–6.

Airenne P. X-linked hypohidrotic ectodermal dysplasia in Finland. Proc Finn Dent Soc 1981; 77 (Suppl 1): 1–107.

Alper JC. The genodermatoses and their significance in pediatric dermatology. Dermatol Clin 1986; 4: 45.

Baab DA, Page RC, Ebersole JL, et al. Laboratory studies of a family manifesting premature exfoliation of deciduous teeth. J Clin Periodontol 1986; 13: 677–83.

Baden E, Jones JR, Khedekar R, Burns WA. Neurofibromatosis of the tongue: a light and electron microscopic study with review of the literature from 1849 to 1981. J Oral Med 1984; 39: 157–64.

Banoczy J, Sugar L, Frithiof L. White sponge nevus, leukoedema exfoliativum mucosae oris: a report on forty-five cases. Swed Dent J 1973; 66: 481–93.

Barabas GM. The Ehlers–Danlos syndrome: abnormalities of the enamel, dentine, cementum and the dental pulp: a histological examination of 24 teeth from 6 patients. Br Dent J 1969; 126: 509–15.

Bjellerup M. Incontinentia pigmenti with dental anomalies: a three-generation study. Acta Dermatovenereol 1982; 62: 262–4.

Bollerslev J. Osteopetrosis: a genetic and epidemiological study. Clin Genet 1987; 31: 86–90.

Braun-Falco O, Hofmann C. Das Goltz–Gorlin-Syndrom: Übersicht und Kasuistik. Hautarzt 1975; 26: 393–400.

Browne RM, Byrne JPH. Dental dysplasia in incontinentia pigmenti achromians (Ito). Br Dent J 1976; 140: 211–4.

Carney RG Jr. Incontinentia pigmenti: a world statistical analysis. Arch Dermatol 1976; 112: 535–42.

Chapple ILC. Hypophosphatasia: dental aspects and mode of inheritance. J Clin Periodontol 1993; 20: 615–22.

Clarke A. Hypohidrotic ectodermal dysplasia. J Med Genet 1987; 24: 659–63.

D'Ambrosio JA, Langlais RP, Young RS. Jaw and skull changes in neurofibromatosis. Oral Surg Oral Med Oral Pathol 1988; 66: 391–6.

Daubeney PEF, Pal K, Stanhope R. Hypomelanosis of Ito and precocious puberty. Eur J Pediatr 1993; 152: 715–6.

El Darouti MA, Al Raubaie SM, Eiada MA. Papillon–Lefèvre syndrome: successful treatment with oral retinoids in three patients. Int J Dermatol 1988; 27: 63–6.

El-Labban NG, Lee KW, Rule D. Permanent teeth in hypophosphatasia: light and electron microscopy study. J Oral Pathol Med 1991; 20: 352–60.

Ellis RWB, Andrew JD. Chondroectodermal dysplasia. J Bone J Surg 1962; 44B: 626–36.

Eronat N, Ucar F, Kiline G. Papillon–Lefèvre syndrome: treatment of two cases with a clinical, microbiological and histopathological investigation. J Clin Pediatr Dent 1993; 17: 99–104.

Freire-Maia N, Pinheiro M. Ectodermal dysplasias: a clinical and genetic study. New York: Liss, 1984.

Gomez MR. Tuberous sclerosis. New York: Raven Press, 1988.

Gorlin RJ. The oral-facial-digital syndrome. Cutis 1968; 4: 1345–9.

Gorlin RJ, Cohen MM, Levin LS. Syndromes of the head and neck. 3rd ed. Oxford: Oxford University Press, 1990.

Haggitt RC, Reid BJ. Hereditary gastrointestinal polyposis syndromes. Am J Surg Pathol 1986; 10: 871–93.

Hall EH, Terezhalmy GT. Focal dermal hypoplasia syndrome: case report and literature review. J Am Acad Dermatol 1983; 9: 443–51.

Haneke E. The Papillon–Lefèvre syndrome: keratosis palmoplantaris with periodontopathy. Hum Genet 1979; 15: 1–35.

Haneke E, Hornstein OP, Lex C. Increased susceptibility to infections in the Papillon–Lefèvre syndrome: successful treatment with oral retinoids in three patients. Int J Dermatol 1988; 27: 63–6.

Hoff M. Dental manifestations in Ehlers–Danlos syndrome. Oral Surg Oral Med Oral Pathol 1977; 44: 707–9.

Ida M, Nakamura T, Utsunomiya J. Osteomatous changes and tooth abnormalities found in the jaws of patients with adenomatosis coli. Oral Surg Oral Med Oral Pathol 1981; 52: 2–11.

Jones EL, Cornell WP. Gardner's syndrome: review of the literature and report of a family. Arch Surg 1966; 92: 287–300.

Koiffmann CP, de Souza DH, Diament A, et al. Incontinentia pigmenti achromians (hypomelanosis of Ito, mim 146150): further evidence of localization at Xp11. Am J Med Genet 1993; 46: 529–33.

Krajewska IA, Moore L, Brown JH. White sponge nevus presenting in the esophagus: case report and literature review. Pathology 1992; 24: 112–5.

Laskaris G, Vareltzidis A, Avgerinou G. Focal palmoplantar and oral mucosa hyperkeratosis syndrome: a report concerning five members of a family. Oral Surg Oral Med Oral Pathol 1980; 50: 250–3.

Laskaris G. Color atlas of oral diseases. 2nd ed. Stuttgart: Thieme, 1994.

Lehner T, Wilton JMA, Ivanyi L, Manson JD. Immunological aspects of juvenile periodontitis (periodontosis). J Periodontol Res 1974; 9: 261–72.

Lipp MJ, Lubit EC. The oral-facial-digital syndrome: case report of a mother and daughter. Cleft Palate 1990; 27: 311–6.

Lygidakis NA, Lindenbaum RH. Oral fibromatosis in tuberous sclerosis. Oral Surg Oral Med Oral Pathol 1989; 68: 725–8.

Milam PE, Griffin TJ, Shapiro RD. A dentofacial deformity associated with incontinentia pigmenti: report of a case. Oral Surg Oral Med Oral Pathol 1990; 70: 420–4.

Mlynarczyk G. Enamel pitting: a common symptom of tuberous sclerosis. Oral Surg Oral Med Oral Pathol 1991; 71: 63–7.

Neville BW, Hann J, Narang R, Garen P. Oral neurofibrosarcoma associated with neurofibromatosis type I. Oral Surg Oral Med Oral Pathol 1991; 72: 456–61.

Pope FM, Komoravska A, Lee KW et al. Ehlers–Danlos syndrome type I with novel dental features. J Oral Pathol Med 1992; 21: 418–21.

Pope FM, Nicholls AC, Palan A, et al. Clinical features of an affected father and daughter with Ehlers–Danlos syndrome type VIIB. Br J Dermatol 1992; 126: 77–82.

Salinas CF, Pai GS, Vera CL, et al. Variability of expression of the oro-facial-digital syndrome type I in black females: six cases. Am J Med Genet 1991; 38: 574–82.

Shapiro SD, Abramovitch K, van Dis ML, et al. Neurofibromatosis: oral and radiographic manifestations. Oral Surg Oral Med Oral Pathol 1984; 58: 493–8.

Steiner M, Gould AR, Graves SM, Kuerschner TW. Klippel–Trenaunay–Weber syndrome. Oral Surg Oral Med Oral Pathol 1987; 63: 208–15.

Steiner M, Gould AR, Means WR. Osteomyelitis of the mandible associated with osteopetrosis. J Oral Maxillofac Surg 1983; 41: 395–405.

Vassilopoulou A, Laskaris G. Papillon–Lefèvre syndrome: report of two brothers. J Dent Child 1989; Sept–Oct: 388–91.

Vogt J, Matheson J. Incontinentia pigmenti (Bloch–Sulzberger syndrome). Oral Surg Oral Med Oral Pathol 1991; 71: 454–6.

Weston SD, Wiener M. Familial polyposis associated with a new type of soft-tissue lesion (skin pigmentation): report of three cases and a review of the literature. Dis Colon Rectum 1967; 10: 311–21.

Winter GB, Geddes M. Oral manifestations of chondroectodermal dysplasia (Ellis–van Creveld syndrome). Br Dent J 1967; 122: 103–7.

Zachariades N. Gardner's syndrome: report of a family. J Oral Maxillofac Surg 1987; 45: 438–40.

Zachariades N, Papanicolaous S, Papadopoulos H, et al. Osteopetrosis: report of a case with maxillary and mandibular involvement. J Oral Med 1987; 12: 97–101.

Chapter 16
Skin Diseases

Aine L, Maki M, et al. Coeliac-type dental enamel defects in patients with dermatitis herpetiformis. Acta Derm Venereol 1992; 72: 25–7.

Alijotas J, Pedragosa R, Bosch J, Vilardell M. Prolonged remission after cyclosporine therapy in pemphigus vulgaris: report of two young siblings. J Am Acad Dermatol 1990; 23: 701–3.

Bauch AM. Kawasaki syndrome: review of new epidemiologic and laboratory developments. Pediatr Infect Dis J 1987; 6: 10–6.

Bazopoulou E, Laskaris G, Katsabas A, Papanicolaou S. Familial benign acanthosis nigricans with predominant early oral manifestations. Clin Genet 1991; 40: 160.

Bhogal B, Wojnarowska F, Marsden RA, et al. Linear IgA bullous dermatosis of adults and children: an immunoelectron microscopic study. Br J Dermatol 1987; 117: 289–96.

Chorzelski TP, Jablonska S. IgA linear dermatosis of childhood (chronic bullous disease of childhood). Br J Dermatol 1979; 101: 535–42.

David M, Zaidenbaum M, Sandbant M. Juvenile pemphigus vulgaris: a 4- to 19-year follow-up for 4 patients. Dermatologica 1988; 177: 165–9.

Elias PM, Jarratt M, Zalitis IE, Catalanotto FA. Childhood pemphigus vulgaris. N Engl J Med 1972; 287: 758–60.

Ermacora E, Prampolini L, Tribbia G, et al. Long-term follow-up of dermatitis herpetiformis in children. J Am Acad Dermatol 1986;15: 24–30.

Esterly NB. Management of vitiligo in children. Pediatr Dermatol 1986; 3: 498–510.

Esterly NB, Wortmann DW. Kawasaki syndrome. Aust J Dermatol 1990; 31: 61–71.

Fabbri P, Panconesi E. Erythema multiforme ("minus" and "maius") and drug intake. Clin Dermatol 1993; 11: 479–89.

Giannetti A, Malmusi M, Girolomoni G. Vesiculobullous drug eruptions in children. Clin Dermatol 1993; 11: 551–5.

Gianotti F, Ermacora E, Prampolini L, et al. Dermatitis herpetiformis in childhood: long-term follow-up of dermatitis herpetiformis in children. J Am Acad Dermatol 1986; 15: 24–30.

Halder RM, Grimes PE, Cowan CA, et al. Childhood vitiligo. J Am Acad Dermatol 1987; 16: 948–54 .

Huff JC, Weston WL, Tonnesen MG. Erythema multiforme: a critical review of characteristics, diagnostic criteria and causes. J Am Acad Dermatol 1983; 8: 763–75.

Kanwar AJ, Kaur S, Rajugopalan M, Dutta BN. Lichen planus in an 8-month-old. Pediatric Dermatol 1989; 6: 358–9.

Kanwar AJ, Handa S, Ghosh S, Kaur S. Lichen planus in childhood: a report of 17 patients. Pediatr Dermatol 1991; 8: 288–91.

Lagrain V, Taieb A, Surleve-Bazeille JE, et al. Linear IgA dermatosis of childhood: case report with an immunoelectron microscopic study. Pediatric Dermatol 1991; 8: 310–3.

Laskaris G. Oral pemphigus vulgaris: an immunofluorescent study of 58 cases. Oral Surg Oral Med Oral Pathol 1981; 51: 626–31.

Laskaris G. Color atlas of oral diseases. 2nd ed. Stuttgart: Thieme, 1994.

Laskaris G, Satriano R. Drug-induced blistering oral lesions. Clin Dermatol 1993; 11: 545–50.

Laskaris G, Stoufi E. Oral pemphigus vulgaris in a 6-year-old girl. Oral Surg Oral Med Oral Pathol 1990; 69: 609–13.

Laskaris G, Sklavounou A, Bovopoulou O. Juvenile pemphigus vulgaris. Oral Surg Oral Med Oral Pathol 1981; 51: 415–20.

Laskaris G, Sklavounou A, Stratigos J. Bullous pemphigoid, cicatricial pemphigoid, and pemphigus vulgaris: a comparative clinical study of 278 cases. Oral Surg Oral Med Oral Pathol 1983; 54: 656–9.

Laskaris G, Triantafyllou A, Economopoulou P. Gingival manifestations of childhood cicatricial pemphigoid. Oral Surg Oral Med Oral Pathol 1988; 66: 349–52.

Lyell A. Drug-induced toxic epidermal necrolysis, 1: an overview. Clin Dermatol 1993; 11: 491–2.

Marsden RA. The treatment of benign chronic bullous dermatosis of childhood, and dermatitis herpetiformis and bullous pemphigoid beginning in childhood. Clin Exp Dermatol 1982; 7: 653–63.

Moy W, Kumar V, Friedman RP, et al. Cicatricial pemphigoid: a case of onset at age 5. J Periodontol 1986; 57: 39–43.

Mutasim DF, Pelc NJ, Anhalt GJ. Cicatricial pemphigoid. Dermatol Clin 1993; 11: 499–510.

Pindborg JJ, Gorlin RJ. Oral changes in acanthosis nigricans (juvenile type). Acta Derm Venereol 1962; 42: 63–71.

Prendiville JS, Esterly NB. Childhood dermatitis herpetiformis. Clin Dermatol 1992; 9: 375–81.

Rauch AM. Kawasaki syndrome: review of new epidemiologic and laboratory developments. Pediatr Infect Dis J 1987; 6: 1016.

Roujeau TC. Drug-induced toxic epidermal necrolysis, 2: current aspects. Clin Dermatol 1993; 11: 493–500.

Scully C, Almeida OPD, Welbury R. Oral lichen planus in childhood. Br J Dermatol 1994; 131: 131–3.

Scully C, Beyli M, Ferreiro M, et al. Update on oral lichen planus: etiopathogenesis and management. Crit Rev Oral Biol Med 1998; 9: 88–122.

Sedano HO, Gorlin RJ. Epidermolysis bullosa. Oral Surg Oral Med Oral Pathol 1989; 67: 555–63.

Sklavounou A, Laskaris G. Childhood cicatricial pemphigoid with exclusive gingival involvement. J Oral Maxillofac Surg 1990; 19: 197–9.

Surbrugg SK, Weston WL. The course of chronic bullous disease of childhood. Pediatr Dermatol 1985; 2: 213–5.

Uitto J, Christiano AM. Inherited epidermolysis bullosa: clinical features, molecular genetics, and pathoetiologic mechanisms. Dermatol Clin 1993; 11: 549–63.

Wright JT. Oral soft tissues in hereditary epidermolysis bullosa. Oral Surg Oral Med Oral Pathol 1991; 71: 440–6.

Chapter 17
Autoimmune Diseases

Alexandridis C, White SC. Periodontal ligament changes in patients with progressive systemic sclerosis. Oral Surg Oral Med Oral Pathol 1984; 58: 113–8.

Ansell BM. Juvenile dermatomyositis. J Rheumatol 1992; 33 (Suppl): 60–2.

Atkinson K. Chronic graft-versus-host disease. Bone Marrow Transpl 1990; 5: 69–82.

Berkowitz RJ, Strandjord S, Jones P, et al. Stomatologic complications of bone marrow transplantation in a pediatric population. Pediatr Dent 1987; 9: 105–10.

Black CM. The aetiopathogenesis of systemic sclerosis. J Intern Med 1993; 234: 3–8.

Calin A. Reiter's syndrome. Med Clin North Am 1977; 61: 365–76.

Cassidy JT, Sullivan DB, Dabich L, et al. Scleroderma in children. Arthritis Rheum 1977; 20: 351–6.

Dahllof G, Heimdahl A, Modeer T, et al. Oral mucous membrane lesions in children treated with bone marrow transplantation. Scand J Dent Res 1989; 97: 268–77.

Deprettere AJ, Van Acker KJ, DeClerck LS, et al. Diagnosis of Sjögren's syndrome in children. Am J Dis Child 1988; 142: 1185–7.

Eversole LR, Jacobsen PL, Stone CE. Oral and gingival changes in systemic sclerosis (scleroderma). J Periodontol 1984; 55: 175–8.

Fox RI, Robinson CA, Curd JG, et al. Sjögren's syndrome: proposed criteria for classification. Arthritis Rheum 1986; 29: 577–85.

Fraga A, Gudino J, Ramos-Niembro F, et al. Mixed connective tissue disease in childhood: relationship with Sjögren's syndrome. Am J Dis Child 1978; 132: 263–5.

George PM, Tunnessen W Jr. Childhood discoid lupus erythematosus. Arch Dermatol 1993; 129: 613–7.

Hiroki A, Nakamura S, Shinohara M, Oka M. Significance of oral examination in chronic graft-versus-host disease. J Oral Pathol Med 1994; 23: 209–15.

Inoue C, Itoh R, Kawa Y, Mizoguchi M. Pathogenesis of mucocutaneous lesions in Behçet's disease. J Dermatol 1994; 21: 474–80.

International Study Group for Behçet's Disease. Criteria for diagnosis of Behçet's disease. Lancet 1990; 335: 1078–80.

Kolbinson DA, Schubert MM, Flournoy N, Truelove EL. Early oral changes following bone marrow transplantation. Oral Surg Oral Med Oral Pathol 1988; 66: 130–8.

Laskaris G. Color atlas of oral diseases. 2nd ed. Stuttgart: Thieme, 1994.

Lee LA. Neonatal lupus erythematosus. J Invest Dermatol 1993; 100: 9S–13S.

Lee LA, Weston WL. Lupus erythematosus in childhood. Dermatol Clin 1986;4: 151–60.

McCurdy FA. Primary Sjögren's syndrome in adolescence: a case report and review. Int Pediatr 1989; 4: 344–8.

Moss JS. Reiter's disease in childhood. Br J Venereol Dis 1964; 40: 166–9.

Nepon BS, Schaller JG. Childhood systemic lupus erythematosus. Prog Clin Rheum 1984; 1: 33.

Oetgen WJ, Boice JA, Lawless OJ. Mixed connective tissue disease in children and adolescents. Pediatrics 1981; 67: 333–7.

Olson NY, Lindsley CB. Neonatal lupus syndrome. Am J Dis Child 1987; 141: 908–10.

Pachman LM. Juvenile dermatomyositis: a clinical overview. Pediatr Rev 1990;12: 117–25.

Provost TT, Watson R, Gaither KK, et al. The neonatal lupus erythematosus syndrome. J Rheumatol 1987; 14 (Suppl 13): 199–205.

Rakover Y, Adar H, Tal I, et al. Behçet's disease: long-term follow-up of three children and review of literature. Pediatrics 1989; 83: 986–92.

Rocco VK, Hurd ER. Scleroderma and scleroderma-like disorders. Semin Arthritis Rheum 1986; 16: 22–69.

Schubert M, Sullivan K, Morton T, et al. Oral manifestations of chronic graft-versus-host disease. Arch Intern Med 1984; 144: 1591–5.

Scully C. Sjögren's syndrome: clinical and laboratory features, immunopathogenesis and management. Oral Surg Oral Med Oral Pathol 1986; 62: 510–23.

Sehgal VN, Koranne RV, Prasad ALS. Unusual manifestations of Reiter's disease in a child. Dermatologica 1985; 170: 77–9.

Siamopoulou-Mavridou L, Drosos LL, Andonopoulos LR. Sjögren's syndrome in childhood: report of two cases. Eur J Pediatr 1989; 148: 523–4.

Stratigos AJ, Laskaris G, Stratigos JD. Behçet's disease. Semin Neurol 1992; 12: 346–57.

Talal N. Immunologic and viral factors in Sjögren's syndrome. Clin Exp Rheumatol 1990; 8 (Suppl 5): 23–6.

Tan EM, Cohen AS, Fries JF, et al. The 1982 revised criteria for the classification of systemic lupus erythematosus. Arthritis Rheum 1982; 25: 1271–5.

Tarpley TM, Anderson LG, White CL. Minor salivary gland involvement in Sjögren's syndrome. Oral Surg Oral Med Oral Pathol 1974; 37: 64–74.

Vermylen C, Meurant A, Noel H, et al. Sjögren's syndrome in a child. Eur J Pediatr 1985; 144: 266–9.

Wallace C, Schaller JG, Emery H et al. Prospective study of childhood systemic lupus erythematosus. Arthritis Rheum 1978; 21: 599–606.

Chapter 18
Gastrointestinal Diseases

Coenen C, Borsch G, Muller KM, Fabry H. Oral inflammatory changes as an initial manifestation of Crohn's disease antedating abdominal diagnosis. Dis Colon Rectum 1988; 31: 548–52.

Ficcara G, Cicchi P, Amorosi A, Piluso S. Oral Crohn's disease and pyostomatitis vegetans. Oral Surg Oral Med Oral Pathol 1993; 75: 220–4.

Field EA, Tyldesley WR. Oral Crohn's disease revisited: a 10-year review. Br J Oral Maxillofac Surg 1989; 27: 114–23.

Ghandour K, Issa M. Oral Crohn's disease with late intestinal manifestations. Oral Surg Oral Med Oral Pathol 1991; 72: 565–7.

Hamilton JR, Bruce GA, Abdourhaman M, et al. Inflammatory bowel disease in children and adolescents. Adv Pediatr 1980; 26: 311–9.

Plouth M, Jenss H, Meyle J. Oral manifestations of Crohn's disease: an analysis of 79 cases. J Clin Gastroenterol 1991; 13: 29–37.

Scully C, Cochran R, Russell H, et al. Crohn's disease of the mouth: an indicator of intestinal involvement. Gut 1982; 23: 198–201.

Tovar JA, Eizaguirre A, Albert A, et al. Peutz–Jeghers syndrome in children: report of two cases and review of the literature. J Pediatr Surg 1983; 18: 1–6.

Chapter 19
Hematological Diseases

Adam E, Pearson HA. Chloramphenicol-responsive congenital neutropenia. N Engl J Med 1983; 309: 1039.

Alter BP, Potter NU. Classification and aetiology of the aplastic anemias. Clin Haematol 1978; 7: 431.

Baehni PC, Payot P, Tsai CC, Cimasoni G. Periodontal status associated with chronic neutropenia. J Clin Periodontol 1983; 10: 222.

Bergmann OJ. Oral infections in haematological patients. Dan Med Bull 1992; 39: 15–29.

Beveridge BR, Bannerman RM, Evanson JM, Witts LJ. Hypochromic anaemia: a retrospective study and follow-up of 378 in patients. Q J Med 1965; 34: 145–61.

Boxer LA, Hutchinson R, Emerson S. Recombinant human granulocyte-colony stimulating factor in the treatment of patients with neutropenia. Clin Immunol Immunopathol 1992; 62: S39–S46.

Dale DC, Hammond WP. Cyclic neutropenia: a clinical review. Blood Rev 1988; 2: 178–85.

Drummond JF, White DK, Damm DD. Megaloblastic anemia with oral lesions: a consequence of gastric bypass surgery. Oral Surg Oral Med Oral Pathol 1985; 59: 149.

Giardina PJ, Hilgartner MW. Update on thalassemia. Pediatr Rev 1992; 13: 55–63.

Greenberg MS. Clinical and histologic changes of the oral mucosa in pernicious anemia. Oral Surg Oral Med Oral Pathol 1981; 52: 38–42.

Kostmann R. Infantile genetic agranulocytosis: a review with presentation of ten new cases. Acta Pediatr Scand 1975; 64: 362.

Lampert F, Fessler A. Periodontal changes during chronic granulocytopenia in childhood: a case report. J Clin Periodontol 1975; 2: 105–10.

Leventhal JM, Silken AB. Oxacillin-induced neutropenia in children. N Engl J Med 1976; 89: 769–72.

Ohishi M, Oobu K, Miyanoshita Y, Yamaguchi K. Acute gingival necrosis caused by drug-induced agranulocytosis. Oral Surg Oral Med Oral Pathol 1988; 66: 194–6.

Orkin SH, Wathan DG. Current concepts: the thalassemias. N Engl J Med 1976; 295: 710.

Palopoli J, Waxman J. Recurrent aphthous stomatitis and vitamin B_{12} deficiency. South Med J 1990; 83: 475–7.

Pearson HA, O'Brien RT. Management of thalassemia major. Semin Hematol 1975; 12: 255–61.

Riggs DR. The thalassemia syndromes. Q Rev Med 1993; 86: 559–64.

Rodenas JM, Ortego N, Herranz MT, et al. Cyclic neutropenia: a cause of recurrent aphthous stomatitis not to be missed. Dermatology 1992; 184: 205–7.

Scully C, McFadyen E, Campbell A. Oral manifestations in cyclic neutropenia. Br J Oral Surg 1982; 230: 96.

Simmons SM, Main CA, Yarsh HM, et al. Idiopathic thrombocytopenic purpura in children. J Pediatr 1975; 87: 16.

Chapter 20
Metabolic Diseases

Arlette JP, Johnston MM. Zinc deficiency dermatitis in premature infants receiving prolonged parenteral alimentation. J Am Acad Dermatol 1981; 5: 37–42.

Barrett AP, Buckley DJ, Katelaris CH. Oral complications in type Ib glycogen storage disease. Oral Surg Oral Med Oral Pathol 1990; 69: 174–6.

Bashan N, Potashnik R, Peleg N, Moran A, Moses SW. Uptake and transport of hexoses into polymorphonuclear leukocytes of patients with glycogen storage disease type Ib. J Inherit Metab Dis 1990; 13: 252–4.

Bergenholtz A, Hofer PA, Ohman J. Oral, pharyngeal and laryngeal manifestations in Urbach–Wiethe disease. Ann Clin Res 1977; 9: 1–7.

Broadbent V, Gardner H, Komp DM, Ladisch S. Histiocytosis syndromes in children, 2: approach to the clinical and laboratory evaluation of children with Langerhans cell histiocytosis (histiocytosis X). Med Pediatr Oncol 1989; 17: 492–5.

Brun A, Sandberg S. Mechanisms of photosensitivity in porphyric patients with special emphasis on erythropoietic protoporphyria. J Photochem Photobiol 1991; 810: 285–302.

Coli AA, Wohl MEB. Cystic fibrosis. Pediatr Rev 1994; 15: 192–200.

Dagenais M, Pharoah MJ, Sikorski PA. The radiographic characteristics of histiocytosis X: a study of 29 cases that involve the jaws. Oral Surg Oral Med Oral Pathol 1992; 74: 230–6.

Gardner DG. The oral manifestations of Hurler's syndrome. Oral Surg Oral Med Oral Pathol 1971; 32: 46–57.

Gilhuus-Moc O, Koppeng H. Oral manifestations of porphyria. Oral Surg Oral Med Oral Pathol 1972; 33: 926–30.

Gorlin RJ, Cohen MM, Levin LS. Syndromes of the head and neck. 3rd ed. Oxford: Oxford University Press, 1990.

Harper JI, Duance VC, Sims TJ, Light ND. Lipoid proteinosis: an inherited disorder of collagen metabolism? Br J Dermatol 1985; 113: 145–9.

Hartman KS. Histiocytosis X: a review of 114 cases with oral involvement. Oral Surg Oral Med Oral Pathol 1980; 49: 38–54.

Hopwood JJ, Morris CP. The mucopolysaccharidoses: diagnosis, molecular genetics and treatment. Mol Biol Med 1990; 7: 381–404.

Kerem B, Rommens JM, Buchanan JA, et al. Identification of the cystic fibrosis gene: genetic analysis. Science 1989; 245: 1073–80.

Kinirons MJ. Increased salivary buffering in association with a low caries experience in children from cystic fibrosis. J Dent Res 1983; 62: 815–7.

McKusick VA, Kaplan D, Wise D, et al. Genetic mucopolysaccharidoses. Medicine 1965; 44: 445–83.

Murphy GM, Hawk JLM, Nickolson DS, Magnus IA. Congenital erythropoietic porphyria (Günther's disease). Clin Exp Dermatol 1987; 12: 61–6.

Novaes AB, Pereira ALA, Moraes ND, Novaes AB. Manifestations of insulin-dependent diabetes mellitus in the periodontium of young Brazilian patients. J Periodontol 1991; 62: 116–22.

Osband ME, Pochedly C. Histiocytosis X: an overview. Hematol Oncol Clin North Am 1987; 1: 1–7.

Rosenbloom AL, Kohrman A, Sperling M. Classification and diagnosis of diabetes mellitus in children and adolescents. J Pediatr 1981; 99: 320–3.

Salapata J, Laskaris G, Drogari E, Harokopos E, Messaritakis J. Oral manifestations in glycogen storage disease type Ib. J Oral Pathol Med 1995; 24: 136–9.

Steiner GA. Successful treatment of acrodermatitis enteropathica with zinc sulfate. Am J Hosp Pharm 1978; 35: 1535–8.

Todd DJ, Nesbitt GS, Lavery TD, Trimble ER, Burrows D. Erythropoietic protoporphyria: the problem of a suitable screening test. Acta Derm Venereol 1990; 70: 347–50.

Tong TK, Adrew LR, Mickell JJ. Childhood AIDS manifesting as acrodermatitis enteropathica. J Pediatr 1986; 108: 424–8.

Tumber-Saini SK, Habbick BF, Oles AM, Schaefer JP, Komiyama K. The role of saliva in aggregation and adherence of *Pseudomonas aeruginosa* in patients with cystic fibrosis. J Oral Pathol Med 1992; 21: 299–304.

Tygstrup I, Haase E, Flensorg EW. The diagnostic value of lip biopsy in mucoviscidosis. Acta Paediatr Scand 1969; 58: 208–9.

Chapter 21
Bacterial Infections

Alvarez S, McCabe WR. Extrapulmonary tuberculosis revisited: a review of experience at Boston city and other hospitals. Medicine 1984; 63: 25–55.

Barnes PF, Hanh QL, Davidson PT. Tuberculosis in patients with HIV infection. Med Clin North Am 1993; 77: 1369–78.

Brignall ID, Gilhooly M. Actinomycosis of the tongue: a diagnostic dilemma. Br J Oral Maxillofac Surg 1989; 27: 249–53.

Burech DL, Koranyi KI, Haynes RE. Serious group A streptococcal diseases in children. J Pediatr 1976; 88: 972–4.

Dimitrakopoulos I, Zouloumis L, Lazaridis N, et al. Primary tuberculosis of the oral cavity. Oral Surg Oral Med Oral Pathol 1991; 72: 712–8.

Drake DD, Holt RJ. Childhood actinomycosis: report of 3 recent cases. Arch Dis Child 1976; 51: 879.

Fiumara NJ, Lesell S. Manifestations of late congenital syphilis: an analysis of 271 patients. Arch Dermatol 1970; 102: 78–83.

Fiumara NJ, Lesell S. The stigmata of late congenital syphilis: an analysis of 100 patients. Sex Transm Dis 1983; 10: 126–9.

Fiumara NJ, Grande DJ, Giunta JL. Papular secondary syphilis of the tongue. Oral Surg Oral Med Oral Surg 1978; 45: 540–2.

Laskaris G. Oral manifestations of infectious diseases. Dent Clin North Am 1996; 40: 395–423.

Phelan JA, Jimenez V, Tompkins DC. Tuberculosis. Dent Clin North Am 1996; 40: 327–41.

Siegel MA. Syphilis and gonorrhea. Dent Clin North Am 1996; 40: 369–83.

Chapter 22
Viral Infections

Badger GR. Oral signs of chickenpox (varicella): report of two cases. J Dent Child 1980; 47: 349–51.

Bagg J. Common infectious diseases. Dent Clin North Am 1996; 40: 385–93.

Cassingham RJ. Infectious mononucleosis: a review of the literature, including recent findings on etiology. Oral Surg Oral Med Oral Pathol 1971; 31: 601–23.

Cawson RA, McSwiggan DA. An outbreak of hand, foot, and mouth disease in a dental hospital. Oral Surg Oral Med Oral Pathol 1969; 27: 451–9.

Cochi SL, Preblud SR, Orenstein WA. Perspectives on the relative resurgence of mumps in the United States. Am J Dis Child 1988; 142): 499–507.

Dunnett WN. Infectious mononucleosis. Br Med J 1963; i: 1187–91.

Farman AG. Clinical and cytological features of the oral lesions caused by chickenpox (varicella). J Oral Med 1976; 6: 396–400.

Goh KT, Doraisingham S, Tan JL, et al. An outbreak of hand, foot, and mouth disease in Singapore. Bull World Health Organ 1982; 60: 965–9.

Greenberg MS. Herpesvirus infections. Dent Clin North Am 1996; 40: 359–68.

Horwitz CA, Henle W, Henle G, et al. Clinical and laboratory evaluation of infants with Epstein–Barr virus–induced infectious mononucleosis: report of 32 patients aged 10 to 48 months. Blood 1981; 57: 933–8.

John TJ, Mauya PP, Jadhav M, et al. Mumps virus meningitis and encephalitis without parotitis. Ind J Med Res 1978; 68: 883.

Johnston JM, Burke JP. Nosocomial outbreak of hand, foot and mouth disease among operating suite personnel. Infect Control 1986; 7: 172–6.

Laskaris G. Oral manifestations of infectious diseases. Dent Clin North Am 1996; 40: 395–423.

Lindenbaum JE, Van Dyck PC, Allen RG. Hand, foot and mouth disease associated with Coxsackie group B. Scand J Infect Dis 1975; 7: 161.

Scully C, Williams G. Oral manifestations of communicable diseases. Dent Update 1978; 5: 295–311.

Suringa BWR, Bank LJ, Ackerman AB. Role of measles virus in skin lesions and Koplik's spots. N Engl J Med 1970; 283: 1139–42.

Chapter 23
HIV Infection and AIDS

Del Toro A, Berkowitz R, Meyerowitz C, Frenkel LM. Oral findings in asymptomatic (P-1) and symptomatic (P-2) HIV-infected children. Pediatr Dent 1996; 18: 117–20.

Don PC, Shen NN, Koestenblatt EK, et al. Mucocutaneous fungal colonization in HIV-infected children. Acta Derm Venereol (Stockh) 1995; 75: 310–1.

EEC Clearinghouse on Oral Problems Related to HIV Infection. Classification and diagnostic criteria for oral lesions in HIV infection. J Oral Pathol Med 1993; 22: 289–91.

Falloon J, Eddy J, Wiener L, Pizzo PA. Human immunodeficiency virus infection in children. J Pediatr 1989; 114: 1–30.

Ferguson FS, Archard H, Nuovo GJ, Nachman S. Hairy leukoplakia in a child with AIDS—a rare symptom: case report. Pediatr Dent 1993; 15: 280–1.

Greenspan JS, Mastrucci MT, Leggott PJ, et al. Hairy leukoplakia in a child. AIDS 1988; 2: 143.

Katchem L, Berkowitz RJ, McIveen L, et al. Oral findings in HIV-seropositive children. Pediatr Dent 1990; 12: 143–6.

Katz MH, Mastrucci MT, Leggott PJ, et al. Prognostic significance of oral lesions in children with perinatally acquired human immunodeficiency virus infection. Am J Dis Child 1993; 147: 45–8.

Laskaris G, Laskari M, Theodoridou M: Oral hairy leukoplakia in a child with AIDS. Oral Surg Oral Med Oral Pathol 1995; 79: 570–1.

Leggott PJ. Oral manifestations of HIV infection in children. Oral Surg Oral Med Oral Pathol 1992; 73: 187–92.

Moniaci D, Cavallari M, Greco D, et al. Oral lesions in children born to HIV-1 positive women. J Oral Pathol Med 1993; 22: 8–11.

Nakou M, Kamma J, Gargalianos P, Laskaris G, Mitsis F. Periodontal microflora of HIV-infected patients with periodontitis. Anaerobe 1997; 3: 97–102.

Pizzo PA. Pediatric AIDS: problems within problems. J Infect Dis 1990; 16: 316–25.

Prose NS. Skin manifestations of HIV-1 infection in children. Clin Dermatol 1991; 9: 59–64.

Ramos-Gomez FJ, Hilton JF, Canchola AJ, et al. Risk factors for HIV-related orofacial soft-tissue manifestations in children. Pediatr Dent 1996; 18: 121–6.

Robinson P. Periodontal diseases and HIV infection: a review of the literature. J Clin Periodontol 1992; 19: 609–14.

Scheutz F, Matee MI, Simon E, et al. Association between carriage of oral yeasts, malnutrition and HIV-1 infection among Tanzanian children aged 18 months to 5 years. Comm Dent Oral Epidemiol 1997; 25: 193–8.

Silverman S Jr, Wara D. Oral manifestations of pediatric AIDS. Pediatrician 1989; 16: 185–7.

Stratigos J, Laskaris G. Skin and oral manifestations of AIDS: color atlas and text. Athens: Zita, 1996.

Chapter 24
Systemic Mycoses

Almeida OP, Scully C. Oral lesions in the systemic mycoses. Curr Opin Dent 1991; 1: 423–8.

Economopoulou P, Laskaris G, Ferekidis E, Kanelis N. Rhinocerebral mucormycosis with severe oral lesions: a case report. J Oral Maxillofac Surg 1995; 53: 215–7.

Laskaris G. Color atlas of oral diseases. 2nd ed. Stuttgart: Thieme, 1994.

Laskaris G. Oral manifestations of infectious diseases. Dent Clin North Am 1996; 40: 395–423.

Myers JD. Fungal infections in bone marrow transplant patients. Semin Oncol 1990; 17 (Suppl 3): 10–3.

Pizzo PA, Walsh TJ. Fungal infections in the pediatric cancer patients. Semin Oncol 1990; 17 (Suppl 3): 6–9.

Samaranayake LP. Oral mycoses in HIV infection. Oral Surg Oral Med Oral Pathol 1992; 73: 171–80.

Scully CM, Welbury EE. Color atlas of oral diseases in children and adolescents. St. Louis: Mosby, 1993.

Sposto MR, Scully C, Almeida OP, et al. Oral paracoccidioidomycosis: a study of 36 South American patients. Oral Surg Oral Med Oral Pathol 1993; 75: 461–5.

Part III Tumors

Chapter 25
Benign Tumors

Aneroth G, Hansen LS. Necrotizing sialometaplasia: the relationship of its pathogenesis to its clinical characteristics. Int J Oral Surg 1982; 11: 283–8.

Angelopoulos AP. Pyogenic granuloma of the oral cavity: statistical analysis of its clinical features. J Oral Surg 1971; 29: 840–7.

Barker DS, Lucas RB. Localized fibrous overgrowths of the oral mucosa. Br J Oral Surg 1967; 5: 86–92.

Bonetti F, Pelosi G, Martignoni G, et al. Peripheral giant cell granuloma: evidence for osteoclastic differentiation. Oral Surg Oral Med Oral Pathol 1990; 70: 471–5.

Brannon RB, Fowler CB, Hartman KS. Necrotizing sialometaplasia: a clinicopathologic study of sixty-nine cases and review of the literature. Oral Surg Oral Med Oral Pathol 1991; 72: 317–25.

Buchner A, Leider AS, Merrell PW, Carpenter WM. Melanocytic nevi of the oral mucosa: a clinicopathologic study of 130 cases from northern California. J Oral Pathol Med 1990; 19: 197–201.

Casso EM, Grin-Jorgensen CM, Grant-Kels JM. Spitz nevi. J Am Acad Dermatol 1992; 27: 901–13.

Chaudry AP, Vickers RA, Gorlin RI. Intraoral minor salivary gland tumors; an analysis of 1414 cases. Oral Surg Oral Med Oral Pathol 1961; 14: 1194–226.

Coffin CM, Dehner LP. Cellular peripheral neural tumors (neurofibromas) in children and adolescents: a clinicopathological and immunohistochemical study. Pediatr Pathol 1990; 10: 351–61.

Cutter LS, Chaudhry AP, Topazian R. Melanotic neuroectodermal tumor of infancy: an ultrastructure study, literature review, and reevaluation. Cancer 1981; 48: 257–70.

Damm DD, Cibull ML, Geissler RH, et al. Investigation into the histogenesis of congenital epulis of the newborn. Oral Surg Oral Med Oral Pathol 1993; 76: 205–12.

Dehner LP, Askin FB. Tumors of fibrous tissue origin in childhood. Cancer 1976; 38: 888–93.

Ellis GL, Auclair PL, Gnepp DR. Surgical pathology of the salivary glands. Philadelphia: Saunders, 1991.

Elzay RP. Traumatic ulcerative granuloma with stromal eosinophilia (Riga–Fede's disease and traumatic eosinophilic granuloma). Oral Surg Oral Med Oral Pathol 1983; 55: 497–506.

Eversole LR, Laipis PJ. Oral squamous papilloma: detection of HPV DNA by in situ hybridization. Oral Surg Oral Med Oral Pathol 1988; 65: 545–50.

Finn MC, Glowacki J, Mulliken JB. Congenital vascular lesions: clinical application of a new classification. J Pediatr Surg 1983; 18: 894–9.

Gardner D. The peripheral odontogenic fibroma: an attempt at clarification. Oral Surg Oral Med Oral Pathol 1982; 54: 40–8.

Hatziotis JC, Asprides H. Neurilemoma (schwannoma) of the oral cavity. Oral Surg Oral Med Oral Pathol 1967; 24: 510–26.

Judd PL, Pedod D, Harrop K, Becker J. Melanotic neuroectodermal tumor of infancy. Oral Surg Oral Med Oral Pathol 1990; 69: 723–6.

Kaiserling E, Ruch P, Xiao JC. Congenital epulis and granular cell tumors: a histologic and immunohistochemical study. Oral Surg Oral Med Oral Pathol 1995; 8: 687–97.

Katsikeris N, Kakarantza-Angelopoulou E, Angelopoulos AP. Peripheral giant cell granuloma: clinicopathologic study of 224 new cases and review of 956 reported cases. Int J Oral Maxillofac Surg 1988; 17: 94–9.

Kaugars GE, Heise AP, Riley WT, et al. Oral melanotic macules: a review of 353 cases. Oral Surg Oral Med Oral Pathol 1993; 76: 59–61.

Kimura K, Yamamoto H. Neurofibroma of the gingiva in a child: report of a case. ASDC J Dent Child 1993; 60: 67–70.

Levin LS, Jorgenson RJ, Jarvey BA. Lymphangiomas of the alveolar ridge in neonates. Pediatrics 1976; 56: 881–4.

Loyola AM, Gatti AF, Pinto DS, et al. Alveolar and extra-alveolar granular cell lesions of the newborn: report of case and review of literature. Oral Surg Oral Med Oral Pathol 1997; 84: 668–71.

Makek MS, Sailer HF. Endothelialer Pseudotumor (sog. pyogenes Granulom). Bericht über 140 Falle. Schweiz Monatsschr Zahnheilkd 1985; 95: 248–60.

Mirchandani R, Sciubba JJ, Mir R. Granular cell lesions of the jaws and oral cavity: a clinicopathologic, immunohistochemical, and ultrastructural study. J Oral Maxillofac Surg 1989; 47: 1248–55.

Monteil RA, Loubière R, Charbit Y, Gillet JY. Gingival granular cell tumor of the newborn: immunoperoxidase investigation with anti–S-100 antiserum. Oral Surg Oral Med Oral Pathol 1987; 64: 78–81.

Pindborg JJ, Harder F. Palatal necrotizing sialometaplasia. Ugeskr Laeger 1977; 139: 657–9.

Powell TG, West CR, Pharaoh POD, Cooke RW. Epidemiology of strawberry haemangioma in low birthweight infants. Br J Dermatol 1987; 116: 635–41.

Rapidis AD, Economidis J, Goumas PD, et al. Tumours of the head and neck in children: a clinicopathological analysis of 1007 cases. J Craniomaxillofac Surg 1988; 16: 276–86.

Shklar G, Meyer I. Vascular tumors of the mouth and jaws. Oral Surg Oral Med Oral Pathol 1965; 19: 335–58.

Shore-Freedman E, Abrahams C, Recant W, et al. Neurilemmomas and salivary gland tumors of the head and neck following childhood irradiation. Cancer 1983; 51: 2159–63.

Slabbert HV, Altini M. Peripheral odontogenic fibroma: a clinicopathologic study. Oral Surg Oral Med Oral Pathol 1991; 72: 86–90.

Slootweg PJ. Heterologous tissue elements in melanotic neuroectodermal tumor of infancy. J Oral Pathol Med 1992; 21: 90–2.

Stewart CM, Watson RE, Eversole LR, et al. Oral granular cell tumors: a clinicopathologic and immunocytochemical study. Oral Surg Oral Med Oral Pathol 1988; 65: 427–35.

Vilmann A, Vilmann P, Vilmann H. Pyogenic granuloma: evaluation of oral conditions. Br J Oral Maxillofac Surg 1986; 24: 376–81.

Waldron CA, El Mofty SK, Gnepp DR. Tumors of the intraoral minor salivary glands: a demographic and histologic study of 426 cases. Oral Surg Oral Med Oral Pathol 1988; 66: 323–33.

Webb DJ, Wescott WB, Correll RW. Firm swelling on the anterior maxillary gingiva of an infant. J Am Dent Assoc 1984; 109: 307–8.

Weedon D, Little JH. Spindle and epithelioid cell nevi in children and adults: a review of 211 cases of the Spitz nevus. Cancer 1977; 40: 217–25.

Chapter 26
Fibro-Osseous and Giant-Cell Lesions

Adekeye EO, Edwards MB, Goubran GF. Fibro-osseous lesions of the skull, face and jaws in Kaduna, Nigeria. Br J Oral Maxillofac Surg 1980; 18: 57–72.

De Pablos PL, Ramos I, De La Calte H. Brown tumor in the palate associated with primary hyperparathyroidism. J Oral Maxillofac Surg 1987; 45: 719–20.

Ficarra G, Kaban LB, Hansen LS. Giant cell lesions of the jaws: a clinicopathologic and cytometric study. Oral Surg Oral Med Oral Pathol 1987; 64: 44–9.

Grunebaum M. Nonfamilial cherubism: report of two cases. J Oral Maxillofac Surg 1973; 31: 632–5.

Peters WJN. Cherubism: a study of twenty cases from one family. Oral Surg Oral Med Oral Pathol 1979; 47: 307–11.

Present D, Bertoni F, Enneking WF. Osteosarcoma of the mandible arising in fibrous dysplasia: a case report. Clin Orthop Related Res 1986; 240: 238–44.

Ragab MA, Mathog RH. Surgery of massive fibrous dysplasia and osteoma of the midface. Head Neck Surg 1987; 9: 202–10.

Ramon Y, Engelberg IS. An unusually extensive case of cherubism. J Oral Maxillofac Surg 1986; 44: 325–8.

Vaillant JM, Romzin P, Divaris M. Cherubism: findings in three cases in the same family. J Craniomaxillofac Surg 1989; 17: 345–9.

Van der Waal I. Diseases of the jaws: diagnosis and treatment. Copenhagen: Munksgaard, 1991.

Wannfors K, Lindskog S, Olander KJ, et al. Fibrous dysplasia of bone and concomitant dysplastic changes in the dentin. Oral Surg Oral Med Oral Pathol 1985; 59: 394–8.

Whitaker SB, Waldron CA. Central giant cell lesions of the jaws: a clinical, radiologic and histopathologic study. Oral Surg Oral Med Oral Pathol 1993; 75: 199–208.

Wold LE, Dobyns JH, Swee RG, et al. Giant cell reaction (giant cell reparative granuloma) of the small bones of the hands and feet. Am J Surg Pathol 1986; 10: 491–6.

Zachariades N, Papanikolaou S, Xypolyta A, et al. Albright syndrome. Int J Oral Maxillofac Surg 1984; 13: 53–8.

Zohar Y, Grausbord R, Shabtai F, Talmi Y. Fibrous dysplasia and cherubism as a hereditary familial disease. J Craniomaxillofac Surg 1989; 17: 340–4.

Chapter 27
Malignant Neoplasms

Batsakis JG. Plasma cell tumors of the head and neck. Ann Otol Rhinol Laryngol 1983; 92: 311–3.

Berk R, Heller A, Heller D, et al. Ewing's sarcoma of the mandible: a case report. Oral Surg Oral Med Oral Pathol 1995; 79: 159–62.

Bayle-Weisgerber C, Lemercier N, Teillet F, et al. Hodgkin's disease in children: results of therapy in a mixed group of 178 clinically and pathologically staged patients over 13 years. Cancer 1984; 54: 215–22.

Bras J, Batsakis JG, Luna MA. Rhabdomyosarcoma of the oral soft tissues. Oral Surg Oral Med Oral Pathol 1987; 64: 585–96.

Burkitt DP. The discovery of Burkitt's lymphoma. Cancer 1983; 51: 1777–86.

Byers RM. Squamous cell carcinoma of the oral tongue in patients less than thirty years of age. Am J Surg 1975; 130: 475–8.

Cheatham BD, Henry RJ. A dental complication involving *Pseudomonas* during chemotherapy for acute lymphoblastic leukemia. J Clin Pediatr Dent 1994; 18: 215–7.

Davis S, Severson RK. Increasing incidence of cancer of the tongue in the United States among young adults. Lancet 1987; ii: 910–1.

De Vries N, Gluckman JL. Multiple primary tumors in the head and neck. Stuttgart: Thieme, 1990.

Epstein JB, Voss NJS, Stevenson-Moore P. Maxillofacial manifestations of multiple myeloma. Oral Surg Oral Med Oral Pathol 1984; 57: 267–71.

Fonseca I, Martins AG, Soares J. Epithelial salivary gland tumors of children and adolescents in southern Portugal. Oral Surg Oral Med Oral Pathol 1991; 72: 696–701.

Groncy P, Finkelstein JZ. Neuroblastoma. Pediatr Ann 1978; 7: 73.

Khanna S, Khanna NN. Primary tumors of the jaws in children. J Oral Maxillofac Surg 1979; 37: 800–4.

Lampkin BC, Woods W, Strauss R, et al. Current status of the end treatment of acute non-lymphocytic leukemia in children (report of the ANLL strategy group of the Children's Study Group). Blood 1983; 61: 215–21.

Millar BG, Browne RM, Flood TR. Juxtacortical osteosarcoma of the jaws. Br J Oral Maxillofac Surg 1990; 28: 73–9.

Murphy SB. Prognostic features and obstacles to cure of childhood non-Hodgkin's lymphoma. Semin Oncol 1977; 4: 265–9.

Nakhleh RE, Swanson PE, Dehner LP. Juvenile (embryonal and alveolar) rhabdomyosarcoma of the head and neck in adults: a clinical, pathologic, and immunohistochemical study of 12 cases. Cancer 1991; 67: 1019–24.

Patel DD, Dave RI. Carcinoma of the anterior tongue in adolescence. Cancer 1976; 37: 917–21.

Patton LL, McMillan CW, Webster WP. American Burkitt's lymphoma: a 10–year review and case study. Oral Surg Oral Med Oral Pathol 1990; 69: 307–16.

Peters E, Cohen M, Altini M, et al. Rhabdomyosarcoma of the oral and paraoral region. Cancer 1989; 63: 963–6.

Pizzo PA. Rhabdomyosarcoma and other soft tissue sarcomas. In: Levine AS, ed. Cancer in the young. New York: Masson, 1982: 615–32.

Pullen DJ, Boyett JM, Crist WM, et al. Utilization of immunologic markers in the designation of acute lymphocytic leukemia subgroups: influence on treatment response (Pediatric Oncology Group). Ann NY Acad Sci 1983; 428: 26–32.

Rapidis AD, Economidis J, Goumas PD, et al. Tumours of the head and neck in children: a clinicopathological analysis of 1007 cases. J Craniomaxillofac Surg 1988; 16: 279–86.

Regezi JA, Zarbo RJ, Batsakis JG. Immunoprofile of mucoepidermoid carcinomas of minor salivary glands. Oral Surg Oral Med Oral Pathol 1991; 71: 189–92.

Russell KL, Donaldson SS, Cox RS, et al. Childhood Hodgkin's disease: patterns of relapse. J Clin Oncol 1984; 2: 80.

Siegal G, Oliver W, Reinus W, et al. Primary Ewing's sarcoma involving the bones of the head and neck. Cancer 1987; 60: 2829–40.

Silverman S Jr. Oral cancer. 3rd ed. Atlantic City, NJ: American Cancer Society, 1990.

Som P, Krespi Y, Hermann G, et al. Ewing's sarcoma of the mandible. Ann Otol Rhinol Laryngol 1981; 89: 20–3.

Spiro RH, Huvos AG, Berk R, Strong EW. Mucoepidermoid carcinoma of salivary gland origin: a clinicopathologic study of 367 cases. Am J Surg 1978; B6: 461–8.

Waldron CA, El Mofty SK, Gnepp DR. Tumors of the intraoral minor salivary glands: a demographic and histologic study of 426 cases. Oral Surg Oral Med Oral Pathol 1988; 66: 323–33.

Warnke RA, Weiss LM, Chan JKC, et al. Tumors of the lymph nodes and spleen. Washington, DC: Armed Forces Institute of Pathology, 1995.

Zachariades N. Neoplasms metastatic to the mouth, jaws and surrounding tissues. J Craniomaxillofac Surg 1989; 17: 283–90.

Index